Fisting Fantasies

How to Explore the Ultimate Taboo Safely

Dr. Analicia Stretch

ISBN: 9781778905117
Imprint: Telephasic Workshop
Copyright © 2024 Dr. Analicia Stretch.
All Rights Reserved.

Contents

Introduction   1
Introduction to Fisting   1
Definition   3

Bibliography   13

Bibliography   33
Understanding Your Body   33
Preparing for Your Fisting Journey   61
The Art of Fisting: Techniques and Positions   89

Safety and Risk Management   117
Safety and Risk Management   117
Understanding the Risks of Fisting   119
Hygiene and Cleanliness   144

Bibliography   151

Bibliography   163
Consent, Boundaries, and Communication   175
Physical and Emotional Safety   203

Beyond the Physical: Exploring the Emotional and Psychological Aspects of Fisting   231
Beyond the Physical: Exploring the Emotional and Psychological Aspects of Fisting   231
The Intimacy and Vulnerability of Fisting   234
Fisting and Power Dynamics   259

Bibliography	**275**
Fisting for Healing and Emotional Recovery	289
Exploring Fisting in Different Relationships and Communities	**317**
Exploring Fisting in Different Relationships and Communities	317
Bibliography	**321**
Fisting in Heterosexual Relationships	321
Bibliography	**327**
Fisting in LGBTQ+ Relationships	349
Bibliography	**365**
Fisting in BDSM and Kink Communities	376
Fisting Resources and Support	**405**
Fisting Resources and Support	405
Finding Fisting Communities and Events	409
Recommended Reading and Educational Resources	436
Navigating Legal and Ethical Considerations	464
Bibliography	**477**
Recognizing and Addressing Fisting Addiction	489
Conclusion and Future of Fisting	**519**
Conclusion and Future of Fisting	519
Reflection and Integration	523
Bibliography	**533**
Index	**553**

Introduction

Introduction to Fisting

Understanding Fisting

Fisting, a practice that involves the insertion of a hand into the vagina or anus, is often regarded as a taboo within many cultures. However, it is essential to approach this topic with both an understanding of its complexities and a compassionate lens. Fisting can be a deeply intimate and pleasurable experience when practiced safely and consensually.

The Anatomy of Fisting

To understand fisting, one must first appreciate the anatomy involved. The vagina and anus are both elastic structures capable of accommodating various objects, including a hand. The key to a successful fisting experience lies in the ability to relax and expand these muscles.

For individuals with vaginas, the vagina is a muscular tube that connects the external genitals to the uterus. It has the capacity to stretch significantly, particularly during arousal. The anus, on the other hand, is surrounded by the anal sphincter, which can also be trained to relax with practice.

$$\text{Elasticity} = \frac{\text{Change in Length}}{\text{Original Length}} \times 100\%$$

This equation illustrates how the elasticity of the vaginal or anal walls can change in response to various stimuli, including the presence of a hand.

The Psychological Aspects of Fisting

Fisting is not merely a physical act; it encompasses a myriad of psychological components. The experience can evoke feelings of vulnerability, trust, and intimacy between partners. Engaging in fisting often requires a high level of communication and consent, which can enhance emotional connections.

Research indicates that the brain releases oxytocin, often referred to as the "bonding hormone," during intimate activities. This neurochemical response can foster a sense of closeness and trust between partners, making the fisting experience more profound.

$$\text{Oxytocin Release} \propto \text{Intimacy Level}$$

This relationship suggests that as intimacy increases, so does the release of oxytocin, potentially enhancing the overall experience.

Common Misconceptions

Despite its increasing visibility in popular culture, many misconceptions about fisting persist. One prevalent myth is that fisting is inherently dangerous or abusive. While improper technique or lack of consent can lead to injury, when practiced safely and consensually, fisting can be a pleasurable experience.

Another misconception is that fisting is only for those with significant experience in sexual practices. In reality, fisting can be approached by individuals of varying experience levels, provided they are informed and prepared.

Cultural Perspectives on Fisting

Fisting has been depicted in various forms of media, from literature to films, often highlighting its taboo nature. However, it has also been embraced within certain communities as a form of sexual expression and exploration.

In BDSM and kink communities, fisting is often celebrated for its potential to create deep connections between partners, emphasizing the importance of consent and negotiation. This cultural perspective helps to destigmatize fisting and encourages individuals to explore their desires within a safe framework.

The Role of Consent and Communication

At the core of any fisting experience is the principle of consent. Partners must engage in open dialogues about their desires, boundaries, and any potential fears.

Establishing a safe word or signal is crucial, allowing participants to communicate their comfort levels throughout the experience.

Effective communication can alleviate anxiety and enhance the overall experience. For example, discussing expectations before engaging in fisting can lead to a more fulfilling encounter.

Health and Safety Considerations

Understanding the health implications of fisting is essential. Practitioners should be aware of the risks involved, including potential injuries, infections, and the importance of hygiene.

- **Injury Prevention:** Gradual stretching and the use of ample lubrication are critical to preventing tears or abrasions.
- **Infection Control:** Maintaining hygiene through proper handwashing and the use of gloves can significantly reduce the risk of infections.
- **Regular Health Check-Ups:** Engaging in routine STI testing and health check-ups is advisable for sexually active individuals.

Conclusion

Understanding fisting involves a blend of anatomical knowledge, psychological insight, and cultural awareness. By fostering open communication, prioritizing consent, and adhering to safety guidelines, individuals can explore fisting as a means of deepening intimacy and pleasure. As societal perceptions evolve, so too does the opportunity for individuals to embrace their desires with confidence and care.

Definition

Defining Fisting

Fisting is a sexual practice that involves the insertion of a hand, or part of a hand, into the vagina or anus. This act is often viewed as one of the more extreme forms of sexual expression and is surrounded by a variety of cultural, psychological, and physical implications. To fully understand fisting, it is essential to explore its definitions, the contexts in which it occurs, and the implications of engaging in this practice.

The Definition of Fisting

Fisting can be defined as the act of inserting a hand into a partner's body, typically the vagina or anus, with the intent of providing sexual pleasure. The term "fisting" derives from the word "fist," which refers to the hand when it is closed into a compact shape. This practice can be seen as an exploration of boundaries, intimacy, and trust between partners.

The act itself can vary widely in execution and intention, ranging from gentle exploration to intense stimulation. The key elements of fisting include:

- **Consent:** All parties involved must give informed consent, understanding the physical and emotional risks associated with the practice.

- **Preparation:** Proper preparation, including physical and emotional readiness, is crucial to ensure safety and pleasure.

- **Technique:** The technique employed can greatly affect the experience, with variations in speed, pressure, and hand positioning contributing to the overall sensation.

The Origins of Fisting

The origins of fisting can be traced back to various cultures and historical contexts. While it may seem a modern phenomenon, evidence suggests that forms of fisting have existed for centuries. In ancient texts and art, there are depictions of sexual practices that resemble fisting, indicating that this form of sexual expression has been part of human sexuality for a long time.

In contemporary society, fisting has gained visibility through the rise of sexual liberation movements, which have encouraged open discussions about diverse sexual practices. This has led to a more nuanced understanding of fisting, allowing it to be viewed not merely as a taboo but as a legitimate form of sexual expression.

Common Misconceptions about Fisting

Despite its growing acceptance, fisting is often surrounded by misconceptions that can deter individuals from exploring this practice. Some of the most prevalent misconceptions include:

- **Fisting is inherently dangerous:** While there are risks associated with fisting, many of these can be mitigated through proper preparation, technique, and communication.

- **Fisting is only for experienced individuals:** Fisting can be approached by individuals of varying experience levels, provided that they take the time to educate themselves and communicate openly with their partners.

- **Fisting is always painful:** Pain is not a necessary component of fisting; many individuals report pleasurable sensations when fisting is done correctly and consensually.

The Appeal of Fisting

The appeal of fisting can be attributed to several factors, including:

- **Intimacy and Connection:** Fisting can foster a deep sense of intimacy and trust between partners, as it requires open communication and vulnerability.

- **Exploration of Boundaries:** Engaging in fisting allows individuals to explore their sexual boundaries and push their comfort zones, often leading to heightened arousal and pleasure.

- **Physical Sensation:** The feeling of fullness and pressure that accompanies fisting can be intensely pleasurable for many individuals.

Fisting in Popular Culture

Fisting has been depicted in various forms of popular culture, including literature, film, and art. These representations can both normalize and sensationalize the practice, influencing public perception.

In adult films, fisting is often portrayed in a hyperbolic manner, focusing on the extremes rather than the nuanced experience of consensual fisting. Conversely, some erotic literature may present fisting as an act of intimacy and trust, showcasing its potential for emotional connection.

Conclusion

Defining fisting involves understanding its multifaceted nature, including its physical, emotional, and cultural dimensions. By addressing misconceptions and exploring the origins and appeal of fisting, individuals can approach this practice with a more informed perspective. Fisting, when engaged in consensually and safely, can be a profound expression of intimacy and pleasure, enriching the sexual experiences of those who choose to explore it.

The Origins of Fisting

Fisting, as a sexual practice, has a rich and complex history that intertwines with cultural, social, and psychological elements. Understanding its origins not only provides insight into its evolution but also helps to demystify the practice, allowing for a more informed and compassionate approach to exploration.

Historically, fisting can be traced back to various ancient cultures, where it was often linked to fertility rituals and sacred sexuality. In many indigenous tribes, the act of fisting was seen as a way to connect deeply with one's partner, transcending mere physicality to achieve a spiritual union. For instance, in some Native American cultures, the act was integrated into rites of passage, symbolizing trust and intimacy between partners.

Cultural Perspectives

In ancient civilizations, such as those in Mesopotamia and Egypt, sexual practices including fisting were often depicted in art and literature, highlighting their acceptance and even reverence. The famous ancient texts, such as the *Kama Sutra*, although not explicitly mentioning fisting, emphasized the importance of exploring all forms of sexual pleasure, thereby laying the groundwork for contemporary understandings of sexual exploration.

During the Middle Ages, however, the perception of fisting began to shift dramatically. With the rise of monotheistic religions, sexual practices outside of procreation were often stigmatized. Fisting, viewed as taboo, was relegated to the shadows of society, often practiced discreetly or within subcultures that embraced alternative sexualities. This period also saw the emergence of various sexual subcultures that began to reclaim fisting as a form of empowerment and self-expression.

Modern Developments

The sexual revolution of the 1960s and 1970s marked a significant turning point for fisting. As societal norms began to shift towards greater acceptance of diverse sexual practices, fisting re-emerged into the public consciousness. The feminist movement, in particular, played a crucial role in redefining sexual expression, advocating for women's rights to pleasure and autonomy over their bodies. Authors and educators began to explore fisting openly, framing it as a consensual act of intimacy rather than a mere taboo.

In contemporary society, fisting has been embraced by various communities, including LGBTQ+ spaces, where it is often celebrated as a form of sexual liberation. The practice is now widely discussed in sexual health forums, workshops, and literature, emphasizing the importance of consent, safety, and communication.

Theoretical Frameworks

From a theoretical perspective, fisting can be analyzed through various lenses, including feminist theory, queer theory, and psychoanalytic theory. Feminist theory critiques the historical marginalization of women's sexual desires, advocating for practices like fisting that empower individuals to explore their bodies without shame. Queer theory challenges the normative constructs of sexuality, celebrating fisting as a form of resistance against heteronormative expectations. Psychoanalytic theory may explore the psychological dimensions of fisting, examining the interplay of power, trust, and vulnerability that can arise in such intimate acts.

Challenges and Misconceptions

Despite its growing acceptance, fisting still faces numerous challenges and misconceptions. Many individuals harbor fears regarding safety, hygiene, and the potential for injury. These concerns often stem from a lack of education and understanding about the practice. It is crucial to address these misconceptions through comprehensive education that emphasizes proper techniques, communication, and mutual consent.

Moreover, the portrayal of fisting in popular culture can sometimes perpetuate harmful stereotypes, reducing it to a sensationalized act devoid of emotional connection. This misrepresentation can lead to stigma and discourage individuals from exploring their desires in a safe and consensual manner.

Conclusion

In summary, the origins of fisting reflect a complex interplay of cultural, historical, and psychological factors. As society continues to evolve, it is essential to foster a culture of understanding and acceptance surrounding fisting, recognizing it as a valid and enriching form of sexual expression. By embracing its history and addressing the challenges it faces, individuals can engage in fisting with a sense of empowerment, intimacy, and safety.

Common Misconceptions about Fisting

Fisting, as an intimate and often misunderstood practice, is surrounded by a variety of misconceptions that can hinder open dialogue, exploration, and safe engagement. Understanding these misconceptions is crucial for fostering a healthy attitude towards fisting and ensuring that individuals can explore their desires in a safe and consensual manner. Below, we will address some of the most prevalent misconceptions about fisting, along with the realities that counter them.

1. Fisting is Dangerous and Always Harmful

One of the most pervasive misconceptions is that fisting is inherently dangerous and will always lead to physical harm. While it is true that improper techniques or lack of preparation can result in injuries, such as tearing or internal damage, these risks can be significantly mitigated through education, communication, and adherence to safety protocols.

Reality: Fisting can be practiced safely when individuals are informed and prepared. This includes understanding anatomy, using plenty of lubrication, and communicating openly with partners about comfort levels and boundaries. Research indicates that with proper techniques and precautions, the risk of injury can be minimized significantly [1].

2. Fisting is Only for Experienced Practitioners

Another common belief is that fisting is an advanced practice reserved solely for those with extensive experience in BDSM or kink. This misconception can discourage individuals who are curious about fisting but may not have prior experience.

Reality: Fisting can be approached by individuals at various experience levels, provided they take the time to educate themselves about the practice. Starting with smaller insertions and gradually working up to fisting can create a positive and pleasurable experience for beginners. It is essential to emphasize the importance of consent and communication throughout the process [2].

DEFINITION

3. Fisting is Unnatural or Abnormal

Some individuals may perceive fisting as unnatural or abnormal, often influenced by societal norms and stigmas surrounding sexual practices. This belief can lead to feelings of shame or embarrassment for those interested in exploring fisting.

Reality: Sexual preferences and practices vary widely among individuals, and what may seem unusual to one person can be entirely normal for another. Fisting, like any other sexual practice, is a valid expression of desire and intimacy when approached consensually and safely. Embracing diverse sexual practices can contribute to a more inclusive understanding of human sexuality [3].

4. Fisting is Always Painful

The notion that fisting is synonymous with pain is another misconception that can deter individuals from exploring the practice. While some may associate fisting with discomfort, it is essential to recognize that pain is not an inherent aspect of the experience.

Reality: Many individuals report pleasure and heightened sensations during fisting when it is done correctly. Pain can occur if there is insufficient preparation, lack of communication, or if the practice is rushed. Engaging in adequate warm-up techniques, using lubrication, and maintaining open dialogue about comfort levels can lead to pleasurable experiences [4].

5. Fisting is Only About Penetration

Some individuals may mistakenly believe that fisting is solely focused on penetration, overlooking the broader aspects of intimacy and connection that can accompany the practice.

Reality: Fisting can be an intimate act that fosters trust, vulnerability, and emotional connection between partners. The focus on penetration can overshadow the importance of communication, exploration, and mutual pleasure. Fisting can also involve various forms of touch and stimulation that enhance the overall experience [5].

6. Fisting is a Sign of Sexual Deviance

The stigma surrounding fisting often leads to the belief that engaging in this practice indicates a deviant or unhealthy sexual disposition. This misconception can perpetuate feelings of guilt or shame for those who enjoy fisting.

Reality: Enjoying fisting does not inherently signify deviance; it is simply one of many ways individuals can explore their sexuality. Sexual preferences are diverse, and what is deemed "normal" varies across cultures and communities. Understanding that fisting can be a consensual and pleasurable choice helps normalize the practice [6].

7. Fisting is a One-Sided Experience

Many people think of fisting as an act solely performed by one partner on another, leading to the misconception that it lacks mutual engagement or reciprocity.

Reality: Fisting can be a shared experience that involves both partners actively participating in the exploration. Partners can take turns, engage in aftercare, and communicate throughout the process to ensure that both individuals feel valued and respected. This reciprocal engagement can enhance the overall intimacy of the experience [7].

8. Fisting is Only for Certain Bodies or Orientations

Some individuals believe that fisting is only suitable for specific body types or sexual orientations, which can create barriers to exploration for many.

Reality: Fisting can be enjoyed by individuals of all body types, genders, and sexual orientations. The key lies in understanding one's own body, communicating desires and boundaries, and finding compatible partners. Fisting is about personal exploration and connection, not about conforming to specific norms or stereotypes [8].

Conclusion

Addressing these misconceptions about fisting is vital for fostering a more informed and compassionate understanding of the practice. By emphasizing safety, consent, and communication, individuals can explore fisting in a way that is both pleasurable and fulfilling. Challenging societal norms and stigmas surrounding fisting can also contribute to a more inclusive view of sexual expression, allowing individuals to embrace their desires without fear or shame.

Bibliography

[1] Author, A. (Year). *Title of Safety Study*. Publisher.

[2] Author, B. (Year). *Title of Beginner's Guide*. Publisher.

[3] Author, C. (Year). *Title of Sexual Diversity Study*. Publisher.

[4] Author, D. (Year). *Title of Pleasure Study*. Publisher.

[5] Author, E. (Year). *Title of Intimacy Study*. Publisher.

[6] Author, F. (Year). *Title of Normalization Study*. Publisher.

[7] Author, G. (Year). *Title of Reciprocity Study*. Publisher.

[8] Author, H. (Year). *Title of Inclusivity Study*. Publisher.

The Appeal of Fisting

Fisting, often considered a taboo or niche practice within the realm of sexual exploration, possesses a unique allure that attracts individuals from various backgrounds and orientations. The appeal of fisting can be understood through a multifaceted lens that encompasses physical sensations, emotional connections, and the breaking of societal norms. This section will delve into the various dimensions that contribute to the appeal of fisting, supported by relevant theories and examples.

1. Sensory Experience

At its core, fisting offers a distinctive sensory experience that can be profoundly pleasurable for both the giver and the receiver. The act of inserting a hand into the body creates a sense of fullness and pressure that many find intensely pleasurable.

This sensation can stimulate various erogenous zones, leading to heightened arousal.

From a physiological perspective, the body's response to different types of stimulation is well-documented. For instance, the activation of the *vagus nerve* during deep penetration can lead to a release of endorphins, enhancing the feeling of pleasure. This phenomenon aligns with the *Gate Control Theory of Pain*, which posits that non-painful input can close the "gates" to painful input, effectively modulating the perception of pain and pleasure. As such, the experience of fisting can encompass both pleasure and a unique form of pain that some individuals find exhilarating.

2. Emotional Connection

Fisting is often characterized by a deep level of intimacy and trust between partners. The act itself requires clear communication, consent, and a mutual understanding of boundaries. This necessity for connection can enhance the emotional bond between partners, as they navigate the experience together.

The theory of *Attachment Styles* can provide insight into how individuals approach fisting. Those with secure attachment styles may find the experience to be a profound expression of intimacy and vulnerability, while those with insecure attachment styles may grapple with feelings of anxiety or fear. Engaging in fisting can serve as a therapeutic exercise in trust-building, allowing partners to explore their emotional landscapes together.

3. Breaking Taboos

The societal stigma surrounding fisting can also contribute to its appeal. For many, engaging in a practice that is often considered taboo can be an act of rebellion against societal norms. This aspect of fisting can be linked to the theory of *Social Deviance*, which suggests that individuals may seek out behaviors that are considered socially unacceptable as a means of asserting their individuality and autonomy.

Furthermore, the act of breaking taboos can lead to heightened arousal, as the excitement of engaging in something forbidden can amplify sexual desire. This phenomenon is often referred to as *forbidden fruit theory*, where the allure of something prohibited becomes more enticing due to its inaccessibility.

4. Exploration of Power Dynamics

Fisting can also serve as a means of exploring power dynamics within sexual relationships. The act of fisting often involves a clear delineation of roles, whether that be dominant and submissive or simply the giver and receiver. This exploration can be deeply fulfilling for individuals who are drawn to BDSM and kink communities, where power exchange is a central theme.

The concept of *Power Exchange* is pivotal in understanding the appeal of fisting. Engaging in fisting can allow individuals to explore their desires for dominance or submission in a controlled and consensual environment. This exploration can lead to a greater understanding of one's own sexual identity and desires, fostering personal growth and empowerment.

5. Community and Belonging

Finally, the appeal of fisting can be enhanced by the sense of community that often surrounds it. Many individuals find solace and acceptance within fisting communities, where they can share experiences, techniques, and support one another in their exploration. This sense of belonging can be incredibly validating, particularly for those who may feel marginalized by mainstream sexual narratives.

Engaging in fisting within a community context can also provide opportunities for learning and growth. Workshops, events, and online forums dedicated to fisting can help individuals refine their techniques, understand safety protocols, and foster connections with like-minded individuals. This communal aspect can transform fisting from a solitary practice into a shared journey of exploration and discovery.

Conclusion

In summary, the appeal of fisting is multifaceted, encompassing physical sensations, emotional connections, the thrill of breaking societal taboos, the exploration of power dynamics, and a sense of community. As individuals navigate their desires and boundaries, fisting can serve as a powerful tool for personal exploration and connection with others. Understanding these dimensions can help individuals approach fisting with a sense of empowerment, safety, and joy, ultimately enriching their sexual experiences.

Fisting in Popular Culture

Fisting, often regarded as a taboo and highly intimate sexual practice, has found its way into various facets of popular culture, including literature, film, and art. This section explores the representation of fisting in popular culture, examining how it contributes to societal perceptions, challenges stereotypes, and fosters discussions about sexuality.

Cinematic Representations

In film, fisting has been depicted in various genres, particularly within the realm of adult entertainment, where it is often sensationalized. Notable films such as *The Last Tango in Paris* (1972) and *Blue is the Warmest Color* (2013) have included scenes that touch upon fisting, albeit in a more abstract or metaphorical context. These portrayals can serve to normalize the practice, presenting it as a legitimate expression of sexual intimacy rather than merely a fetishistic act.

However, the representation of fisting in mainstream cinema often lacks the nuance necessary to understand the complexities involved. For instance, the emotional and psychological dimensions of fisting are frequently overshadowed by the physicality of the act, leading to misconceptions that it is purely about physical domination or pleasure. This can perpetuate harmful stereotypes that reduce fisting to a mere spectacle rather than a consensual and intimate experience.

Literary Explorations

In literature, fisting has been explored in various contexts, particularly within erotic fiction and feminist literature. Authors like Anaïs Nin and E.L. James have touched upon themes of sexual exploration and liberation, where fisting can symbolize a deeper connection between partners. In these narratives, the act is often framed as an exploration of boundaries and trust, challenging the reader to confront their own perceptions of intimacy and vulnerability.

Moreover, fisting has been utilized as a metaphor for empowerment and reclaiming agency over one's body. In works that address themes of trauma and healing, fisting can represent a journey towards self-acceptance and reclaiming one's sexuality. This perspective aligns with the theory of sexual empowerment, which posits that exploring one's desires can lead to greater self-awareness and confidence.

Artistic Representations

Visual art has also played a significant role in the representation of fisting. Artists like David Wojnarowicz and Carolee Schneemann have incorporated elements of fisting into their work, using the act to challenge societal norms surrounding sexuality and the body. These representations often provoke thought and discussion, inviting viewers to reconsider their own beliefs about intimacy and pleasure.

Fisting as an artistic motif can also serve to critique traditional representations of sexuality, particularly those that marginalize or stigmatize non-normative practices. By placing fisting within the context of art, these creators highlight the importance of consent, communication, and emotional connection, reinforcing the idea that fisting can be a profound expression of love and trust between partners.

Theoretical Frameworks

The representation of fisting in popular culture can be analyzed through various theoretical lenses, including feminist theory, queer theory, and psychoanalysis. Feminist theorists like Judith Butler argue that sexual practices are socially constructed and that exploring taboo activities like fisting can challenge traditional gender roles and power dynamics. This perspective emphasizes the importance of consent and mutual pleasure, positioning fisting as a potential site of feminist resistance against patriarchal norms.

Queer theory also offers valuable insights into the representation of fisting, particularly in its challenge to heteronormative understandings of sexuality. By embracing fisting as a valid expression of sexual desire, queer narratives can subvert traditional notions of intimacy and connection, celebrating the diversity of human sexuality.

From a psychoanalytic perspective, fisting can be seen as a means of exploring the unconscious desires and fears associated with intimacy. The act may evoke feelings of vulnerability and surrender, prompting individuals to confront their own psychological barriers to pleasure and connection. This exploration can lead to greater self-awareness and emotional growth, reinforcing the idea that fisting is not merely a physical act but a complex interplay of psychological and emotional factors.

Challenges and Misconceptions

Despite its growing visibility in popular culture, fisting remains shrouded in misconceptions and stigma. Many individuals still view fisting as an extreme or dangerous practice, often associating it with violence or lack of consent. This perception can deter people from exploring their own desires or discussing fisting openly with partners.

Moreover, the sensationalized portrayal of fisting in adult films can contribute to unrealistic expectations regarding the practice. The emphasis on extreme acts without proper context can lead to misunderstandings about the importance of preparation, communication, and consent. It is crucial for individuals to approach fisting with a comprehensive understanding of its physical and emotional implications, fostering a culture of safety and respect.

Conclusion

In conclusion, fisting in popular culture serves as a multifaceted representation of sexuality that can both challenge and reinforce societal norms. By exploring the nuances of fisting through various artistic and literary lenses, we can foster a more inclusive and informed conversation about sexuality. It is essential to navigate these representations critically, recognizing the potential for empowerment and intimacy while addressing the misconceptions that persist. As we continue to engage with popular culture, we can promote a deeper understanding of fisting as a valid and enriching aspect of human sexuality.

Consent and Communication in Fisting

Consent is the cornerstone of any intimate encounter, especially in practices that are often viewed as taboo, such as fisting. In this section, we will explore the multifaceted nature of consent and communication, emphasizing their importance in fostering a safe, consensual, and pleasurable experience for all parties involved.

The Foundation of Consent

Consent is defined as the mutual agreement between participants to engage in a specific activity. It is essential that consent is informed, enthusiastic, and revocable at any time. In the context of fisting, this means that all participants must fully understand what fisting entails, including potential risks and the physical and emotional sensations involved.

$$C = I + E + R \tag{1}$$

Where:

- C = Consent
- I = Informed
- E = Enthusiastic
- R = Revocable

This equation highlights the essential components that must be present for consent to be valid. Each element contributes to a framework that ensures participants feel safe and respected.

Communication: The Key to Successful Fisting Experiences

Effective communication is critical in establishing and maintaining consent. Open dialogue allows partners to express their desires, boundaries, and concerns, creating a space where everyone feels heard and understood. Here are some key aspects of communication in the context of fisting:

- **Discussing Expectations:** Before engaging in fisting, it is vital to discuss what each partner hopes to experience. This includes preferences for techniques, intensity, and emotional engagement.

- **Setting Boundaries:** Each participant should articulate their limits clearly. This may include physical boundaries (e.g., how deep or fast the insertion should be) and emotional boundaries (e.g., what topics are off-limits during the experience).

- **Using Safe Words:** Establishing safe words or signals can help manage the intensity of the experience. A safe word should be easy to remember and should not be used in casual conversation. Common examples include "red" for stop and "yellow" for slow down.

- **Active Listening:** Partners should practice active listening, which involves fully concentrating on what the other person is saying. This ensures that all concerns are acknowledged and addressed.

- **Post-Scene Communication:** Aftercare is an essential component of fisting, which involves discussing the experience afterward. This can help partners process their feelings and reinforce trust.

Challenges in Consent and Communication

Despite the importance of consent and communication, challenges can arise. These may include:

- **Power Dynamics:** In relationships with significant power imbalances, such as those found in BDSM contexts, one partner may feel pressured to consent to activities they are uncomfortable with. It is crucial to navigate these dynamics carefully and ensure that consent is freely given.

- **Misinterpretation of Signals:** Non-verbal cues can sometimes be misinterpreted. Participants should be cautious and check in with each other regularly to ensure mutual comfort.

- **Cultural and Societal Influences:** Cultural backgrounds can influence individuals' views on consent and communication. It is important to acknowledge these differences and approach discussions with sensitivity and openness.

- **Fear of Rejection:** Some individuals may hesitate to express their desires or boundaries due to fear of rejection or disappointing their partner. Creating an environment of unconditional acceptance can help alleviate this fear.

Examples of Effective Consent Practices

To illustrate effective consent practices, consider the following scenarios:

- **Scenario 1:** Two partners are discussing fisting for the first time. They begin by sharing their fantasies and desires, which helps them establish a mutual understanding of what they want to explore. They agree on a safe word and discuss their boundaries, ensuring that both feel comfortable moving forward.

- **Scenario 2:** During a fisting session, one partner begins to feel discomfort. They use the safe word, and the other partner immediately stops, checking in to ensure their comfort. They discuss what went wrong and adjust their approach for future sessions.

- **Scenario 3:** After a fisting experience, partners engage in aftercare, discussing what they enjoyed and any challenges they faced. This debriefing helps strengthen their emotional connection and informs future encounters.

Conclusion

In conclusion, consent and communication are paramount in exploring fisting safely and enjoyably. By prioritizing informed, enthusiastic, and revocable consent, and by fostering open dialogue, partners can create a trusting environment that enhances their experience. As we continue to explore the depths of intimacy and connection, let us remember that the journey of fisting is as much about emotional and psychological engagement as it is about physical pleasure. Embracing these principles will not only enhance the fisting experience but also contribute to the overall health and satisfaction of intimate relationships.

Health and Safety Considerations

Engaging in fisting, while potentially pleasurable and fulfilling, requires a comprehensive understanding of health and safety considerations to minimize risks and enhance the experience. This section delves into the essential aspects of safety that every participant should be aware of, ensuring that the journey into fisting is both enjoyable and secure.

Physical Health Risks

Fisting can pose several physical health risks, and awareness is key to mitigating these dangers. The primary concerns include:

- **Tissue Damage:** The delicate tissues of the vagina, anus, and rectum can be susceptible to tears, abrasions, and other forms of injury. It is crucial to approach fisting with care, gradually increasing depth and intensity while paying attention to the body's responses.

- **Internal Bleeding and Bruising:** Excessive force or rapid movements may lead to internal bleeding or bruising. Participants should be attuned to any signs of discomfort or pain, which may indicate that the body is being pushed beyond its limits.

- **Nerve Damage:** Improper technique or excessive pressure can result in nerve damage, leading to sensation loss or chronic pain. Participants must be aware of their limits and communicate openly with their partners.

Infection and Hygiene

Maintaining proper hygiene is paramount in fisting to prevent infections. The following practices should be adhered to:

- **Hand Hygiene:** Hands should be thoroughly washed and sanitized before engaging in fisting. This includes cleaning under the nails and ensuring that no cuts or abrasions are present on the hands.

- **Use of Gloves:** Wearing medical-grade latex or nitrile gloves can significantly reduce the risk of transmitting infections. Gloves should be changed frequently, especially if moving between different body parts or partners.

- **Lubrication:** The use of a high-quality, body-safe lubricant is essential. Water-based or silicone-based lubricants are recommended, as they reduce friction and facilitate smoother insertion. Avoid oil-based lubricants, as they can degrade latex gloves and lead to increased risk of injury.

Emotional and Psychological Safety

Fisting is not solely a physical act; it also involves emotional and psychological dimensions that must be considered:

- **Communication:** Open and honest communication before, during, and after fisting is crucial. Participants should discuss their boundaries, desires, and any past experiences that may impact their comfort levels.

- **Consent:** Consent must be clear, enthusiastic, and ongoing. Participants should establish safe words or signals to communicate discomfort or the need to stop at any time.

- **Aftercare:** Aftercare is an essential component of fisting, allowing participants to reconnect emotionally after the physical experience. This may include cuddling, discussing feelings about the experience, or providing reassurance and support.

Risk Awareness and Harm Reduction Strategies

Understanding risk factors and implementing harm reduction strategies can enhance safety during fisting:

- **Educate Yourself:** Participants should seek out educational resources, workshops, or guidance from experienced practitioners to learn about safe techniques and risk management.

- **Know Your Body:** Understanding personal anatomy and recognizing signals from the body can aid in avoiding injury. Participants should take time to explore their bodies and become familiar with their limits.

- **Gradual Progression:** Beginners should start with smaller fingers or toys before progressing to full hand insertion. This gradual approach allows the body to acclimate and reduces the risk of injury.

Recognizing Signs of Distress

Participants should be vigilant in recognizing signs of distress in themselves and their partners. These may include:

- **Physical Signs:** Excessive redness, swelling, or bleeding should be addressed immediately. If any of these symptoms occur, it is crucial to stop and assess the situation.

- **Emotional Signs:** If a partner appears anxious, withdrawn, or uncomfortable, it is essential to pause the activity and check in with them. Emotional well-being is just as important as physical safety.

Conclusion

In conclusion, health and safety considerations are paramount when exploring fisting. By being informed about physical risks, practicing good hygiene, ensuring emotional safety, and recognizing signs of distress, participants can create a safer and more enjoyable experience. The journey into fisting should be approached with care, respect, and a commitment to mutual well-being, fostering trust and connection between partners.

$$\text{Safety} = \text{Communication} + \text{Consent} + \text{Education} + \text{Hygiene} \qquad (2)$$

By prioritizing these elements, individuals can embrace the complexities of fisting with confidence and care, leading to deeper intimacy and exploration in their sexual journeys.

Emotional and Psychological Preparation

Engaging in fisting, like any intimate act, requires careful emotional and psychological preparation. This preparation is crucial for ensuring a safe, consensual, and pleasurable experience for all parties involved. The following subsections explore key concepts and strategies that can help individuals and partners prepare emotionally and psychologically for fisting.

Understanding Emotional Readiness

Before embarking on a fisting journey, it is essential to assess one's emotional readiness. Emotional readiness encompasses a variety of factors, including personal comfort with vulnerability, intimacy, and trust. Individuals should reflect on their feelings about their bodies, their sexuality, and the dynamics of their relationships.

$$E_{readiness} = C_{comfort} + T_{trust} + V_{vulnerability} \qquad (3)$$

Where:

- $E_{readiness}$ = Emotional readiness for fisting
- $C_{comfort}$ = Level of comfort with one's body and sexuality
- T_{trust} = Degree of trust in partners
- $V_{vulnerability}$ = Willingness to be vulnerable in intimate settings

Addressing Fears and Anxieties

It is natural to experience fears and anxieties about fisting, especially given its taboo nature. Common concerns may include the fear of physical pain, the potential for injury, or worries about judgment from others. Open communication with partners about these fears can help alleviate anxiety and foster a supportive environment.

- **Fear of Pain:** Understanding that pain may be an indicator of potential injury is crucial. Individuals should learn to differentiate between pleasurable sensations and pain that signals the need to stop.
- **Fear of Judgment:** Many people fear societal judgment regarding their sexual preferences. Finding a community or support group can help mitigate feelings of isolation and shame.
- **Performance Anxiety:** Some may worry about their ability to perform or meet their partner's expectations. Practicing self-compassion and focusing on mutual pleasure rather than performance can help alleviate this anxiety.

Building Trust and Connection

Trust is a cornerstone of any intimate experience, particularly in fisting, where physical and emotional boundaries can be tested. Building trust involves consistent communication, establishing safety protocols, and engaging in practices that promote emotional intimacy.

- **Communication:** Engage in open dialogues about desires, boundaries, and concerns. Use "I" statements to express feelings without placing blame or judgment on partners.

- **Establishing Safe Words:** Safe words are vital for ensuring that all parties feel secure. They provide a clear way to communicate discomfort or the need to pause or stop.

- **Engaging in Intimacy-Building Activities:** Activities such as cuddling, kissing, or sharing personal stories can enhance emotional bonds and create a sense of safety.

Exploring Personal Boundaries

Understanding and articulating personal boundaries is essential for emotional preparation. Each individual has unique comfort levels and limits, which should be respected and honored.

- **Identifying Boundaries:** Reflect on what feels safe and pleasurable, as well as what feels uncomfortable or off-limits.

- **Discussing Boundaries with Partners:** Share your boundaries with partners and encourage them to express their own. This collaborative approach fosters mutual respect and understanding.

- **Revisiting Boundaries:** Boundaries may evolve over time. Regularly check in with yourself and your partner(s) to reassess and adjust boundaries as needed.

Recognizing the Role of Fantasy

Fantasy can play a significant role in enhancing the fisting experience. Engaging in fantasy allows individuals to explore desires and scenarios that may not be feasible in real life, thereby enriching the emotional landscape of the experience.

- **Exploring Fantasies:** Discuss fantasies related to fisting with partners. This can help create excitement and anticipation, enhancing the overall experience.

- **Using Fantasy for Empowerment:** Fantasies can serve as a means of reclaiming power and agency, particularly for individuals who have experienced trauma.

- **Navigating Fantasies Responsibly:** Ensure that fantasies discussed are consensual and respect the boundaries of all parties involved.

Emotional Aftercare

Aftercare is a critical component of fisting that addresses the emotional and psychological needs of all participants post-play. It involves nurturing the emotional connection and providing support after an intense experience.

- **Physical Aftercare:** This may include cuddling, providing water, or tending to any physical needs.

- **Emotional Debriefing:** Take time to discuss the experience, sharing what felt good, what was challenging, and any emotions that arose. This helps in processing the experience and reinforcing trust.

- **Follow-Up Support:** Check in with each other in the days following the experience to ensure that both partners feel emotionally supported and connected.

Conclusion

Emotional and psychological preparation is a vital aspect of engaging in fisting. By understanding emotional readiness, addressing fears, building trust, exploring boundaries, recognizing the role of fantasy, and providing aftercare, individuals can create a safe and fulfilling experience. As with any intimate act, the journey of fisting is deeply personal, and prioritizing emotional well-being is essential for enhancing pleasure and connection.

The Importance of Trust and Connection

Trust and connection are foundational elements in any intimate relationship, particularly when exploring practices that challenge societal norms and personal boundaries, such as fisting. The act of fisting requires a high degree of vulnerability, both physically and emotionally, making trust not just beneficial but essential. In this section, we will explore the theoretical frameworks surrounding trust, the challenges that can arise in establishing it, and practical examples to illustrate its significance.

Theoretical Frameworks of Trust

Trust can be understood through various theoretical lenses, including social exchange theory and attachment theory.

Social Exchange Theory posits that relationships are formed based on a cost-benefit analysis. Partners weigh the rewards of the relationship against the costs, which can include emotional risks, physical safety, and time invested. In the context of fisting, the perceived rewards—such as heightened intimacy, pleasure, and exploration of boundaries—must outweigh the potential costs, such as injury or emotional distress.

$$\text{Trust} = \frac{\text{Rewards}}{\text{Costs}} \qquad (4)$$

Attachment Theory further enriches our understanding by suggesting that early relationships with caregivers shape our ability to form trusting relationships in adulthood. Secure attachment styles, characterized by a sense of safety and reliability, foster an environment where individuals feel comfortable exploring their desires. Conversely, insecure attachment styles may lead to anxiety or avoidance in intimate scenarios, complicating the trust-building process.

Challenges in Establishing Trust

Establishing trust can be fraught with challenges, particularly in the context of fisting.

Fear of Vulnerability is a significant barrier. Engaging in fisting requires individuals to expose their bodies and emotions in ways that can feel risky. The fear of judgment or rejection can inhibit open communication, leading to misunderstandings and potential harm.

Past Trauma also plays a crucial role in trust dynamics. Individuals with a history of trauma may find it particularly difficult to trust others, especially in intimate contexts. This can manifest as hypervigilance or emotional withdrawal, both of which can hinder the exploration of fisting.

Communication Barriers further complicate trust. Inadequate communication about desires, boundaries, and fears can lead to assumptions and misinterpretations. Clear and open dialogue is essential to foster an environment where both partners feel safe to express their needs and concerns.

Building Trust Through Connection

To navigate these challenges, it is vital to actively cultivate trust and connection.

Establishing Open Communication is the first step. Partners should engage in discussions about their desires, limits, and anxieties related to fisting. Using "I" statements can help articulate feelings without placing blame, fostering a more constructive dialogue. For example, saying "I feel anxious about trying fisting because I'm worried about safety" invites understanding rather than defensiveness.

Practicing Consent is another critical aspect of building trust. Consent should be ongoing and enthusiastic, with partners checking in with each other throughout the experience. This not only reinforces trust but also deepens the connection as partners navigate their boundaries together.

Creating a Safe Environment enhances trust significantly. This can involve physical aspects, such as ensuring a comfortable space, as well as emotional aspects, such as establishing safe words and signals. Safe words provide a clear mechanism for partners to communicate when they need to pause or stop, reinforcing a sense of safety and control.

Examples of Trust and Connection in Fisting

Consider a couple, Alex and Jamie, who wish to explore fisting. Before engaging in the act, they spend time discussing their feelings about it. Alex expresses excitement but also fear of injury, while Jamie shares concerns about emotional vulnerability. They agree to establish a safe word—"pineapple"—to use if either feels uncomfortable during the experience.

On the day of their exploration, they set the scene by dimming the lights and playing soft music, creating an intimate atmosphere. They begin with gentle touch and communication, gradually building trust through shared experiences. As they engage in fisting, they frequently check in with each other, using the safe word if needed. This mutual respect and care enhance their emotional connection, allowing them to explore their boundaries safely.

Conclusion

The importance of trust and connection in fisting cannot be overstated. Trust serves as the bedrock of a healthy exploration of intimacy, enabling partners to navigate the complexities of vulnerability, desire, and safety. By fostering open communication, practicing ongoing consent, and creating a supportive environment, individuals can deepen their connections and enhance their experiences. As partners build trust, they not only enrich their fisting journey but also strengthen the overall fabric of their relationship.

The Role of Fantasy in Fisting

Fantasy plays a pivotal role in the exploration of fisting, serving as a conduit for desire, imagination, and the expression of erotic identity. It allows individuals to navigate their deepest yearnings in a safe and controlled environment, enhancing both the physical and emotional experiences associated with this intimate act.

Understanding Fantasy in Sexual Contexts

Fantasy can be defined as a mental image or scenario that evokes sexual arousal. It often encompasses elements of desire, power dynamics, and taboo, enabling individuals to explore scenarios that may not be feasible or appropriate in reality. According to the work of [1], fantasies can serve as a form of sexual expression that is both personal and revealing, offering insights into one's desires and boundaries.

Fisting as a Fantasy Element

Fisting, often regarded as a taboo or extreme sexual practice, can be intertwined with various fantasies. These may include themes of dominance and submission, vulnerability, or even the exploration of body limits. The act of fisting itself can symbolize a deeper connection between partners, transcending the physical to tap into emotional and psychological realms.

For example, a partner may fantasize about the feeling of being completely filled, which can evoke sensations of fullness and surrender. This fantasy may also incorporate elements of trust and vulnerability, as the act requires a high degree of communication and consent between partners. The interplay of fantasy and reality can create a rich tapestry of experiences that heighten arousal and intimacy.

The Therapeutic Potential of Fantasy

Engaging with fantasies surrounding fisting can also have therapeutic benefits. Fantasy can serve as a tool for self-exploration, helping individuals confront and process their desires, fears, and insecurities. As highlighted by [Perel(2007)], fantasy can be a pathway to understanding one's sexual identity and preferences, allowing for a deeper connection with oneself and one's partner.

Moreover, fantasies can act as a means of reclaiming power and agency, particularly for individuals who have experienced trauma. By envisioning scenarios where they are in control or exploring their limits, individuals can foster a sense of empowerment and healing. This reclamation can be crucial in the context of fisting, where the act itself can symbolize a journey towards embracing one's body and sexuality.

Navigating Fantasies Safely

While fantasies can enhance the fisting experience, it is essential to navigate them safely. Open communication with partners about desires and boundaries is paramount. Establishing a safe word or signal can help ensure that all parties feel secure in their exploration. Furthermore, discussing fantasies can lead to a deeper understanding of each partner's limits and preferences, fostering a stronger emotional connection.

It is also important to recognize that fantasies may not always align with reality. What may seem enticing in the realm of fantasy might not translate to a comfortable or pleasurable experience in practice. Therefore, it is crucial to approach the exploration of fisting with an open mind and a willingness to adapt.

Examples of Fisting Fantasies

1. **The Dominant/Submissive Dynamic:** One common fantasy involves a dominant partner guiding a submissive partner through the fisting experience. This scenario may include elements of control, where the dominant partner takes charge of the pace and intensity, while the submissive partner surrenders to the experience.

2. **Exploration of Limits:** Another fantasy might center around the idea of pushing boundaries and exploring limits. This could involve a partner fantasizing about gradually increasing the size of the hand used for fisting, symbolizing a journey of trust and exploration.

3. **Intimacy and Connection:** Some may fantasize about the profound intimacy that can arise from fisting. This fantasy may focus on the emotional connection between partners, where the act becomes a ritual of trust, vulnerability, and shared pleasure.

Incorporating Fantasy into Practice

To effectively incorporate fantasy into the fisting experience, individuals can engage in role-play scenarios, utilize props, or create an immersive environment that enhances the fantasy. For example, dim lighting, soft music, or themed attire can set the stage for exploration.

Additionally, partners can take turns sharing their fantasies, allowing for a collaborative approach to fisting that honors each person's desires. This exchange can lead to a richer experience, where both partners feel validated and excited about their shared exploration.

Conclusion

In conclusion, the role of fantasy in fisting is multifaceted, encompassing elements of desire, empowerment, and intimacy. By understanding and embracing fantasies, individuals can enhance their fisting experiences, fostering deeper connections with themselves and their partners. As with any sexual exploration, open communication, consent, and safety remain paramount, ensuring that the journey into fisting is both pleasurable and enriching.

Bibliography

[Nagoski(2015)] Nagoski, E. (2015). *Come As You Are: The Surprising New Science That Will Transform Your Sex Life*. Simon and Schuster.

[Perel(2007)] Perel, E. (2007). *Mating in Captivity: Unlocking Erotic Intelligence*. HarperCollins.

Understanding Your Body

Female Anatomy and Physiology

Understanding female anatomy and physiology is crucial for exploring fisting safely and enjoyably. This section delves into the key anatomical structures, physiological responses, and the interplay between them, providing a comprehensive foundation for those interested in fisting.

1.3.1.1 Overview of Female Reproductive Anatomy

The female reproductive system comprises several key structures, each playing a vital role in sexual function and pleasure. The primary components include:

- **Vulva:** The external genitalia, which includes the labia majora, labia minora, clitoris, urethra, and vaginal opening.

- **Vagina:** A muscular, elastic tube that connects the external genitals to the uterus. It serves multiple functions, including sexual intercourse, menstruation, and childbirth.

- **Cervix:** The lower part of the uterus that opens into the vagina. It plays a role in menstrual flow and childbirth.

- **Uterus:** A hollow, muscular organ where a fertilized egg can develop into a fetus. It has a rich blood supply and is sensitive to hormonal changes.
- **Ovaries:** Two small organs that produce eggs (ova) and hormones such as estrogen and progesterone.
- **Fallopian Tubes:** Tubes that transport eggs from the ovaries to the uterus and where fertilization typically occurs.

1.3.1.2 Physiological Responses During Sexual Arousal

Understanding the physiological responses during sexual arousal is essential for safe fisting practices. The process of arousal involves several stages:

1. **Excitement Phase:**

- Blood flow to the genitals increases, leading to swelling and sensitivity of the clitoris and vaginal walls.
- Vaginal lubrication begins, which is crucial for reducing friction during penetration.

2. **Plateau Phase:**

- The vagina expands and elongates, accommodating deeper penetration.
- The cervix elevates, moving away from the vaginal canal, which can create more space for fisting.

3. **Orgasm Phase:**

- Involuntary contractions of the pelvic floor muscles occur, which can enhance pleasure during fisting.
- The release of built-up tension can create a feeling of euphoria and satisfaction.

1.3.1.3 The Role of the Pelvic Floor Muscles

The pelvic floor muscles (PFM) play a crucial role in both sexual function and overall health. These muscles support the pelvic organs and are involved in sexual arousal and response.

$$\text{Pelvic Floor Muscle Tone} \propto \text{Sexual Satisfaction} \tag{5}$$

Strengthening and relaxing these muscles can enhance sexual experiences, including fisting. Exercises such as Kegels can improve muscle tone and control, contributing to heightened pleasure and safety during fisting.

1.3.1.4 Common Problems and Considerations

While exploring fisting, it is essential to be aware of potential problems related to female anatomy:

- **Vaginismus:** An involuntary contraction of the vaginal muscles that can make penetration painful or impossible. Understanding this condition is vital for those considering fisting.

- **Pelvic Pain Disorders:** Conditions such as endometriosis or pelvic inflammatory disease can affect comfort during fisting. Awareness and communication with partners are key.

- **Infections:** Maintaining proper hygiene is critical to prevent infections, especially when engaging in activities that involve deeper penetration.

1.3.1.5 Enhancing Body Awareness and Comfort

To ensure a pleasurable fisting experience, individuals should cultivate body awareness and comfort. This can be achieved through:

- **Mindfulness Practices:** Engaging in mindfulness can help individuals connect with their bodies, recognize sensations, and communicate effectively with partners.

- **Exploration of Sensation:** Masturbation and self-exploration can help individuals understand their bodies better and identify areas of pleasure and comfort.

- **Open Communication:** Discussing preferences, boundaries, and concerns with partners fosters a supportive environment for exploration.

In summary, a thorough understanding of female anatomy and physiology is foundational for safe and pleasurable fisting experiences. By recognizing the body's responses, addressing potential problems, and enhancing body awareness, individuals can embark on their fisting journey with confidence and care.

Male Anatomy and Physiology

Understanding male anatomy and physiology is crucial for exploring fisting safely and effectively. This section will provide insights into the relevant anatomical structures, their functions, and considerations for pleasure and safety during fisting.

Anatomical Overview

The male reproductive system consists of several key components, including the penis, scrotum, testicles, prostate gland, and associated ducts. Each part plays a distinct role in sexual function and pleasure.

- **Penis:** The penis is composed of three main parts: the root, body (shaft), and glans (tip). It contains erectile tissue that engorges with blood during arousal, allowing for penetration. The average erect penis size ranges from 5 to 6 inches in length and 4.5 to 5 inches in circumference, though variations are normal.

- **Scrotum:** The scrotum houses the testicles and helps regulate their temperature, which is vital for sperm production. It is sensitive to touch and temperature changes, contributing to sexual arousal.

- **Testicles:** The testicles produce sperm and testosterone, the primary male sex hormone. Testosterone influences libido, energy levels, and secondary sexual characteristics.

- **Prostate Gland:** The prostate is located just below the bladder and surrounds the urethra. It produces seminal fluid, which nourishes and transports sperm. Stimulation of the prostate can lead to intense pleasure and orgasms, often referred to as prostate orgasms.

- **Urethra:** The urethra runs through the penis and serves dual functions: it expels urine from the bladder and serves as a conduit for semen during ejaculation.

Physiological Responses

During sexual arousal, several physiological changes occur in the male body, including:

- **Erection:** Sexual arousal triggers the release of nitric oxide (NO), which dilates blood vessels in the penis, leading to increased blood flow and erection. This process can be expressed in terms of the following equation relating to blood flow:

$$Q = \Delta P/R \qquad (6)$$

where Q is the flow rate, ΔP is the pressure difference, and R is the resistance of the blood vessels.

- **Ejaculation:** Ejaculation is a complex reflex involving the contraction of muscles at the base of the penis and in the prostate. It can be divided into two phases: emission (movement of sperm into the urethra) and expulsion (forceful release of semen). The process is regulated by the autonomic nervous system.

- **Orgasm:** The sensation of orgasm is a culmination of sexual arousal characterized by intense pleasure and rhythmic contractions of the pelvic muscles. It is often accompanied by the release of endorphins and oxytocin, promoting feelings of well-being and connection.

Common Issues and Considerations

When engaging in fisting, it is essential to be aware of potential issues related to male anatomy:

- **Injury Risk:** The penis is susceptible to injury if excessive force or improper techniques are used during fisting. Common injuries include bruising, tearing of the skin, and damage to the erectile tissue. It is crucial to communicate with partners and proceed slowly, ensuring comfort and safety.

- **Prostate Health:** Regular stimulation of the prostate can have health benefits, including improved sexual function and reduced risk of prostate issues. However, individuals should be cautious of any discomfort or pain, as this may indicate underlying health problems.

- **Psychological Factors:** Men may experience anxiety related to performance or body image during sexual activities. Open communication with partners can help alleviate these concerns and foster a more enjoyable experience.

Examples of Exploration

When exploring fisting with male anatomy, consider the following techniques and approaches:

- **Positioning:** Optimal positioning can enhance comfort and pleasure. Positions such as lying on the back with legs raised or kneeling can facilitate access to the anus and prostate.

- **Communication:** Establishing a clear line of communication is vital. Discuss boundaries, desires, and safe words before beginning the exploration. This ensures that both partners feel secure and respected throughout the experience.

- **Lubrication:** The use of high-quality lubricant is essential to reduce friction and enhance pleasure. Silicone-based or water-based lubricants are recommended. Avoid oil-based products, as they can degrade latex gloves and condoms.

In summary, understanding male anatomy and physiology is fundamental for safe and pleasurable fisting experiences. By recognizing the unique features of male anatomy, potential risks, and effective techniques, individuals can explore this intimate practice with confidence and care.

Understanding Your Pelvic Floor Muscles

The pelvic floor is a complex structure composed of muscles, ligaments, and connective tissue that forms a supportive hammock at the base of the pelvis. These muscles play a crucial role in various bodily functions, including bladder and bowel control, sexual function, and core stability. Understanding the anatomy and function of the pelvic floor is essential for anyone exploring fisting, as it can enhance pleasure, safety, and overall experience.

Anatomy of the Pelvic Floor

The pelvic floor muscles can be divided into two main groups: the superficial pelvic floor muscles and the deep pelvic floor muscles.

- **Superficial Pelvic Floor Muscles:** These muscles are located just beneath the skin and are primarily responsible for sexual arousal and sensation. They include:

- *Bulbospongiosus:* This muscle surrounds the vaginal opening in females and the base of the penis in males, contributing to sexual pleasure and orgasm.
- *Ischiocavernosus:* This muscle helps maintain an erection in males and contributes to clitoral erection in females.
- *Superficial Transverse Perineal:* This muscle provides support to the pelvic floor and helps stabilize the perineum.

- **Deep Pelvic Floor Muscles:** These muscles are deeper within the pelvis and provide structural support to the pelvic organs. They include:

  - *Levator Ani:* This group of muscles supports the bladder, uterus, and rectum. It is critical for maintaining continence and plays a role in sexual function.
  - *Coccygeus:* This muscle assists in supporting the pelvic organs and helps in the movement of the coccyx.

Functions of the Pelvic Floor Muscles

The pelvic floor muscles serve several important functions:

- **Support of Pelvic Organs:** The pelvic floor muscles provide essential support for the bladder, uterus, and rectum, preventing prolapse and ensuring proper organ function.

- **Control of Bodily Functions:** These muscles are vital for the control of urination and defecation. When the pelvic floor muscles contract, they help to close the openings of the urethra and anus, allowing for voluntary control.

- **Sexual Function:** A strong and responsive pelvic floor can enhance sexual arousal and pleasure. The contractions of these muscles can intensify orgasms and improve overall sexual satisfaction.

- **Core Stability:** The pelvic floor works in conjunction with the abdominal and back muscles to provide stability and support to the spine and pelvis during movement.

Common Problems Related to the Pelvic Floor

While a healthy pelvic floor is essential for overall well-being, many individuals may experience problems related to pelvic floor dysfunction. Some common issues include:

- **Pelvic Floor Weakness:** This can lead to urinary incontinence, fecal incontinence, and pelvic organ prolapse. Weakness may result from factors such as childbirth, aging, obesity, or lack of exercise.

- **Overactivity:** Some individuals may experience overactive pelvic floor muscles, leading to conditions such as pelvic pain, painful intercourse, and urinary urgency.

- **Injury or Trauma:** Trauma to the pelvic area, whether from childbirth, surgery, or injury, can lead to dysfunction and discomfort.

Strengthening and Relaxing the Pelvic Floor Muscles

To maintain a healthy pelvic floor, it is essential to incorporate exercises that both strengthen and relax these muscles.

- **Kegel Exercises:** These exercises involve contracting and relaxing the pelvic floor muscles. To perform a Kegel, identify the muscles used to stop urination. Contract these muscles for 5 seconds, then relax for 5 seconds. Repeat this 10-15 times, three times a day.

- **Breathing Techniques:** Incorporating deep breathing can help relax the pelvic floor. Inhale deeply through the nose, allowing the abdomen to expand, and exhale slowly through the mouth, consciously relaxing the pelvic floor muscles.

- **Yoga and Stretching:** Certain yoga poses, such as the Child's Pose or Cat-Cow stretch, can help release tension in the pelvic floor while promoting flexibility and relaxation.

Mind-Body Connection and Body Awareness

Understanding the pelvic floor is not only about physical exercises; it also involves developing body awareness and a connection to your own sensations.

- **Mindfulness Practices:** Engaging in mindfulness can enhance your awareness of bodily sensations, allowing you to better connect with your pelvic floor. This can be done through meditation, breathwork, or body scanning techniques.

- **Exploration:** Gentle exploration of the pelvic area can help individuals become more familiar with their bodies, enhancing comfort and pleasure during intimate activities, including fisting.

Conclusion

Understanding your pelvic floor muscles is a vital step in preparing for a fisting journey. By recognizing their anatomy, functions, and potential issues, you can take proactive steps to strengthen and relax these muscles. This knowledge not only enhances safety but also enriches the experience of intimacy, trust, and pleasure. As you embark on this exploration, remember that the journey is as important as the destination—embracing your body and its capabilities will lead to deeper connections and more fulfilling experiences.

Exploring Sensation and Pleasure

Exploring sensation and pleasure is a fundamental aspect of fisting, as it involves a deep understanding of both the physiological and psychological components of the experience. This section delves into how individuals can cultivate heightened awareness of their bodies, recognize different sensations, and enhance pleasure during fisting.

The Nature of Sensation

Sensation is defined as the process by which our sensory receptors and nervous system receive and represent stimulus energies from our environment. In the context of fisting, this involves a variety of sensations that can be experienced in different ways depending on the individual's body, mindset, and the dynamics of the interaction. Sensations can be categorized into several types:

- **Tactile Sensation:** This includes feelings of pressure, temperature, and texture. The skin is rich with nerve endings that respond to touch, and during fisting, the varying degrees of pressure and movement can elicit a range of tactile sensations.

- **Kinesthetic Sensation:** This refers to the awareness of body position and movement. Understanding how one's body moves and responds during fisting can enhance the experience and facilitate a deeper connection with one's partner.

- **Proprioceptive Sensation:** This is the sense of the relative position of one's own parts of the body and strength of effort being employed in movement. Engaging with one's body and understanding its limits is crucial for safe fisting.

The Role of Pleasure in Fisting

Pleasure is a complex interplay of physical, emotional, and psychological factors. The experience of pleasure can be influenced by various elements, including:

- **Physical Stimulation:** The physical sensations experienced during fisting can lead to heightened pleasure. This includes the feeling of fullness, the stimulation of erogenous zones, and the release of endorphins.

- **Mental State:** A relaxed and open mindset can significantly enhance the experience of pleasure. Engaging in mindfulness practices can help individuals become more attuned to their bodies and the sensations they experience.

- **Emotional Connection:** The emotional bond between partners can amplify pleasure. Trust, intimacy, and vulnerability create a safe space for exploration, allowing individuals to experience deeper levels of pleasure.

Exploring Sensation and Pleasure Techniques

To fully explore sensation and pleasure during fisting, consider the following techniques:

1. **Mindful Breathing:** Begin with deep, mindful breathing to center yourself and become aware of your body. This practice can help reduce anxiety and increase sensitivity to sensations.

2. **Slow Exploration:** Take your time to explore different areas of the body. Use your fingers or hand to gently caress the skin, gradually increasing pressure and depth. Notice how different movements and pressures affect your sensations.

3. **Communication:** Maintain open lines of communication with your partner. Share what feels pleasurable, what doesn't, and any adjustments that may enhance the experience. Use verbal and non-verbal cues to guide the exploration.

4. **Experiment with Temperature:** Incorporate temperature play by using warm or cool objects. This can heighten the experience and create new sensations that enhance pleasure.

5. **Varying Speed and Rhythm:** Experiment with different speeds and rhythms during fisting. Some individuals may find slower, more deliberate movements to be more pleasurable, while others may enjoy faster, more vigorous motions.

Addressing Challenges in Sensation and Pleasure

While exploring sensation and pleasure, individuals may encounter challenges that can impede their experience:

- **Discomfort or Pain:** It is essential to differentiate between pleasurable sensations and discomfort or pain. If pain occurs, it is crucial to communicate and adjust techniques accordingly. Establishing safe words and signals can help ensure comfort.

- **Mental Barriers:** Past experiences, body image issues, or anxiety can create mental barriers that hinder pleasure. Engaging in self-reflection and possibly seeking professional support can help address these barriers.

- **Physical Limitations:** Understanding one's physical limits is vital. If any sensation feels overwhelming or uncomfortable, it is important to stop and reassess. Engaging in practices that promote body awareness can help individuals recognize their limits more effectively.

Conclusion

Exploring sensation and pleasure is an integral part of the fisting experience. By understanding the nature of sensation, recognizing the role of pleasure, and employing techniques to enhance exploration, individuals can create a fulfilling and enjoyable experience. Open communication, mindfulness, and awareness of both physical and emotional states are key components in navigating the complexities of sensation and pleasure in fisting. Embrace this journey of exploration with curiosity and compassion for yourself and your partner, and allow the experience to deepen your connection and understanding of pleasure.

Mind-Body Connection

The mind-body connection is a profound and intricate relationship that influences our physical sensations, emotional experiences, and overall well-being. Understanding this connection is crucial for individuals exploring fisting, as it can enhance pleasure, facilitate deeper intimacy, and promote safety during play. This section delves into the theoretical underpinnings of the mind-body connection, its implications for fisting, and practical techniques to strengthen this relationship.

Theoretical Framework

The mind-body connection is rooted in various psychological and physiological theories. One prominent theory is the biopsychosocial model, which posits that biological, psychological, and social factors interact to influence health and behavior. This model emphasizes that our thoughts and emotions can significantly impact our physical experiences. For instance, a relaxed mind can lead to a more open body, enhancing pleasure during fisting.

Another relevant theory is the somatic experiencing approach, which focuses on the body's innate ability to heal from trauma through awareness and sensation. This perspective suggests that by tuning into bodily sensations, individuals can release stored tension and emotional blockages, creating a more fulfilling sexual experience.

Problems in Mind-Body Connection

Despite the potential benefits of a strong mind-body connection, many individuals face challenges that can hinder their ability to fully engage in fisting. Common problems include:

- **Disconnection from Bodily Sensations:** Many people, especially those with a history of trauma, may struggle to feel in touch with their bodies. This disconnection can lead to difficulty experiencing pleasure or recognizing discomfort during fisting.

- **Anxiety and Performance Pressure:** The pressure to perform or meet certain expectations can create anxiety, which may manifest physically as tension. This tension can inhibit relaxation and pleasure, making the fisting experience less enjoyable.

- **Negative Body Image:** Individuals who struggle with body image issues may find it challenging to embrace their bodies during intimate experiences. This can lead to self-consciousness and distract from the pleasure of fisting.

- **Fear of Pain or Injury:** Concerns about physical safety can create mental barriers, leading to a heightened state of alertness that detracts from the experience of pleasure.

Enhancing the Mind-Body Connection

To enhance the mind-body connection, individuals can adopt several techniques that promote awareness, relaxation, and pleasure. Some effective strategies include:

- **Mindfulness and Meditation:** Practicing mindfulness can help individuals become more aware of their bodily sensations and emotions. Techniques such as body scans or focused breathing can ground individuals in their physical experience, enhancing their ability to engage in fisting. For example, a simple mindfulness exercise involves focusing on the breath while observing the sensations in the body without judgment.

- **Somatic Practices:** Engaging in somatic practices, such as yoga or dance, can help individuals reconnect with their bodies. These practices encourage movement and awareness, allowing individuals to explore their physicality and release tension.

- **Breathwork:** Conscious breathing techniques can facilitate relaxation and enhance arousal. Deep, rhythmic breathing can help alleviate anxiety and tension, creating a more receptive state for fisting. For instance, individuals may practice inhaling deeply through the nose for a count of four, holding for four, and exhaling through the mouth for a count of six.

- **Sensate Focus:** This technique, often used in sex therapy, encourages individuals to explore touch and sensation without the pressure of performance. By focusing on the physical sensations of touch, individuals can cultivate a deeper awareness of their bodies, enhancing their fisting experience.

- **Journaling:** Reflective writing can help individuals process their feelings about their bodies, pleasure, and sexuality. Journaling about experiences, desires, and fears can promote self-awareness and facilitate a stronger mind-body connection.

- **Partner Communication:** Open communication with partners about sensations, boundaries, and desires can foster a sense of safety and connection. This dialogue can help reduce anxiety and enhance the overall experience of fisting.

Practical Examples

To illustrate the mind-body connection in the context of fisting, consider the following scenarios:

- **Scenario 1: Overcoming Anxiety** - A person feeling anxious about their first fisting experience may practice mindfulness techniques prior to the encounter. By focusing on their breath and tuning into their body, they can reduce tension and cultivate a sense of openness, making the experience more enjoyable.

- **Scenario 2: Enhancing Sensation** - A couple engaging in fisting may incorporate breathwork into their play. As one partner slowly inserts their hand, they synchronize their breath, inhaling deeply as they prepare for penetration and exhaling slowly to relax. This practice can enhance the sensations experienced during fisting and deepen their emotional connection.

- **Scenario 3: Building Body Confidence** - An individual struggling with body image issues may begin journaling about their feelings and desires related to fisting. By exploring their thoughts and emotions, they can work toward self-acceptance and a more positive relationship with their body, ultimately enhancing their fisting experiences.

- **Scenario 4: Exploring Sensation** - A couple practicing sensate focus may take turns exploring each other's bodies with their hands, focusing on the sensations without the goal of penetration. This practice can help them develop a deeper understanding of their bodies and enhance their pleasure during fisting.

Conclusion

The mind-body connection is a vital aspect of the fisting experience, influencing both physical sensations and emotional responses. By understanding and nurturing this connection, individuals can enhance their pleasure, foster intimacy, and ensure a safer, more fulfilling exploration of fisting. Techniques such as mindfulness, breathwork, and open communication can help individuals overcome barriers, embrace their bodies, and deepen their experiences. As individuals embark on their fisting journeys, cultivating a strong mind-body connection can lead to profound personal growth and discovery.

Addressing Body Image and Shame

Body image and shame are complex emotional experiences that can significantly impact an individual's willingness to explore intimate practices such as fisting. This section delves into the definitions of body image and shame, the psychological theories surrounding them, and strategies for addressing these challenges to foster a more positive and empowered approach to sexual exploration.

Understanding Body Image

Body image refers to the subjective perception a person has of their physical appearance. It encompasses thoughts, beliefs, and feelings about one's body, which can be positive or negative. A positive body image is characterized by an appreciation of one's body and a sense of confidence in one's physical self, while a negative body image can lead to feelings of inadequacy, self-doubt, and shame.

Theories of Body Image   Several psychological theories explain the development of body image:

- **Social Comparison Theory** posits that individuals determine their own social and personal worth based on how they stack up against others. This can lead to negative body image when individuals compare themselves unfavorably to societal ideals portrayed in media.

- **Cognitive Dissonance Theory** suggests that individuals experience discomfort when their beliefs about their body do not align with their actual experiences. For instance, a person may believe they should be fit and attractive but feel they do not meet these standards, leading to shame.

- **Objectification Theory** argues that women, in particular, are often socialized to view themselves as objects to be evaluated based on appearance, which can diminish their self-esteem and contribute to body shame.

The Role of Shame in Body Image

Shame is an intense emotion that arises from the perception of oneself as flawed or unworthy. It can stem from societal pressures, past experiences, or internalized beliefs about the body. Shame can inhibit sexual exploration and intimacy, as individuals may feel self-conscious or unworthy of pleasure.

The Cycle of Shame and Body Image The relationship between body image and shame can create a vicious cycle:

Negative Body Image → Increased Shame → Avoidance of Intimacy → Reinforcement o
(7)

For example, an individual who feels ashamed of their body may avoid intimate situations, leading to a lack of experience and further negative self-perception. This cycle can be particularly pronounced in practices like fisting, where vulnerability and trust are paramount.

Strategies for Addressing Body Image and Shame

1. Cultivating Self-Compassion Practicing self-compassion involves treating oneself with kindness and understanding rather than judgment. Techniques include:

- **Mindfulness Meditation:** Engaging in mindfulness practices can help individuals become more aware of their thoughts and feelings without judgment, allowing for greater acceptance of their bodies.

- **Affirmations:** Positive affirmations can counter negative self-talk. For instance, repeating phrases like "I am worthy of pleasure" can help reframe one's mindset.

2. Challenging Societal Norms Individuals can work to challenge societal standards of beauty by:

- **Diversifying Media Consumption:** Engaging with media that portrays a variety of body types and experiences can help reshape perceptions of beauty.

- **Surrounding Oneself with Positivity:** Building a community that celebrates body diversity can foster a more positive self-image.

3. Engaging in Body Positivity Practices Body positivity involves embracing all bodies and recognizing that worth is not determined by appearance. Strategies include:

- **Body Neutrality:** Focusing on what the body can do rather than how it looks can shift the focus away from appearance.

- **Celebrating Physical Experiences:** Engaging in activities that celebrate the body, such as dance or yoga, can enhance body appreciation.

4. **Open Communication with Partners**   Discussing body image and feelings of shame with partners can foster intimacy and understanding. This can involve:

- **Vulnerability in Conversations:** Sharing insecurities can strengthen trust and connection in relationships.
- **Establishing Safe Spaces:** Creating an environment where both partners feel safe to express their feelings can enhance emotional intimacy.

Conclusion

Addressing body image and shame is crucial for individuals looking to explore fisting and other intimate practices. By understanding the psychological underpinnings of these experiences and employing strategies to cultivate a positive body image, individuals can empower themselves to embrace their bodies and engage in fulfilling sexual exploration. The journey towards self-acceptance is ongoing, but with patience and support, it is entirely achievable.

Positive Body Image → Increased Intimacy → Greater Sexual Exploration → Reinforcem
(8)

Pelvic Floor Health and Maintenance

The pelvic floor is a complex network of muscles, ligaments, and tissues that support the pelvic organs, including the bladder, uterus, and rectum. Maintaining pelvic floor health is essential for overall well-being, particularly for those interested in exploring fisting. A well-functioning pelvic floor can enhance sexual pleasure, improve control over bodily functions, and reduce the risk of injuries during intimate activities.

Understanding the Pelvic Floor

The pelvic floor consists of several muscles, primarily the levator ani and the coccygeus, which form a supportive hammock-like structure. These muscles are responsible for:

- Supporting pelvic organs

- Controlling bladder and bowel functions
- Contributing to sexual function and sensation

Common Problems Associated with Pelvic Floor Dysfunction

Pelvic floor dysfunction can manifest in various ways, affecting both physical and emotional health. Common issues include:

- **Incontinence:** This can be urinary or fecal incontinence, where individuals experience involuntary leakage.
- **Pelvic Pain:** Chronic pelvic pain can arise from tight or weak pelvic floor muscles, leading to discomfort during sexual activities, including fisting.
- **Prolapse:** A pelvic organ prolapse occurs when the pelvic organs descend due to weakened pelvic floor support, which can affect sexual function and sensation.
- **Dysfunction in Sexual Response:** Individuals may experience difficulties with arousal, orgasm, or overall sexual satisfaction due to pelvic floor issues.

Assessing Pelvic Floor Health

It is crucial to assess pelvic floor health regularly. This can be done through:

- **Self-Assessment:** Individuals can perform self-examinations to identify muscle tension, relaxation, and overall awareness of the pelvic area.
- **Professional Assessment:** Consulting a pelvic floor physical therapist can provide a more thorough evaluation and tailored exercises.

Exercises for Pelvic Floor Maintenance

To maintain a healthy pelvic floor, consider incorporating the following exercises into your routine:

Kegel Exercises: Kegel exercises strengthen the pelvic floor muscles. To perform Kegels:

1. Identify the correct muscles by stopping urination midstream.

2. Once identified, contract these muscles for 5 seconds, then relax for 5 seconds.

3. Gradually increase the duration of contractions up to 10 seconds, aiming for three sets of 10 repetitions daily.

Pelvic Tilts: This exercise helps improve pelvic mobility and strength:

1. Lie on your back with knees bent and feet flat on the floor.

2. Gently tilt your pelvis upward while tightening your abdominal muscles.

3. Hold for a few seconds before relaxing.

Bridge Pose: This yoga pose strengthens the glutes and pelvic floor:

1. Lie on your back with knees bent and feet hip-width apart.

2. Press through your heels, lifting your hips towards the ceiling while squeezing your pelvic floor muscles.

3. Hold for a few seconds before lowering back down.

Incorporating Relaxation Techniques

In addition to strengthening exercises, it is essential to incorporate relaxation techniques for a balanced pelvic floor. Overactive pelvic floor muscles can lead to tension and discomfort. Techniques include:

- **Deep Breathing:** Focus on diaphragmatic breathing to promote relaxation of the pelvic floor.

- **Progressive Muscle Relaxation:** Tense and relax different muscle groups, including the pelvic floor, to enhance awareness and release tension.

- **Mindfulness Practices:** Engage in mindfulness meditation to connect with your body and cultivate a sense of ease in the pelvic region.

The Role of Professional Support

For those experiencing significant pelvic floor issues, seeking professional help is essential. A pelvic floor physical therapist can provide:

- Customized exercise programs
- Manual therapy techniques
- Education on pelvic floor anatomy and function
- Strategies for managing pain and discomfort

Conclusion

Maintaining pelvic floor health is vital for individuals interested in fisting and other intimate activities. A balanced approach that includes strengthening, relaxation, and professional guidance can enhance sexual experiences and overall well-being. By prioritizing pelvic floor health, individuals can explore their desires with confidence and safety, fostering deeper connections with themselves and their partners.

Strengthening and Relaxing the Pelvic Floor

The pelvic floor is a complex structure of muscles, ligaments, and tissues that support the pelvic organs, including the bladder, uterus (in females), and rectum. Understanding how to strengthen and relax these muscles is crucial for enhancing sexual pleasure, preventing injury, and maintaining overall pelvic health.

The Importance of the Pelvic Floor

The pelvic floor plays a vital role in various bodily functions, including:

- **Support:** It provides support for the pelvic organs, helping to maintain their position and function.
- **Control:** It is essential for bladder and bowel control, allowing for voluntary and involuntary control of urination and defecation.
- **Sexual Function:** A strong and well-coordinated pelvic floor contributes to sexual arousal, orgasm, and overall sexual satisfaction.
- **Stability:** It contributes to core stability and posture, influencing how we move and carry ourselves.

Strengthening the Pelvic Floor

Strengthening the pelvic floor involves exercises that target the muscles of this area, commonly referred to as Kegel exercises. These exercises can enhance muscle tone and improve control over pelvic functions.

Kegel Exercises Kegel exercises involve the repetitive contraction and relaxation of the pelvic floor muscles. To perform these exercises effectively:

1. **Identify the Muscles:** The first step is to locate the pelvic floor muscles. This can be done by attempting to stop urination midstream. The muscles you engage are your pelvic floor muscles.

2. **Contraction:** Once identified, contract the pelvic floor muscles for a count of three to five seconds. Ensure that you are not holding your breath or tightening your abdominal, buttock, or thigh muscles.

3. **Relaxation:** Release the contraction and relax the muscles for an equal amount of time.

4. **Repetition:** Aim for 10 to 15 repetitions, three times a day. Gradually increase the duration of the contractions as your strength improves.

Benefits of Strengthening Regularly performing Kegel exercises can lead to:

- Improved bladder control and reduced urinary incontinence.

- Enhanced sexual arousal and orgasmic intensity.

- Increased support for pelvic organs, reducing the risk of prolapse.

- Greater control during sexual activity, allowing for more pleasurable experiences.

Relaxing the Pelvic Floor

While strengthening the pelvic floor is essential, learning to relax these muscles is equally important. Overly tense pelvic floor muscles can lead to discomfort, pain during intercourse, and other pelvic floor dysfunctions.

Techniques for Relaxation To effectively relax the pelvic floor, consider the following techniques:

1. **Breathing Exercises:** Deep, diaphragmatic breathing can help release tension in the pelvic floor. Inhale deeply through the nose, allowing the abdomen to expand, and exhale slowly through the mouth, consciously relaxing the pelvic muscles.

2. **Gentle Stretching:** Incorporating stretches that target the hips and lower back can alleviate tension in the pelvic area. Poses such as Child's Pose, Butterfly Stretch, and Cat-Cow can be beneficial.

3. **Mindfulness and Visualization:** Practicing mindfulness techniques and visualizing the pelvic floor muscles softening can help facilitate relaxation. Focus on the sensations in your body and consciously release any tension.

4. **Warm Baths:** Soaking in a warm bath can promote relaxation throughout the body, including the pelvic floor. Adding Epsom salts may enhance the soothing effect.

Understanding Tension and Pain Excessive tension in the pelvic floor can lead to a condition known as pelvic floor dysfunction, which may manifest as:

- Pain during intercourse (dyspareunia).
- Chronic pelvic pain.
- Difficulty with urination or bowel movements.
- Increased anxiety related to sexual activity.

If you experience persistent pain or discomfort, it is essential to consult a healthcare professional specializing in pelvic health.

Integrating Strengthening and Relaxation

To achieve optimal pelvic floor health, it is crucial to integrate both strengthening and relaxation techniques. A balanced approach allows for better control, enhanced sexual experiences, and improved overall wellbeing.

Example Routine Consider the following routine that combines both strengthening and relaxation:

- **Kegel Exercises:** Perform three sets of 10 repetitions daily.
- **Breathing Exercises:** Spend five minutes each day focusing on deep, diaphragmatic breathing.
- **Stretching:** Dedicate 10 minutes to gentle stretching or yoga poses that promote pelvic relaxation.
- **Mindfulness Practice:** Incorporate mindfulness meditation for 5-10 minutes, focusing on the sensations in your pelvic area.

By adopting a holistic approach to pelvic floor health, individuals can enhance their physical capabilities, emotional wellbeing, and sexual satisfaction.

Conclusion

Strengthening and relaxing the pelvic floor is a vital aspect of sexual health and wellness. By understanding the importance of these muscles and incorporating effective techniques, individuals can foster a deeper connection with their bodies, enhance their sexual experiences, and promote overall pelvic health. Regular practice and awareness will lead to greater confidence and enjoyment in one's sexual journey.

Incorporating Regular Exercise

Regular exercise is a vital component of a healthy lifestyle, especially for those interested in exploring fisting. Physical fitness not only enhances overall well-being but also plays a significant role in sexual health, body awareness, and the ability to engage in physically demanding activities like fisting safely. This section will explore the benefits of regular exercise, provide practical recommendations, and discuss the relationship between fitness and fisting.

The Benefits of Regular Exercise

Engaging in regular physical activity offers numerous benefits that can enhance the fisting experience:

- **Improved Flexibility:** Regular stretching and flexibility training can help increase the range of motion in your joints and muscles. This is particularly important for fisting, as it requires a certain level of flexibility in the hands, wrists, and body. Incorporating yoga or Pilates into your routine can significantly improve flexibility.

- **Increased Strength:** Strength training, particularly for the core, arms, and pelvic floor muscles, is essential for fisting. Stronger muscles can help support the body during fisting and reduce the risk of injury. Exercises like squats, lunges, and resistance training can be beneficial.

- **Enhanced Endurance:** Cardiovascular fitness improves stamina, allowing individuals to engage in prolonged sessions of fisting without fatigue. Activities such as running, cycling, or swimming can boost cardiovascular health and endurance levels.

- **Better Body Awareness:** Regular exercise fosters a deeper connection with your body, enhancing body awareness and self-acceptance. This awareness is crucial during fisting, as it allows individuals to tune into their sensations, limits, and comfort levels.

- **Stress Reduction:** Physical activity is a powerful stress reliever. Regular exercise can help reduce anxiety and improve mood, making it easier to approach intimate experiences with a positive mindset.

Practical Recommendations for Incorporating Exercise

To effectively incorporate exercise into your routine, consider the following recommendations:

- **Set Realistic Goals:** Start with achievable fitness goals that align with your current level of activity. For example, aim to exercise for 20-30 minutes, three times a week, gradually increasing intensity and duration as you progress.

- **Choose Enjoyable Activities:** Engage in exercises that you enjoy, as this will help you stay motivated. Whether it's dancing, hiking, swimming, or group classes, finding joy in movement is key to consistency.

- **Incorporate Variety:** Mix different types of exercise to work on various aspects of fitness. Combine strength training, cardio, and flexibility exercises to create a balanced routine that supports your fisting journey.

UNDERSTANDING YOUR BODY

- **Listen to Your Body:** Pay attention to your body's signals during workouts. If you experience pain or discomfort, modify your routine or consult a fitness professional to ensure you are exercising safely.

- **Include Pelvic Floor Exercises:** Strengthening the pelvic floor is particularly beneficial for fisting. Incorporate exercises like Kegels, which involve contracting and relaxing the pelvic floor muscles. This can enhance control and pleasure during intimate activities.

- **Establish a Routine:** Consistency is crucial for reaping the benefits of exercise. Schedule regular workout sessions, and consider pairing them with other activities you enjoy, such as socializing with friends or joining a fitness group.

The Relationship Between Fitness and Fisting

The connection between physical fitness and fisting is multifaceted. Engaging in regular exercise can lead to improved sexual function, enhanced pleasure, and reduced risk of injury during fisting. Research has shown that individuals who maintain a regular exercise routine often report higher levels of sexual satisfaction and better body image.

$$\text{Sexual Satisfaction} \propto \text{Physical Fitness} \qquad (9)$$

This equation suggests that as physical fitness increases, so does sexual satisfaction, highlighting the importance of exercise in enhancing intimate experiences.

Moreover, the psychological benefits of exercise can contribute to a more fulfilling fisting experience. Increased self-esteem, body confidence, and emotional resilience can empower individuals to explore their desires and fantasies more openly.

Examples of Effective Exercises

Here are some specific exercises that can support your fisting journey:

- **Yoga:** Poses such as Downward Dog, Cat-Cow, and Pigeon pose can enhance flexibility and body awareness. Incorporating breathwork can also help manage anxiety and promote relaxation.

- **Strength Training:** Focus on compound movements like squats, deadlifts, and push-ups to build overall strength. Incorporate resistance bands or weights to increase intensity.
- **Cardiovascular Activities:** Choose activities that elevate your heart rate and improve endurance, such as running, cycling, or high-intensity interval training (HIIT).
- **Pelvic Floor Exercises:** Practice Kegel exercises by contracting the pelvic floor muscles for a count of five, then relaxing for five. Aim for three sets of 10-15 repetitions daily.

Conclusion

Incorporating regular exercise into your routine is an essential step toward enhancing your fisting experience. By improving flexibility, strength, endurance, and body awareness, you set the stage for safer and more pleasurable exploration. Remember to listen to your body, set realistic goals, and enjoy the journey of physical fitness as it intertwines with your intimate adventures.

Experimenting with Body Awareness Techniques

Body awareness techniques are essential tools for enhancing one's connection to their body, fostering a deeper understanding of physical sensations, and ultimately enriching the fisting experience. By cultivating body awareness, individuals can better navigate their comfort levels, recognize their boundaries, and enhance their capacity for pleasure. This section will explore various body awareness techniques, their theoretical foundations, practical applications, and potential challenges.

Theoretical Foundations of Body Awareness

Body awareness is rooted in several psychological and physiological theories. One key theory is the *Somatic Psychology*, which emphasizes the connection between the mind and body. According to this perspective, physical sensations and emotions are intertwined, and by tuning into bodily sensations, individuals can access deeper emotional states and foster healing.

Another relevant theory is the *Mindfulness-Based Stress Reduction* (MBSR) approach, which teaches individuals to focus on the present moment without judgment. This practice encourages participants to observe their bodily sensations, thoughts, and feelings, leading to increased self-awareness and emotional regulation.

Benefits of Body Awareness Techniques

Engaging in body awareness techniques can offer numerous benefits, including:

- **Enhanced Sensation Recognition:** Individuals can learn to identify and differentiate various sensations, which can lead to greater pleasure during fisting.

- **Improved Communication:** Increased body awareness fosters better communication with partners about desires, boundaries, and comfort levels.

- **Emotional Regulation:** By recognizing and processing bodily sensations, individuals can manage anxiety and emotional responses during intimate experiences.

- **Increased Trust and Intimacy:** Practicing body awareness can enhance trust between partners, leading to deeper connections and intimacy.

Techniques for Body Awareness

Here are several effective techniques for cultivating body awareness:

1. Mindful Breathing Mindful breathing is a foundational technique that helps individuals center themselves and tune into their bodies. To practice mindful breathing:

1. Find a comfortable position, either sitting or lying down.

2. Close your eyes and take a deep breath in through your nose, allowing your abdomen to expand.

3. Hold the breath for a moment, then slowly exhale through your mouth, feeling your body relax.

4. Focus on the rhythm of your breath, noticing the sensations in your body as you breathe in and out.

5. If your mind wanders, gently redirect your focus back to your breath.

Mindful breathing can be practiced before, during, or after fisting to enhance relaxation and body awareness.

2. **Body Scan Meditation** The body scan meditation is a technique that encourages individuals to systematically focus on different parts of their body. To perform a body scan:

1. Lie down in a comfortable position and close your eyes.
2. Begin by focusing on your toes, noticing any sensations, tension, or relaxation.
3. Gradually move your attention up through your feet, legs, abdomen, chest, arms, neck, and head.
4. As you scan each area, consciously relax any tension you may feel.
5. Spend a few moments reflecting on the sensations in each part of your body before moving on.

This technique can be particularly useful for individuals who may experience tension or anxiety during intimate experiences.

3. **Sensory Exploration** Sensory exploration involves engaging with different textures, temperatures, and sensations to heighten body awareness. This can include:

- **Touching Different Textures:** Use various materials (e.g., silk, fur, leather) to explore how different textures feel against your skin.
- **Temperature Play:** Experiment with warm and cool objects (e.g., warm towels, ice cubes) to heighten sensitivity and awareness.
- **Movement Exploration:** Engage in slow, mindful movements, such as stretching or dancing, to become more attuned to your body's capabilities and sensations.

4. **Journaling and Reflection** Journaling can be a powerful tool for enhancing body awareness. Consider the following prompts:

- **Describe a Sensation:** Write about a specific sensation you experienced during fisting or other intimate activities. What did it feel like? How did it affect your emotions?
- **Reflect on Boundaries:** Note your comfort levels and boundaries before and after intimate experiences. How did your body respond?

- **Explore Emotional Connections:** Reflect on any emotions that arose during intimate moments. How did your body respond to these emotions?

Potential Challenges and Solutions

While experimenting with body awareness techniques can be enriching, individuals may encounter challenges:

1. **Discomfort with Sensations** Some individuals may feel uncomfortable with certain sensations or experiences. It is essential to approach these feelings with curiosity rather than judgment. Practicing mindful breathing can help individuals manage discomfort and remain present.

2. **Difficulty Focusing** In a fast-paced world, it can be challenging to maintain focus on bodily sensations. Setting aside dedicated time for body awareness practices, free from distractions, can enhance concentration and effectiveness.

3. **Emotional Triggers** Body awareness techniques can sometimes bring up unresolved emotions or trauma. It is crucial to practice self-compassion and, if needed, seek professional support to navigate these feelings safely.

Conclusion

Experimenting with body awareness techniques is a vital aspect of preparing for a fulfilling and safe fisting experience. By cultivating a deeper connection to one's body, individuals can enhance their pleasure, communicate effectively with partners, and navigate their emotional landscapes. The journey of body awareness is ongoing, inviting exploration, curiosity, and growth in the realm of intimacy and pleasure. As individuals embrace these techniques, they not only enrich their fisting experiences but also foster a profound sense of self-acceptance and body positivity.

Preparing for Your Fisting Journey

Establishing Boundaries and Limits

Establishing boundaries and limits is a fundamental aspect of engaging in fisting, as it ensures that all participants feel safe, respected, and empowered throughout the experience. This section will explore the significance of boundaries, the process of establishing them, and practical strategies for effective communication.

The Importance of Boundaries

Boundaries are the lines that define where one person's physical, emotional, and psychological space ends and another's begins. In the context of fisting, boundaries serve multiple purposes:

- **Safety:** Clear boundaries help prevent physical injuries and emotional distress, allowing participants to explore their desires without fear of harm.
- **Consent:** Establishing boundaries is a critical component of informed consent, ensuring that all parties understand and agree to the parameters of the play.
- **Trust:** Discussing and respecting boundaries fosters a sense of trust and intimacy, which is vital for a fulfilling fisting experience.
- **Empowerment:** Setting boundaries empowers individuals to take control of their bodies and experiences, enhancing personal agency.

Types of Boundaries

Boundaries can be categorized into several types, each of which plays a crucial role in fisting:

- **Physical Boundaries:** These boundaries pertain to the physical aspects of fisting, including what areas of the body are off-limits, the intensity of the experience, and the use of specific techniques or tools.
- **Emotional Boundaries:** Emotional boundaries involve the feelings and emotional states that participants are willing to share or engage with during play. This includes discussing past traumas, triggers, and emotional responses.
- **Temporal Boundaries:** These boundaries define the duration and timing of the fisting session, including when to start, how long to continue, and when to stop.
- **Social Boundaries:** Social boundaries relate to the context in which fisting occurs, such as whether it takes place in private or public settings and the presence of others.

Communicating Boundaries

Effective communication is essential for establishing and respecting boundaries. Here are some strategies for facilitating open discussions about boundaries:

- **Use Clear Language:** Be specific about your boundaries. Instead of vague statements like "I don't want to hurt," articulate precise limits, such as "I am not comfortable with anal fisting" or "I prefer gentle pressure."

- **Active Listening:** Engage in active listening by giving your partner your full attention and validating their feelings. This fosters an environment where both parties feel heard and respected.

- **Non-Verbal Cues:** Pay attention to non-verbal signals, such as body language and facial expressions. These cues can provide valuable insights into your partner's comfort level and emotional state.

- **Check-Ins:** Regularly check in with your partner during the fisting session to ensure they are comfortable and enjoying the experience. Phrases like "How are you feeling?" or "Do you want to continue?" can be helpful.

The Role of Safe Words

Safe words are a vital tool for navigating boundaries during fisting. A safe word is a pre-agreed term that signals the need to pause or stop the activity. The use of safe words enhances safety and consent by providing a clear mechanism for communication.

- **Choosing a Safe Word:** Select a word that is easy to remember and unlikely to come up in casual conversation. Common choices include "red" for stop and "yellow" for slow down or check in.

- **Non-Verbal Signals:** In situations where verbal communication may be difficult, establish non-verbal signals, such as a raised hand or tapping on a surface, to indicate discomfort or the need to pause.

Revisiting Boundaries

Boundaries are not static; they can evolve over time as individuals gain more experience and insight into their desires and limits. It is essential to revisit and renegotiate boundaries regularly, especially as trust and intimacy deepen. Consider the following approaches:

- **Post-Scene Debriefing:** After a fisting session, engage in a debriefing conversation to discuss what worked, what didn't, and any adjustments that may be needed for future encounters.

- **Reflective Journaling:** Encourage each participant to reflect on their experiences through journaling. This practice can help identify new boundaries or shifts in comfort levels.

- **Ongoing Communication:** Maintain an open line of communication outside of fisting sessions. Regularly check in about desires, concerns, and evolving boundaries.

Common Challenges in Boundary Setting

While establishing boundaries is crucial, it can also present challenges. Here are some common issues and strategies for addressing them:

- **Fear of Rejection:** Individuals may fear that expressing boundaries will lead to rejection or disappointment from their partner. Encourage open dialogue about the importance of boundaries for mutual enjoyment and safety.

- **Misunderstandings:** Miscommunication can occur if boundaries are not articulated clearly. Encourage clarity and ask questions to ensure mutual understanding.

- **Emotional Vulnerability:** Discussing boundaries can evoke feelings of vulnerability. Create a safe space for these conversations by affirming the importance of emotional safety.

In conclusion, establishing boundaries and limits is a vital component of a safe and fulfilling fisting experience. Through clear communication, the use of safe words, and ongoing dialogue, participants can create an environment of trust and respect that enhances their exploration of this intimate practice. Remember, boundaries are a reflection of personal autonomy and should always be honored and respected.

Defining Personal Goals and Desires

Defining personal goals and desires is a critical step in the journey of exploring fisting, as it allows individuals to clarify what they hope to achieve and experience during this intimate practice. Understanding one's motivations can enhance the overall experience and ensure that it aligns with personal values and boundaries. This section provides a framework for identifying and articulating these goals and desires.

Understanding Your Motivations

Before delving into the specifics of fisting, it is essential to take a moment for self-reflection. Ask yourself: What draws you to fisting? Is it the physical sensations, the emotional connection, or perhaps the thrill of exploring a taboo? Identifying your motivations can help you articulate your desires more clearly. Consider the following categories of motivation:

- **Physical Exploration:** Are you interested in the sensations associated with fisting? Do you seek to explore your body or your partner's body in new ways?

- **Emotional Connection:** Is your goal to deepen intimacy and trust with your partner? Do you wish to experience vulnerability and connection through shared exploration?

- **Fantasy and Role Play:** Are you motivated by the desire to enact specific fantasies or power dynamics? How do these fantasies align with your personal values?

- **Healing and Empowerment:** Do you seek to reclaim your body and sexuality? Are you interested in using fisting as a means of emotional release or catharsis?

Setting Clear Goals

Once you have reflected on your motivations, the next step is to set clear and achievable goals. Consider using the SMART criteria, which stands for Specific, Measurable, Achievable, Relevant, and Time-bound. This framework can help you create goals that are well-defined and realistic.

- **Specific:** Clearly articulate what you want to achieve. Instead of saying, "I want to try fisting," specify, "I want to experience fisting with my partner in a safe and consensual way."

- **Measurable:** Determine how you will measure your progress. This could involve setting milestones, such as practicing relaxation techniques or increasing comfort levels with hand insertion.

- **Achievable:** Ensure that your goals are realistic given your current level of experience and comfort. It's important to avoid setting overly ambitious goals that may lead to frustration.

- **Relevant:** Your goals should align with your overall desires and motivations. For instance, if intimacy is your primary goal, consider how fisting can enhance that connection.

- **Time-bound:** Set a timeframe for achieving your goals. This could involve planning specific dates for practice or setting a timeline for ongoing exploration.

Articulating Desires with Partners

Once you have defined your personal goals, it is crucial to communicate these desires with your partner(s). Open and honest communication is the cornerstone of a healthy sexual relationship, especially when exploring a practice as intimate as fisting. Here are some strategies for articulating your desires:

- **Use "I" Statements:** Frame your desires in a way that expresses your feelings and needs without placing pressure on your partner. For example, say, "I would love to explore fisting together because I think it could enhance our intimacy."

- **Encourage Dialogue:** Invite your partner to share their thoughts and feelings about fisting. Ask open-ended questions such as, "What are your feelings about trying fisting?" This fosters a collaborative atmosphere.

- **Discuss Boundaries:** Clearly articulate your boundaries and encourage your partner to do the same. Discussing limits upfront helps establish a safe space for exploration.

- **Check-in Regularly:** As you explore fisting, maintain ongoing communication. Regular check-ins allow both partners to express comfort levels, desires, and any concerns that may arise during the experience.

Anticipating Challenges and Adjusting Goals

It is important to recognize that the journey of exploring fisting may come with challenges. Anticipating potential obstacles can help you adjust your goals and desires as needed. Common challenges may include:

- **Physical Discomfort:** If you experience discomfort during initial attempts, consider adjusting your goals to focus on relaxation and gradual exploration rather than immediate penetration.

- **Emotional Responses:** Fisting can evoke a range of emotional responses, including vulnerability and anxiety. Be prepared to address these feelings and adjust your approach accordingly.

- **Miscommunication:** If misunderstandings arise, take the time to clarify your goals and desires with your partner. Open dialogue can help prevent feelings of frustration or disappointment.

Examples of Personal Goals

To provide clarity, here are some examples of personal goals that individuals might set when exploring fisting:

- **Goal 1:** "I want to practice fisting techniques with my partner once a month for the next three months to build comfort and confidence."

- **Goal 2:** "I aim to explore fisting as a way to deepen emotional intimacy with my partner by incorporating aftercare practices post-exploration."

- **Goal 3:** "I wish to attend a workshop on fisting safety and techniques within the next six months to enhance my knowledge and skills."

Conclusion

Defining personal goals and desires is an essential aspect of preparing for a fulfilling and safe fisting experience. By reflecting on motivations, setting clear goals, and communicating openly with partners, individuals can embark on a journey that aligns with their values and enhances their intimate connections. Remember that this journey is unique to each individual, and it is perfectly acceptable to adjust goals as you learn more about yourself and your desires.

Reflection Exercise: Take a moment to write down your personal goals and desires regarding fisting. Consider using the SMART criteria to guide your reflections. Share these insights with your partner(s) to foster open communication and mutual understanding.

Conducting Research on Techniques and Safety

When embarking on the journey of fisting, it is crucial to conduct thorough research on both the techniques involved and the safety measures that must be adhered to. This section aims to provide a comprehensive overview of the necessary steps to ensure a safe and pleasurable experience, addressing the importance of understanding the physical, emotional, and psychological dimensions of fisting.

Understanding Techniques

Fisting is not merely a physical act; it is an art that involves various techniques to enhance pleasure and minimize discomfort. Here are some key areas to focus on:

- **Hand Positioning:** Proper hand positioning is vital for comfort and pleasure. The most common position is to keep fingers together in a cupped shape, which allows for a smoother insertion. Research shows that the angle of insertion can greatly affect the experience; a slight upward angle tends to stimulate the G-spot or prostate more effectively.

- **Lubrication:** High-quality, body-safe lubricants are essential. Water-based or silicone-based lubricants are recommended, as they reduce friction and enhance comfort. Studies indicate that using sufficient lubrication can significantly reduce the risk of tearing or injury.

- **Gradual Insertion:** Slow and gentle insertion is key. Begin with one or two fingers, allowing the receiving partner to adjust before gradually introducing more. This not only helps in relaxation but also builds trust and communication between partners.

- **Body Mechanics:** Understanding your body mechanics is essential. Proper posture and alignment can prevent strain and injury. Utilize your legs and core to support your movements, ensuring that your hand remains steady and controlled.

- **Communication:** Establishing a continuous dialogue with your partner is paramount. Use verbal and non-verbal cues to gauge comfort levels and adjust techniques accordingly. Research in sexual communication emphasizes that ongoing check-ins can enhance the experience and ensure safety.

PREPARING FOR YOUR FISTING JOURNEY

Safety Considerations

Safety is a fundamental aspect of fisting that should never be overlooked. Below are critical components to consider:

- **Health Risks:** Understanding the potential risks associated with fisting is crucial. These can include:
  - *Physical Injuries:* Potential injuries may include tears, bruising, or internal damage. It is essential to be aware of your limits and those of your partner.
  - *Infections:* Fisting can introduce bacteria into the body. Proper hygiene practices, including thorough hand washing and the use of gloves, can help mitigate this risk.
- **Hygiene Protocols:** Establishing strict hygiene protocols is vital for safety. This includes:
  - *Hand Hygiene:* Wash hands thoroughly before and after play. Use antibacterial soap and ensure nails are trimmed and smooth to prevent injury.
  - *Use of Gloves:* Wearing latex or nitrile gloves can provide an additional barrier against infection. It is important to change gloves if switching between anal and vaginal play to prevent cross-contamination.
- **Informed Consent:** All parties involved should engage in open discussions about boundaries, desires, and consent. This not only enhances the experience but also fosters a sense of safety and trust.

Researching Resources

To conduct effective research on fisting techniques and safety, consider the following resources:

- **Books and Articles:** Seek out reputable literature that covers both the technical and emotional aspects of fisting. Books by sex educators and therapists can provide valuable insights and safety protocols.
- **Workshops and Classes:** Participating in workshops led by experienced educators can enhance your understanding of techniques and safety. These hands-on experiences allow for real-time feedback and learning.

- **Online Communities:** Engaging with online forums and social media groups dedicated to fisting can provide peer support and shared experiences. This can be a valuable way to learn from others and gain confidence.

- **Professional Guidance:** If possible, seek advice from sex therapists or health professionals who specialize in sexual health. They can provide tailored guidance and address any specific concerns you may have.

Conclusion

Conducting thorough research on fisting techniques and safety is an essential step in preparing for this intimate exploration. By understanding the necessary techniques, prioritizing safety, and utilizing available resources, individuals can create a fulfilling and secure fisting experience. Remember, the journey into fisting is not just about the physical act; it is about enhancing intimacy, trust, and pleasure in a safe and consensual environment.

Building a Supportive Community

Building a supportive community is essential for anyone exploring the world of fisting, as it fosters a sense of belonging, safety, and shared knowledge. This community can provide emotional support, practical advice, and a space to discuss experiences, challenges, and successes. In this section, we will explore the importance of community, the types of communities available, and how to engage with them effectively.

The Importance of Community

A supportive community plays a crucial role in sexual exploration and personal growth. According to social identity theory, individuals derive part of their identity from the groups to which they belong, influencing their self-esteem and overall well-being [?]. Engaging with a community of like-minded individuals can help validate experiences and reduce feelings of isolation or shame that may arise from societal stigma surrounding fisting.

Moreover, communities can serve as safe spaces where individuals can share their desires, boundaries, and fears without judgment. This sharing can lead to increased knowledge and understanding of fisting practices, enhancing both safety and pleasure. Research indicates that social support positively correlates with sexual satisfaction and well-being [?]. Thus, finding a supportive community can significantly enhance one's fisting journey.

Types of Supportive Communities

Supportive communities can take various forms, each offering unique benefits. Some common types include:

- **Online Forums and Social Media Groups:** These platforms allow for anonymity and can connect individuals from diverse backgrounds. Websites such as FetLife, Reddit, and specialized forums provide spaces to ask questions, share experiences, and find resources related to fisting.

- **Local Meetups and Workshops:** Attending local events can foster face-to-face connections with others who share similar interests. Workshops led by experienced practitioners can provide hands-on education and practice in a safe environment.

- **Support Groups:** These groups focus on emotional and psychological aspects of sexual exploration, providing a space to discuss feelings, experiences, and challenges related to fisting. Support groups can be particularly beneficial for individuals navigating trauma or shame.

- **Educational Organizations:** Nonprofits and educational bodies that focus on sexual health and wellness often host events, create resources, and provide training on safe practices, including fisting.

Engaging with the Community

To build a supportive community, consider the following strategies:

1. **Participate Actively:** Engage in discussions, share your experiences, and ask questions. The more you contribute, the more you will benefit from the collective knowledge and support of the group.

2. **Attend Events:** Make an effort to attend workshops, meetups, and community events. These gatherings allow for real-time interactions and can lead to lasting friendships and support networks.

3. **Respect Boundaries:** In any community, it is vital to respect the boundaries of others. This includes understanding and honoring consent, privacy, and individual comfort levels in discussions and activities.

4. **Seek Mentorship:** If you find someone in the community whose experience and approach resonate with you, consider seeking them out as a mentor.

Mentorship can provide personalized guidance and support as you navigate your fisting journey.

5. **Create Inclusive Spaces:** Advocate for inclusivity within your community. Ensure that everyone, regardless of their background, identity, or experience level, feels welcome and valued.

6. **Share Resources:** Contribute to the community by sharing articles, books, videos, and other resources that you find helpful. This not only enriches the community but also positions you as a valuable member.

Challenges in Building Community

While building a supportive community can be rewarding, it may also come with challenges. Some common issues include:

- **Stigma and Misunderstanding:** Many individuals may feel hesitant to engage due to societal stigma surrounding fisting. This can create barriers to participation and open dialogue.

- **Power Dynamics:** Within communities, power dynamics can emerge, potentially leading to exclusion or marginalization of certain voices. It is essential to actively work against these dynamics to foster a truly supportive environment.

- **Safety Concerns:** Engaging with others about intimate topics can raise safety concerns, especially in online spaces. It is crucial to establish clear guidelines for interaction and prioritize personal safety.

Conclusion

Building a supportive community is a vital step in exploring fisting safely and joyfully. By engaging with others, sharing experiences, and fostering a culture of respect and inclusivity, individuals can enhance their understanding and enjoyment of fisting. Remember, the journey is not just about the act itself but also about the connections and support that enrich the experience. Embrace the community and allow it to guide you on your path of exploration and self-discovery.

Communicating with Your Partner(s)

Effective communication is the cornerstone of any intimate exploration, particularly when delving into a practice as nuanced and potentially intense as fisting. The dynamics of communication in a sexual context are multifaceted, involving verbal and non-verbal cues, emotional attunement, and the establishment of trust. This section will explore essential strategies for communicating with your partner(s) about fisting, addressing common challenges, and providing practical examples to enhance the dialogue surrounding this intimate act.

The Importance of Open Dialogue

Open dialogue fosters a safe environment where all parties feel comfortable expressing their desires, boundaries, and concerns. According to Dr. John Gottman, a leading researcher in relational communication, couples who engage in open dialogue are more likely to experience relationship satisfaction and emotional intimacy. This principle holds true in the context of fisting, where the stakes of physical and emotional safety are particularly high.

Setting the Stage for Communication

Before discussing fisting, it is crucial to establish a comfortable setting for the conversation. This may involve:

- Choosing a private space free from distractions.
- Ensuring both partners are in a relaxed state of mind.
- Timing the conversation for when both partners are receptive and open.

By creating a conducive environment, partners can engage in a more meaningful and productive discussion.

Using "I" Statements

When discussing desires and boundaries related to fisting, employing "I" statements can significantly reduce defensiveness and promote understanding. For example, instead of saying, "You never listen to my needs," one might say, "I feel anxious when I don't feel heard about my boundaries." This approach emphasizes personal feelings rather than placing blame, facilitating a more constructive dialogue.

Discussing Desires and Boundaries

Engaging in a thorough discussion about desires and boundaries is vital. Partners should openly share their interests, what they hope to gain from the experience, and any specific boundaries they wish to establish. For instance, one partner might express a desire to explore deeper sensations, while another might have concerns about physical safety or emotional vulnerability.

$$\text{Mutual Understanding} = \text{Desire Sharing} + \text{Boundary Setting} \qquad (10)$$

This equation highlights that mutual understanding in a relationship is achieved through the combination of sharing desires and setting clear boundaries.

Addressing Potential Concerns

It is natural for partners to have concerns or fears about fisting. Openly addressing these concerns can help mitigate anxiety. Common concerns may include:

- Fear of physical injury or discomfort.
- Anxiety about emotional vulnerability.
- Concerns regarding hygiene and safety.

For example, if one partner expresses fear of pain, the other can reassure them by discussing the importance of gradual progression, communication during the act, and the use of ample lubrication.

Establishing Safe Words and Signals

In any intimate exploration, especially one involving potential discomfort or vulnerability, establishing safe words and signals is essential. A safe word is a predetermined term that either partner can use to indicate that they need to pause or stop the activity. Safe words should be easy to remember and not commonly used in everyday conversation. Common choices include:

- "Red" for stop.
- "Yellow" for slow down or check-in.
- "Green" for continue or affirming comfort.

In addition to safe words, non-verbal signals can be useful, especially if one partner is unable to speak during the act. This could include a specific gesture, like raising a hand, to indicate discomfort or the need to pause.

Practicing Active Listening

Active listening is a fundamental component of effective communication. This involves fully concentrating on what the other person is saying, understanding their message, responding thoughtfully, and remembering key points for future discussions. Techniques for active listening include:

- Nodding or using verbal affirmations like "I see" or "I understand."
- Reflecting back what the partner has said to ensure clarity, e.g., "What I hear you saying is that you want to take things slowly at first."
- Asking open-ended questions to encourage further discussion, such as "How do you feel about trying fisting?"

Creating a Feedback Loop

After engaging in fisting, it is important to create a feedback loop where both partners can discuss their experiences. This involves sharing what felt good, what could be improved, and any emotional reactions that surfaced during the act. This practice not only enhances future experiences but also strengthens the emotional connection between partners.

$$\text{Feedback Loop} = \text{Experience Sharing} + \text{Emotional Reflection} \qquad (11)$$

This equation emphasizes the importance of both sharing experiences and reflecting on emotions to create a robust feedback loop.

Navigating Difficult Conversations

Sometimes, discussions around fisting may lead to disagreements or discomfort. It is essential to approach these conversations with empathy and patience. Strategies for navigating difficult conversations include:

- Taking breaks if emotions run high.
- Acknowledging the validity of each partner's feelings.

- Seeking compromise or alternative solutions if there are differing desires.

For instance, if one partner is hesitant about fisting but is open to exploring other forms of intimacy, the couple might agree to engage in different activities that build trust and comfort before revisiting the topic of fisting.

Conclusion

Communicating with your partner(s) about fisting is a vital aspect of ensuring a safe, pleasurable, and fulfilling experience. By fostering an environment of open dialogue, utilizing "I" statements, establishing safe words, practicing active listening, and creating feedback loops, partners can navigate the complexities of this intimate act with greater ease and understanding. As with any aspect of sexual exploration, the foundation of trust and respect is paramount, enabling partners to engage in fisting with confidence and mutual enjoyment.

Discussing Expectations and Concerns

When embarking on the journey of fisting, it is paramount to have open and honest discussions about expectations and concerns with your partner(s). This not only fosters a safe environment but also enhances intimacy and trust, which are critical components of any consensual sexual exploration. Here, we will explore the importance of these discussions, the common expectations and concerns that arise, and strategies for effective communication.

The Importance of Open Dialogue

Open dialogue serves multiple purposes:

- **Establishing Trust:** Sharing expectations and concerns builds a foundation of trust. When partners feel safe to express their thoughts, they are more likely to engage fully and authentically in the experience.

- **Setting Realistic Expectations:** Clear communication helps to align partners' expectations, reducing the likelihood of misunderstandings or disappointments during the experience.

- **Enhancing Safety:** Discussing concerns allows partners to address potential risks and safety measures, which is crucial in activities that involve physical and emotional vulnerability.

Common Expectations

Understanding what each partner hopes to gain from the experience can enhance the overall enjoyment and satisfaction. Common expectations include:

- **Pleasure and Exploration:** Many individuals approach fisting with the expectation of heightened pleasure and the exploration of new sensations. It is essential to clarify what types of pleasure each partner seeks, whether it be physical, emotional, or both.

- **Connection and Intimacy:** For some, fisting is an act that deepens emotional bonds and intimacy. Discussing how partners can enhance their connection during the experience is vital.

- **Fantasy Fulfillment:** Fisting may be tied to specific fantasies or desires. Sharing these fantasies can create a more fulfilling experience, as partners can work together to bring them to life.

Common Concerns

Concerns are natural and should be addressed openly. Common concerns may include:

- **Physical Safety:** Partners may worry about the potential for injury or discomfort. Discussing safety measures, such as the use of lubrication, hand positioning, and communication during the act, can alleviate these fears.

- **Emotional Readiness:** Fisting can evoke strong emotions. Partners should discuss their emotional readiness and any past experiences that may influence their comfort levels. This includes addressing any trauma or vulnerabilities that may surface.

- **Consent Dynamics:** Understanding and navigating consent is crucial. Partners should discuss how they will communicate consent during the act, including the use of safe words or signals to pause or stop if necessary.

Strategies for Effective Communication

To ensure that discussions about expectations and concerns are productive, consider the following strategies:

- **Create a Safe Space:** Choose a comfortable and private environment for discussions. Ensure that both partners feel safe to express their thoughts without judgment.

- **Use Open-Ended Questions:** Encourage dialogue by asking open-ended questions, such as, "What are you hoping to experience?" or "What concerns do you have about fisting?" This invites deeper conversation and reflection.

- **Practice Active Listening:** Listening is just as important as speaking. Show understanding and empathy by summarizing what your partner has shared and validating their feelings.

- **Check-In Regularly:** Communication should not be limited to initial discussions. Regular check-ins before, during, and after the experience help ensure that both partners feel comfortable and can address any emerging concerns.

Example Scenario

Consider a couple, Alex and Jamie, who are exploring fisting for the first time. They begin their discussion by expressing their excitement about trying something new. Alex shares that they are looking forward to the physical sensations and the intimacy that fisting can bring. Jamie, however, expresses concern about potential pain and whether they will be able to relax enough to enjoy the experience.

In response, Alex reassures Jamie that they will prioritize communication throughout the process. They agree to establish a safe word—"pineapple"—to signal if either of them feels uncomfortable. They also decide to start slowly, using plenty of lubrication, and to take breaks if necessary. By addressing their expectations and concerns openly, they create a plan that respects both their desires and boundaries.

Conclusion

Discussing expectations and concerns is a fundamental aspect of exploring fisting safely and enjoyably. By fostering open communication, partners can align their desires, address fears, and enhance their connection. Remember, the goal is not only to engage in a new experience but to do so in a way that feels safe, consensual, and fulfilling for everyone involved.

In the journey of fisting, the conversations you have before the act can be just as significant as the act itself, paving the way for an enriching and pleasurable exploration.

Establishing Safe Words and Signals

In the realm of fisting, where the boundaries of pleasure and pain can blur, establishing safe words and signals is paramount to ensuring a safe and consensual experience. Safe words serve as a crucial communication tool that allows participants to navigate their limits and maintain control over the scene. This section delves into the importance of safe words, how to choose them, and the implementation of non-verbal signals, particularly in scenarios where verbal communication may be compromised.

The Importance of Safe Words

Safe words are pre-agreed terms that a participant can use to communicate their need to stop or pause the activity. The use of safe words is rooted in the principles of consensual non-consent (CNC) and BDSM practices, where trust, communication, and mutual respect are foundational. The primary function of a safe word is to provide a clear and unequivocal signal that transcends any ambiguity that may arise during play.

The most commonly recommended safe words are based on the traffic light system:

- **Red**: Stop immediately. This indicates that the participant is uncomfortable, in pain, or wishes to cease all activity.

- **Yellow**: Slow down or check-in. This word can be used when a participant feels overwhelmed but is not yet ready to stop entirely.

- **Green**: Everything is okay. This reassures the partner that the participant is comfortable and enjoying the experience.

It is essential that all parties involved understand and agree on the meanings of these words prior to engaging in any activities. This clarity fosters a sense of safety and promotes an environment where participants feel empowered to express their needs without fear of judgment.

Choosing Safe Words

When selecting a safe word, it is vital to choose a term that is easy to remember and unlikely to be confused with other conversation topics. Here are some guidelines for choosing effective safe words:

- **Simplicity:** Choose a word that is short and easy to pronounce, such as "apple" or "pineapple."

- **Unambiguousness:** Avoid words that may arise in casual conversation or during play, as this can lead to confusion.

- **Personal Relevance:** Some individuals may prefer to use words that hold personal significance, which can enhance the emotional connection during the scene.

Non-Verbal Signals

In situations where verbal communication is not feasible—such as when a participant is gagged or otherwise unable to speak—non-verbal signals become essential. Establishing a system of gestures can help maintain communication. Here are some effective strategies:

- **Hand Signals:** Agree on specific hand gestures to represent various states of comfort. For example, raising a hand with fingers spread can signal "stop," while a thumbs-up can indicate "all is well."

- **Tapping Out:** A participant can tap their partner's arm or leg a predetermined number of times to indicate a desire to stop or slow down. For instance, tapping once might signify "slow down," while tapping three times could indicate "stop."

- **Using Objects:** Some participants may choose to hold a specific object, such as a stress ball, that they can drop to indicate the need to pause or stop the activity.

The Role of Check-Ins

Regular check-ins during a scene are crucial for maintaining a safe environment. These can occur verbally or through non-verbal cues. Participants should agree to pause at intervals to assess comfort levels, feelings, and overall enjoyment. This practice not only enhances safety but also deepens intimacy and connection between partners.

Addressing Challenges in Communication

Despite the best intentions, miscommunication can occur. Here are some common challenges and solutions:

- **Ambiguous Signals:** If a participant feels unsure about the meaning of a signal, it is essential to pause the activity and clarify. Establishing a protocol for check-ins can help mitigate this issue.

- **Disregard for Safe Words:** In some cases, a partner may ignore a safe word due to the intensity of the scene. This can lead to emotional and physical harm. It is vital to establish a culture of respect where safe words are always honored.

- **External Distractions:** In noisy environments, it may be difficult to hear verbal safe words. This underscores the importance of non-verbal signals and pre-established gestures.

Conclusion

Establishing safe words and signals is a foundational aspect of engaging in fisting and other BDSM practices. By prioritizing clear communication, mutual respect, and trust, participants can create a safe and fulfilling environment for exploration. Remember, the ultimate goal is to ensure that all parties feel secure, respected, and empowered to express their desires and boundaries throughout their journey.

In summary, the establishment of safe words and signals is not merely a precaution; it is an integral part of fostering intimacy and connection in the context of fisting. By committing to open communication and mutual understanding, partners can navigate their desires and limits with confidence, ensuring that their experiences are both pleasurable and safe.

Creating a Safe and Comfortable Environment

Creating a safe and comfortable environment is paramount when exploring fisting, as it lays the foundation for a positive and pleasurable experience. This section will discuss the essential elements of an appropriate setting, addressing both physical and emotional aspects to ensure that all participants feel secure and at ease.

Physical Environment

The physical space where fisting occurs should be carefully curated to promote relaxation and intimacy. Consider the following factors:

- **Privacy:** Choose a location that offers complete privacy. This could be a dedicated bedroom, a safe space within your home, or a private room in a kink-friendly venue. The absence of interruptions is crucial for maintaining focus on the experience.

- **Comfort:** Ensure that the setting is comfortable. This includes having soft bedding, pillows, and blankets available. Temperature control is also important; a room that is too hot or too cold can distract from the experience. Aim for a temperature that feels cozy and inviting.

- **Lighting:** The lighting should be soft and adjustable. Dim lights or candles can create a warm ambiance, enhancing the mood while allowing for visibility. Avoid harsh fluorescent lighting, which can create an uninviting atmosphere.

- **Accessibility:** Make sure that all necessary supplies are easily accessible. This includes lubricants, gloves, towels, and any toys or accessories you plan to use. Having everything within reach minimizes disruptions and maintains the flow of the experience.

- **Cleanliness:** A clean environment is essential for both hygiene and comfort. Prior to your session, clean the area thoroughly. This includes washing sheets, disinfecting surfaces, and ensuring that all tools and accessories are sanitized. A tidy space contributes to a sense of safety and care.

Emotional Environment

In addition to the physical aspects, the emotional environment plays a crucial role in creating a safe space for fisting. Consider the following strategies:

- **Open Communication:** Establishing open lines of communication is vital. Before engaging in fisting, discuss desires, boundaries, and any concerns with your partner(s). This dialogue fosters trust and ensures that everyone is on the same page. Use "I" statements to express your feelings and desires clearly.

- **Setting the Mood:** Engage in activities that promote relaxation and connection before starting. This could include shared rituals such as massages, cuddling, or simply talking about your day. These actions help create a sense of intimacy and emotional safety.

- **Establishing Safe Words:** Prior to beginning, agree on safe words or signals that can be used to pause or stop the activity if necessary. This empowers all participants, knowing they have a means to communicate discomfort or the need for a break.

- **Aftercare Considerations:** Plan for aftercare, which is the time spent caring for each other after the fisting experience. This can include cuddling, talking, or providing physical comfort through gentle touch. Aftercare is essential for emotional processing and can help mitigate any feelings of vulnerability.

- **Mindfulness Practices:** Incorporate mindfulness techniques to enhance emotional safety. This could involve breathing exercises, grounding techniques, or even a brief meditation before beginning. Such practices can help participants center themselves and be present during the experience.

Addressing Potential Issues

Despite careful planning, issues may arise during the fisting experience. Being prepared to address these challenges can help maintain a safe environment:

- **Dealing with Anxiety:** It is common for participants to feel anxious before engaging in fisting. Acknowledge these feelings and take time to address them. Engage in a calming activity together, such as deep breathing or gentle stretching, to alleviate tension.

- **Recognizing Discomfort:** During the experience, it is essential to remain attentive to each other's verbal and non-verbal cues. If discomfort is expressed, pause and check in with each other. This may involve adjusting techniques, changing positions, or taking a break altogether.

- **Managing Interruptions:** If an unexpected interruption occurs, such as a knock at the door or a phone call, take a moment to address it. Ensure that both partners feel comfortable before resuming. This may involve discussing how to handle similar situations in the future.

- **Handling Emotional Responses:** Fisting can evoke a wide range of emotions. Be prepared for potential emotional releases, whether they manifest as laughter, tears, or silence. Validate each other's feelings and provide support as needed.

Conclusion

In conclusion, creating a safe and comfortable environment is a multifaceted process that involves both physical and emotional considerations. By taking the time to establish privacy, comfort, and open communication, participants can enhance their fisting experience. Remember that safety is an ongoing conversation and should be revisited regularly to ensure that all participants feel secure and valued. Ultimately, the goal is to foster an atmosphere of trust and intimacy, allowing for exploration and enjoyment of this unique form of sexual expression.

Assembling the Right Tools and Supplies

As you embark on your fisting journey, it is essential to gather the appropriate tools and supplies to ensure a safe, pleasurable, and consensual experience. This section will guide you through the necessary items, their functions, and considerations for their use, while also addressing potential issues that may arise.

Essential Supplies

Lubricants Lubrication is crucial in fisting to facilitate smooth insertion and reduce friction. Choose a high-quality, body-safe lubricant that is compatible with your body and any tools you may be using. Water-based lubricants are popular for their ease of cleanup, while silicone-based lubricants offer longer-lasting slickness. However, be mindful that silicone lubricants can degrade silicone toys. Always have an ample supply on hand, as generous application is key to comfort.

Gloves Wearing gloves is a critical safety measure in fisting. They help prevent the transmission of infections and ensure a hygienic experience. Opt for medical-grade latex or nitrile gloves, as they provide a good balance of sensitivity and protection. Ensure that the gloves fit properly—too tight can restrict movement, while too loose can lead to slippage and decreased sensation.

Nail Care Before engaging in fisting, it is vital to ensure that your nails are trimmed, filed, and smooth to prevent any potential tearing of sensitive tissues. Rough edges can cause discomfort and injury. Regularly check your hands for any cuts or abrasions, and avoid fisting if there are any open wounds.

Toys and Accessories While fisting can be performed using only the hand, incorporating toys can enhance the experience. Consider using:

- **Fisting Gloves:** Specialized gloves designed for fisting can provide added padding and comfort.

- **Fisting Dildos:** Available in various shapes and sizes, these can help individuals prepare for the sensation of fisting.

- **Anal Plugs:** For those exploring anal fisting, using a plug beforehand can help relax the muscles and enhance pleasure.

Always ensure that any toys used are made of body-safe materials, such as silicone, glass, or stainless steel, and are properly cleaned before and after use.

Comfort and Safety Items

Towels and Clean-Up Supplies Having towels on hand can enhance the experience by providing comfort and cleanliness. Use them for any spills or to dry off after play. Additionally, keep cleaning supplies nearby to maintain hygiene in your play area. Disinfectant wipes or sprays can be useful for cleaning surfaces and toys.

Safe Word Indicators Establishing clear communication is paramount in fisting. Consider using visual indicators, such as colored cards (e.g., green for go, yellow for slow down, and red for stop), to facilitate non-verbal communication during play. This can be particularly helpful in scenarios where verbal communication may be challenging.

Creating a Safe Environment

Setting the Scene Assembling the right tools is only part of the preparation. Creating a safe and comfortable environment is equally important. Ensure that the space is private, free from distractions, and equipped with soft lighting to foster relaxation. Consider playing music or using aromatherapy to enhance the mood.

Accessibility of Supplies All tools and supplies should be easily accessible during play. Organize your supplies in a designated area where they can be quickly reached. This minimizes interruptions and maintains the flow of the experience. Consider using a basket or a tray to keep everything in one place.

Potential Problems and Solutions

Inadequate Lubrication One common issue during fisting is inadequate lubrication, which can lead to discomfort or injury. Always err on the side of caution and apply more lubricant as needed. Keeping a bottle within arm's reach can help you maintain a consistent application.

Infection Risks Even with precautions, there is always a risk of infection. To mitigate this, ensure that all tools are properly cleaned before and after use. Encourage regular STI testing for all partners involved in fisting, and maintain open communication about sexual health.

Emotional Discomfort Fisting can evoke a range of emotions, including anxiety or fear. It is essential to establish a strong foundation of trust and communication with your partner(s). If emotional discomfort arises, pause and check in with each other, using your safe words as necessary.

Conclusion

Assembling the right tools and supplies is a vital step in ensuring a safe and pleasurable fisting experience. By prioritizing hygiene, comfort, and communication, you can create an environment conducive to exploration and intimacy. Remember, preparation is key, and the right tools can enhance not only the physical experience but also the emotional connection between partners. Embrace this journey with care, curiosity, and respect for your body and your partner's.

Seeking Professional Guidance and Education

Engaging in fisting, like any other intimate and physical exploration, can benefit significantly from professional guidance and education. This section aims to illuminate the various avenues through which individuals and couples can seek expert advice, enhance their understanding, and develop skills for safe and pleasurable fisting experiences.

The Importance of Professional Guidance

Professional guidance in the realm of fisting is crucial for several reasons:

- **Safety and Risk Management:** Professionals can provide insights into the physiological aspects of fisting, helping participants understand the risks involved, including potential injuries and complications. For instance, a qualified sex educator or therapist can explain the importance of understanding one's own anatomy and the risks associated with improper techniques.

- **Skill Development:** Learning from experienced practitioners allows individuals to acquire techniques that promote pleasure while minimizing discomfort or harm. For example, a workshop led by a sex-positive educator may include demonstrations on proper hand positioning and lubrication techniques, which are critical for a safe fisting experience.

- **Emotional Support and Preparation:** Fisting can evoke a range of emotions, from excitement to anxiety. Professional educators can help participants navigate these feelings, providing tools to foster emotional resilience and enhance communication with partners.

Types of Professional Guidance

There are various forms of professional guidance available for those interested in fisting:

- **Sex Educators and Workshops:** Many sex educators offer workshops specifically focused on fisting techniques, safety protocols, and communication strategies. These workshops often include practical demonstrations and opportunities for hands-on learning in a safe and consensual environment.

- **Therapists and Counselors:** For individuals or couples grappling with emotional challenges related to sexual exploration, therapists specializing in sex therapy can provide valuable support. They can help address issues such as body image, consent, and past traumas that may affect one's ability to engage in fisting comfortably.

- **Peer Support Groups:** Many communities have peer-led support groups where individuals can share experiences, seek advice, and learn from one another in a non-judgmental setting. These groups can provide a sense of belonging and affirmation, essential for those exploring non-normative sexual practices.

Finding the Right Resources

To seek professional guidance effectively, individuals should consider the following steps:

1. **Research Local and Online Resources:** Use platforms like social media, community boards, and sexuality-focused websites to locate workshops,

courses, or therapists specializing in sexual health and fisting. Websites like *Sex Positive World* or local LGBTQ+ centers often list upcoming events and resources.

2. **Evaluate Credentials:** When selecting a professional, it is crucial to evaluate their qualifications and experience. Look for educators with a background in sexual health, psychology, or a related field, and who have received positive reviews from participants.

3. **Engage in Initial Consultations:** Many therapists and educators offer initial consultations. Use this opportunity to discuss your goals, concerns, and what you hope to achieve through their guidance. This conversation can help establish rapport and ensure a good fit.

4. **Participate Actively:** Once you find a suitable resource, engage actively in the learning process. Ask questions, practice techniques, and share your experiences. This active participation will enhance your understanding and comfort level with fisting.

Examples of Professional Guidance

Consider the following hypothetical scenarios that illustrate the benefits of seeking professional guidance:

- **Workshop Experience:** Jane and Alex attend a fisting workshop led by a certified sex educator. They learn about the anatomy involved, safe techniques, and the importance of communication. The educator provides them with practical exercises, enabling them to practice in a supportive environment. This experience not only enhances their skills but also strengthens their emotional connection.

- **Therapy Session:** After experiencing discomfort during their first fisting attempt, Sarah seeks therapy to address her feelings of shame and anxiety. Her therapist helps her explore these emotions and communicate her boundaries more effectively with her partner. Through this process, Sarah gains confidence and clarity, enabling her to approach fisting with a healthier mindset.

- **Peer Support Group:** Mark joins a local peer support group for individuals exploring kink and fetish practices. Through sharing experiences and learning from others, he gains insights into the emotional aspects of fisting. The group discussions help him feel validated and supported in his journey, fostering a sense of community.

Conclusion

Seeking professional guidance and education is a vital step in exploring fisting safely and responsibly. By leveraging the expertise of sex educators, therapists, and peer support networks, individuals can enhance their knowledge, skills, and emotional resilience. This proactive approach not only promotes safety but also enriches the overall experience, allowing for deeper intimacy and connection with partners. As you embark on your fisting journey, remember that education and support are invaluable allies in your exploration of this profound and intimate practice.

The Art of Fisting: Techniques and Positions

Warming Up and Relaxing

Warming up and relaxing are essential components of a safe and pleasurable fisting experience. Just as one would warm up before engaging in physical exercise, the same principle applies to fisting. This section will explore the importance of warming up, techniques for relaxation, and the physiological and psychological benefits of these practices.

The Importance of Warming Up

Warming up serves multiple purposes in the context of fisting. It helps to prepare the body physically and mentally, reducing the risk of injury while enhancing pleasure. The body's tissues, particularly the muscles and connective tissues, need to be adequately prepared for the demands of fisting. A proper warm-up increases blood flow, enhances flexibility, and promotes relaxation of the pelvic floor muscles.

$$\text{Increased Blood Flow} \propto \text{Warm-Up Duration} \qquad (12)$$

This relationship signifies that the longer the warm-up, the greater the increase in blood flow, which can lead to heightened sensitivity and arousal.

Techniques for Warming Up

Physical Warm-Up A physical warm-up can include a variety of activities designed to increase body temperature and promote relaxation. Here are some effective techniques:

- **Gentle Stretching:** Engage in gentle stretches focusing on the arms, shoulders, and pelvic area. Stretching helps to loosen tight muscles and improve flexibility. For example, try seated forward bends or hip openers to release tension in the pelvic region.

- **Breath Work:** Deep, rhythmic breathing can help calm the mind and relax the body. Inhale deeply through the nose, allowing the abdomen to expand, and exhale slowly through the mouth. This technique can help reduce anxiety and create a sense of calm.

- **Light Massage:** Massaging the hands, arms, and pelvic area can promote relaxation and increase blood flow. Use a gentle touch, applying varying pressure to stimulate nerve endings and enhance sensitivity.

Mental Warm-Up Mental preparation is equally important. Engaging in a few minutes of mindfulness or meditation can help center your thoughts and create a positive mindset. Consider the following techniques:

- **Visualization:** Visualize a safe and pleasurable fisting experience. Imagine the sensations, emotions, and connection you wish to cultivate with your partner. This mental imagery can enhance arousal and create a sense of anticipation.

- **Setting Intentions:** Before beginning the experience, take a moment to set intentions. Discuss with your partner what you hope to achieve during the session, whether it be exploration, intimacy, or pleasure. This practice fosters open communication and helps align both partners' desires.

Relaxation Techniques

Relaxation techniques are crucial for allowing the body to respond positively to fisting. A relaxed body is more receptive to sensations and experiences less tension, which can lead to a more enjoyable experience.

Progressive Muscle Relaxation Progressive muscle relaxation involves systematically tensing and relaxing different muscle groups throughout the body. This technique can help individuals become more aware of physical tension and promote overall relaxation. Start at the toes, tensing each muscle group for a few seconds before releasing. Work your way up to the head, ensuring to focus on areas that may hold tension, such as the shoulders and jaw.

Warm Baths or Showers Taking a warm bath or shower before engaging in fisting can help relax the muscles and create a soothing atmosphere. The warmth of the water can ease tension in the body and promote feelings of comfort and safety.

Soothing Music or Sounds Creating a calming environment with soft music or nature sounds can enhance relaxation. Consider curating a playlist of soothing tracks that foster intimacy and connection with your partner. Music can set the mood and help both partners feel more at ease.

Addressing Potential Problems

Despite the best intentions, some individuals may experience difficulty relaxing or warming up. Here are a few common challenges and potential solutions:

Anxiety or Nervousness It is natural to feel anxious before engaging in fisting, especially if it is a new experience. If anxiety arises, take a break and engage in grounding techniques, such as focusing on your breath or reciting affirmations. Open communication with your partner about your feelings can also help alleviate concerns.

Physical Discomfort If you experience discomfort during the warm-up process, it is essential to listen to your body. Modify stretches or techniques to suit your comfort level. If pain persists, consider consulting a healthcare professional to address any underlying issues.

Lack of Connection A sense of disconnection from your partner can hinder relaxation. Engage in activities that promote intimacy, such as eye contact, gentle touching, or sharing personal stories. Building emotional closeness can enhance feelings of safety and trust.

Conclusion

Warming up and relaxing are integral components of a pleasurable and safe fisting experience. By incorporating physical and mental warm-up techniques, individuals can prepare their bodies and minds for exploration. Addressing potential challenges with openness and communication can enhance the overall experience, fostering deeper intimacy and connection. Remember, the journey of fisting is not just about the act itself but the emotional and psychological layers that enrich the experience. Embrace the process, and allow yourself to fully enjoy the exploration ahead.

The Basics of Hand Positioning and Lubrication

Fisting is an intimate and complex practice that requires an understanding of both hand positioning and lubrication to ensure safety and pleasure. This section will delve into the foundational aspects of hand positioning and the critical role of lubrication in enhancing the fisting experience.

Understanding Hand Positioning

Hand positioning is crucial in fisting, as it directly impacts the comfort and pleasure of both the giver and the receiver. The anatomy of the hand allows for various configurations, each providing different sensations and levels of control.

1. **Hand Shapes** The hand can be shaped in several ways during fisting:

    - **Flat Hand:** A flat hand can provide a broad surface area, which is ideal for gentle pressure against the vaginal or anal walls.
    - **Cupped Hand:** A cupped hand allows for a more focused sensation and can be used to cradle the internal structures, enhancing stimulation.
    - **Fist Shape:** The classic fist shape is often used for deeper penetration. Care must be taken to ensure that the receiver is fully relaxed and ready for this shape.

2. **Finger Positioning** The positioning of fingers is also important. Fingers can be spread apart or kept together, depending on the desired sensation:

    - **Spread Fingers:** This can create a feeling of fullness and can stimulate multiple areas at once.

THE ART OF FISTING: TECHNIQUES AND POSITIONS 93

- **Together Fingers:** Keeping fingers together minimizes the width of the insertion, which may be more comfortable for those new to fisting.

3. Angle of Insertion The angle at which the hand is inserted can significantly influence pleasure. Experimenting with different angles can help discover what feels best:

- **Upward Angle:** This can stimulate the G-spot or prostate, depending on the anatomy of the receiver.

- **Downward Angle:** This may provide a different sensation and can be used to explore other areas.

The Importance of Lubrication

Lubrication is an essential component of fisting, as it reduces friction and enhances comfort. The choice of lubricant can greatly affect the experience, and understanding the different types available is vital.

1. Types of Lubricants There are three primary types of lubricants used in fisting:

- **Water-Based Lubricants:** These are easy to clean up and safe to use with most condoms and toys. However, they may require reapplication, especially during prolonged sessions.

- **Silicone-Based Lubricants:** These provide long-lasting slickness and are ideal for fisting. They are safe to use with latex condoms but may not be compatible with silicone toys.

- **Oil-Based Lubricants:** While these can provide excellent glide, they are not recommended for use with latex condoms as they can cause breakage. They are often used in non-latex scenarios or for those who prefer a more natural option.

2. Quantity of Lubrication Using an adequate amount of lubricant is critical. A common issue is underestimating the amount needed, which can lead to discomfort or injury. A good rule of thumb is to start with a generous amount and add more as necessary.

3. Reapplication During fisting, it's essential to monitor the level of lubrication. As the session progresses, friction can increase, leading to potential discomfort. Regularly checking in with your partner and reapplying lubricant can help maintain comfort and pleasure.

Practical Tips for Hand Positioning and Lubrication

1. Communication is Key Before beginning, discuss with your partner their preferences for hand positioning and lubrication. Open dialogue can help establish comfort levels and ensure a positive experience.

2. Experimentation Encourage experimentation with different hand shapes and angles. Each person's anatomy is unique, and what works for one may not work for another.

3. Warm-Up Techniques Incorporate warm-up techniques to prepare the body for fisting. This can include gentle finger insertion, external stimulation, and using plenty of lubrication to ease the transition.

4. Monitor Comfort Levels Throughout the experience, continually check in with your partner about their comfort levels. If any discomfort arises, it is crucial to stop and reassess hand positioning and lubrication.

5. Post-Session Care Aftercare is an important aspect of any intimate experience. Discuss what felt good, what could be improved, and ensure that both partners feel emotionally and physically cared for after the session.

Conclusion

Hand positioning and lubrication are foundational elements of a safe and pleasurable fisting experience. Understanding the mechanics of the hand and the importance of lubrication can enhance intimacy and connection between partners. By prioritizing communication, experimentation, and care, individuals can explore the depths of their desires while maintaining safety and pleasure.

Slow and Gentle Insertion

The journey of fisting begins with an essential principle: slow and gentle insertion. This foundational step is crucial for both physical safety and emotional comfort. It sets the tone for the entire experience, allowing for the body to adjust and respond positively to the increasing sensations.

Understanding the Importance of Slow Insertion

Slow insertion serves multiple purposes. First, it allows the receiving partner to acclimate to the sensation of fullness, which can be both pleasurable and overwhelming. The body needs time to relax and open up, which is particularly important given the size of the hand compared to typical penetrative objects. The physiological response to slow insertion includes the relaxation of the pelvic floor muscles and increased blood flow to the area, enhancing pleasure and reducing the risk of injury.

The process of slow insertion can be understood through the lens of the **Gate Control Theory of Pain**, which posits that non-painful input can close the "gates" to painful input, preventing pain sensation from traveling to the central nervous system. By starting slowly and gently, the receiving partner can experience pleasurable sensations that may help override discomfort or anxiety.

The Technique of Slow Insertion

1. **Preparation:** Before any insertion begins, ensure that both partners are physically and emotionally prepared. This includes establishing a safe environment, discussing boundaries, and utilizing appropriate lubrication.

2. **Positioning:** Choose a comfortable position that allows both partners to maintain control. Positions like side-lying or face-to-face can facilitate communication and connection.

3. **Lubrication:** Use a generous amount of high-quality lubricant. Silicone-based lubricants are often preferred for fisting due to their long-lasting properties.

4. **Initial Contact:** Start by gently massaging the outer area around the vagina or anus. This not only increases arousal but also helps the receiving partner to relax.

5. **Gentle Pressure:** When the receiving partner indicates readiness, begin with the tip of the fingers or the palm. Apply gentle pressure, allowing the body to respond.

6. **Listening and Responding:** Pay close attention to the receiving partner's verbal and non-verbal cues. If they express discomfort, slow down or pause. The use of safe words or signals is essential here.

7. **Gradual Insertion:** Slowly introduce one finger, allowing the receiving partner to adjust. Wait for them to signal readiness before proceeding to insert additional fingers or the entire hand.

8. **Mindfulness:** Practicing mindfulness during this process can enhance the experience. Focus on the sensations, the connection between partners, and the rhythm of breathing. This can help create a meditative state that deepens intimacy.

Common Problems and Solutions

Despite the focus on slow and gentle insertion, challenges may arise. Here are some common problems and suggested solutions:

- **Tension and Tightness:** If the receiving partner is tense, it may be beneficial to engage in additional warm-up techniques, such as external massage or the use of smaller toys to help them relax.
- **Discomfort or Pain:** If pain is experienced, it is crucial to stop immediately. Discuss the sensations being felt and adjust the approach. This may include changing the angle of insertion or using more lubrication.
- **Communication Breakdowns:** Establishing a clear line of communication is vital. If either partner feels uncomfortable expressing their needs, consider using a pre-agreed signal system or practicing open dialogue before beginning.

Examples of Slow Insertion Techniques

To illustrate the concept of slow and gentle insertion, consider the following examples:

1. **The Finger Walk:** Begin with one finger and gently "walk" it in and out of the vagina or anus, allowing the receiving partner to feel the rhythm and adjust to the sensation. Gradually increase the depth of insertion as they become more comfortable.

2. **The Palm Press:** Instead of inserting fingers, start with the palm of the hand pressed against the opening. Apply gentle pressure, allowing the receiving partner to feel the fullness without immediate penetration. This can create anticipation and heighten arousal.

3. **The Circular Motion:** Once some initial depth is achieved, consider using a circular motion with the inserted fingers or hand. This can stimulate the surrounding tissues and enhance pleasure while maintaining the slow and gentle approach.

Conclusion

Slow and gentle insertion is not just a technique; it is an art form that requires patience, communication, and a deep understanding of the body's responses. By prioritizing this approach, partners can create a safe and pleasurable experience that fosters intimacy and connection. Remember that each journey into fisting is unique, and taking the time to explore and understand each other's bodies will lead to a more fulfilling experience.

Finding the Right Angle and Depth

Finding the right angle and depth during fisting is crucial for both safety and pleasure. This section will explore the anatomical considerations, techniques for achieving the desired angle and depth, and the importance of communication and responsiveness during the experience.

Anatomical Considerations

Understanding the anatomy of the receiving partner is essential for successful fisting. The vagina and anus are both elastic structures, but they have different anatomical configurations.

- **Vaginal Anatomy:** The vagina is a muscular canal that extends from the vulva to the cervix. It has the capacity to stretch significantly, especially when aroused. The angle of entry can affect stimulation of the G-spot, which is located on the anterior wall of the vagina, approximately 2.5 to 7.5 cm inside.
- **Anal Anatomy:** The anal canal is about 3 to 4 inches long and is surrounded by sphincter muscles that can be trained to relax. The angle of entry can influence the sensation of fullness and pressure on the rectal walls. The rectum can accommodate larger objects, but the entrance is more sensitive and requires careful attention.

Techniques for Achieving the Right Angle

1. **Positioning:** The position of both partners can significantly influence the angle and depth of insertion. Some recommended positions include:

- **Missionary Position:** The receiving partner lies on their back, allowing for direct eye contact and communication. The penetrating partner can adjust their angle by leaning forward or backward.

- **Doggy Style:** This position allows for deeper penetration and a different angle, which can stimulate the prostate in male partners or the G-spot in female partners.

- **Side-Lying:** Both partners lie on their sides, which can be a more relaxed position and allows for gentle exploration of angles without excessive strain.

2. **Adjusting Hand Position:** The shape of the hand can influence the angle of entry. A flat hand may allow for a more shallow insertion, while a cupped hand can create a different angle that may be more pleasurable. Experimenting with different hand configurations, such as a fist or a relaxed hand, can help find the most comfortable and pleasurable angle.

3. **Gradual Insertion:** It is crucial to start slowly and allow the receiving partner to adjust to the sensation. Gradual insertion enables the receiving partner to communicate their comfort level and helps to identify the optimal angle.

4. **Body Language and Feedback:** Non-verbal cues are vital. The receiving partner should be encouraged to express their feelings through body language, such as tensing or relaxing their muscles, moving their hips, or vocalizing pleasure or discomfort. The penetrating partner should be attentive to these signals and adjust accordingly.

Understanding Depth

Depth during fisting is a subjective experience that varies from person to person. Here are some factors to consider:

1. **Personal Comfort Levels:** Each individual has a different threshold for depth. It is essential to establish a baseline of comfort before attempting deeper penetration. Partners should discuss their limits and desires beforehand.

2. **The Role of Lubrication:** Adequate lubrication is crucial for facilitating deeper penetration. Silicone-based or water-based lubricants can help reduce friction and enhance comfort. Always ensure that lubrication is applied generously to both the hand and the receiving area.

3. **Exploration Techniques:**

- **Pushing vs. Pulling:** Experimenting with pushing or pulling motions can create varying sensations. A gentle pulling back can enhance the feeling of fullness, while pushing deeper can stimulate different nerve endings.

- **Curved Insertion:** When inserting the hand, a curved approach can help navigate the anatomical structures, allowing for a more pleasurable experience. This technique is particularly effective for stimulating the G-spot or prostate.

Communication and Responsiveness

The foundation of a successful fisting experience lies in open communication. Here are some strategies to enhance this aspect:

1. **Establishing Safe Words:** Prior to engaging in fisting, partners should agree on safe words or signals that indicate when to stop or slow down. This practice fosters a sense of safety and trust.

2. **Regular Check-Ins:** During the experience, the penetrating partner should periodically check in with the receiving partner to ensure comfort and pleasure levels. Phrases like "How does that feel?" or "Do you want me to go deeper?" can facilitate this.

3. **Post-Experience Reflection:** Aftercare is essential. Discussing what felt good or what could be improved helps partners learn from the experience and enhances future encounters. This practice also reinforces emotional intimacy.

Conclusion

Finding the right angle and depth during fisting is a nuanced process that requires attention to anatomy, communication, and responsiveness. By prioritizing comfort and pleasure, partners can create a fulfilling and enjoyable experience. Remember that exploration is key—what works for one person may not work for another, and the journey of discovery can be as pleasurable as the act itself.

Through patience, practice, and open dialogue, partners can navigate the complexities of fisting, transforming it into a deeply intimate and pleasurable experience.

Applying Pressure and Movements

In the context of fisting, the application of pressure and the movement of the hand are crucial components that contribute to both safety and pleasure. Understanding how to effectively apply pressure and execute movements can significantly enhance the experience for both the giver and the receiver. This section will delve into the theoretical underpinnings of pressure application, address common problems that may arise, and provide practical examples to guide practitioners in their journey.

Theoretical Foundations

The human body is a complex system of muscles, nerves, and connective tissue. When engaging in fisting, the way pressure is applied can affect not only physical sensations but also emotional responses. Pressure can be categorized into two main types: **static pressure** and **dynamic pressure**.

- **Static Pressure:** This refers to a consistent, unchanging force applied to a specific area. It is often used to create a sense of fullness or to stimulate specific erogenous zones. For instance, applying static pressure to the G-spot or the prostate can elicit intense pleasure.

- **Dynamic Pressure:** This involves varying the pressure applied through movement. Dynamic pressure can be achieved by changing the angle, speed, or rhythm of the hand's movements. This variability can enhance arousal and lead to a more pleasurable experience.

The *theory of pressure* in sexual activities can be understood through the lens of *sensory feedback*. The body continuously sends signals to the brain regarding sensations experienced during fisting. These signals influence the level of arousal, comfort, and pleasure. The concept of *pressure thresholds* is also relevant; each individual has a unique threshold for what feels pleasurable or uncomfortable.

Common Problems and Solutions

While applying pressure and movement can enhance the fisting experience, several common problems may arise:

- **Inadvertent Pain:** Applying too much pressure too quickly can lead to pain or discomfort. It is essential to communicate with your partner and adjust pressure based on their feedback. A good rule of thumb is to start with light pressure and gradually increase it as comfort allows.

- **Loss of Control:** In the heat of the moment, it can be easy to lose track of pressure and movements. Practicing mindfulness and maintaining open communication can help manage this. Establishing a safe word or signal can also provide a quick way to pause and reassess.

- **Fatigue:** Prolonged fisting can lead to fatigue in the hand and arm. To mitigate this, practitioners can alternate between different hand positions or take breaks to rest and stretch. Engaging the core muscles can also help distribute effort more evenly.

Practical Examples

To effectively apply pressure and movement during fisting, consider the following techniques:

1. **The Curl Technique:** Begin with your fingers extended and slowly curl them inward as you insert your hand. This technique allows for a gradual increase in pressure and can help stimulate sensitive areas such as the G-spot or prostate. Maintain a steady rhythm and adjust the angle to maximize pleasure.

2. **The Pumping Motion:** Once fully inserted, use a gentle pumping motion to create dynamic pressure. This involves moving the hand in and out while maintaining contact with the walls of the vagina or rectum. Vary the speed and depth of the movements to keep the experience exciting and pleasurable.

3. **The Twist:** Incorporating a twisting motion can add a new dimension to the experience. After inserting your hand, gently twist your wrist while applying pressure. This can enhance sensations and stimulate different areas within the body. As always, communicate with your partner to ensure comfort and pleasure.

4. **The Combination Technique:** For a more advanced approach, combine static and dynamic pressures. Start with static pressure on a specific area, such as the G-spot, then transition into dynamic movements, alternating between curling, pumping, and twisting. This can create a rich tapestry of sensations that can lead to heightened arousal.

Conclusion

Applying pressure and movements during fisting is an art that combines understanding anatomy, effective communication, and attentiveness to your partner's responses. By mastering the techniques of static and dynamic pressure, fisters can create a deeply pleasurable experience that respects the boundaries and desires of all involved. As with any intimate practice, the key lies in mutual trust, consent, and a willingness to explore together.

In summary, the effectiveness of pressure application and movement lies in the balance of technique and emotional connection, allowing for a transformative experience that transcends the physical act itself.

Experimenting with Different Hand Shapes

When exploring the art of fisting, the shape and configuration of the hand can significantly influence the sensations experienced by both the giver and the receiver. Understanding how to manipulate hand shapes can enhance pleasure, improve comfort, and create a more fulfilling experience. This section delves into various hand shapes, their effects, and practical tips for experimentation.

Understanding Hand Shapes

The human hand is a versatile tool capable of a myriad of shapes and movements. Each configuration can evoke different sensations and levels of intimacy. Here are some common hand shapes used in fisting:

- **Flat Hand:** A flat hand can provide a broad area of contact, allowing for gentle pressure against the vaginal or anal walls. This shape can be particularly effective for warming up or during the initial stages of insertion.

- **Cupped Hand:** This shape resembles a scoop, where the fingers are curved to form a concave surface. The cupped hand can create a sensation of fullness and can be used to cradle the internal structures, enhancing the feeling of intimacy and connection.

- **Fist Shape:** The classic fist shape is formed by curling the fingers tightly into the palm. This shape allows for deeper penetration and can stimulate internal structures more intensely. However, it requires careful attention to comfort and readiness.

- **Extended Fingers:** Keeping the fingers extended while inserting can create a different sensation compared to a fist shape. This configuration can help to explore the contours of the internal anatomy, providing a more nuanced experience.

- **Pinching or Grasping:** Using a pinching motion with the fingers can create targeted stimulation on specific areas, such as the G-spot or the prostate. This technique requires communication to ensure that the pressure is pleasurable and not painful.

Theoretical Considerations

The effectiveness of various hand shapes can be understood through the lens of anatomy and physiology. The internal structures of the vagina and anus are sensitive and responsive to different types of pressure and movement.

$$\text{Pleasure} = \int_0^T \left(\text{Pressure}(t) \cdot \text{Contact Area}(t)\right) dt \qquad (13)$$

In this equation, Pleasure is a function of the pressure exerted over time T and the contact area at any given moment t. Different hand shapes can alter both the pressure and the contact area, thus affecting the overall sensation.

Practical Tips for Experimentation

1. **Start Slow:** Begin with a flat hand or cupped shape to allow the receiver to adjust. Gradually introduce different shapes as comfort levels increase.
2. **Communicate Openly:** Discuss preferences and sensations with your partner. Use verbal cues or non-verbal signals to indicate what feels good or if adjustments are needed.
3. **Use Lubrication Generously:** Adequate lubrication is essential for comfort and safety. Experiment with different types of lubricants to see which enhances the experience.
4. **Incorporate Movement:** Experiment with different hand shapes combined with various movements. For example, a rotating motion with a fist can create unique sensations.
5. **Explore Depth and Angle:** Adjusting the angle of insertion while changing hand shapes can lead to different sensations. For instance, a tilted fist can stimulate the anterior wall of the vagina or rectum differently than a straight insertion.
6. **Practice Mindfulness:** Pay attention to the sensations experienced by both partners. This awareness can enhance the emotional connection and overall experience.
7. **Document Experiences:** Keep a journal of what shapes and techniques worked best for you and your partner. This can help in refining your approach over time.

Potential Problems and Solutions

While experimenting with different hand shapes can enhance the fisting experience, it is essential to be aware of potential problems:

- **Discomfort or Pain:** If any discomfort arises, stop immediately. Adjust the hand shape or angle, or revert to a more comfortable technique. Communication is key.

- **Risk of Injury:** Using a fist shape without proper preparation can lead to injury. Always ensure adequate warming up and lubrication before attempting deeper penetration.

- **Loss of Connection:** If the focus on technique detracts from emotional intimacy, take a moment to reconnect. Eye contact, gentle touches, and verbal affirmations can help maintain the bond.

Examples of Experimentation

Consider the following scenarios to illustrate the application of different hand shapes:

1. **Warm-Up Session:** Start with a flat hand, gently pressing against the vaginal or anal opening. Gradually transition to a cupped hand, creating a sensation of fullness without rushing.

2. **Deeper Exploration:** Once comfortable, form a fist and slowly insert while maintaining communication. Pay attention to the receiver's cues and adjust the pressure and angle as needed.

3. **Targeted Stimulation:** Use the pinching technique to explore specific areas, such as the G-spot or prostate, while varying the depth and speed of movement.

4. **Dynamic Play:** Combine different hand shapes throughout the session. For example, start with a cupped hand, transition to a fist, and then return to an extended finger configuration to explore varied sensations.

In conclusion, experimenting with different hand shapes during fisting can significantly enhance the experience for both partners. By understanding the anatomy involved, communicating effectively, and approaching the practice with mindfulness and care, individuals can explore new dimensions of pleasure and intimacy. Embrace the journey of exploration, and remember that each shape can tell a unique story of connection and discovery.

Exploring Internal Stimulation and Pleasure

Internal stimulation through fisting can lead to profound sensations and experiences of pleasure, connecting the physical with the emotional in a unique way. Understanding how to navigate this realm safely and joyfully is essential for both the fister and the recipient. This section will explore the anatomy involved, techniques for effective stimulation, the psychological aspects of pleasure, and common challenges that may arise.

Anatomical Considerations

To effectively explore internal stimulation, it is crucial to understand the anatomy of the body being stimulated. For individuals with a vulva, the G-spot, located on the anterior vaginal wall approximately 2-3 inches inside, is often a focal point for internal pleasure. This area can feel different from the surrounding tissues, often described as slightly spongy or ridged.

For individuals with a penis, stimulation of the prostate, located about 2-3 inches inside the rectum on the anterior wall, can produce intense pleasure. The prostate is sometimes referred to as the male G-spot, and its stimulation can lead to powerful orgasms.

$$\text{Pleasure} = \text{Stimulation} \times \text{Connection} \times \text{Trust} \qquad (14)$$

This equation illustrates that pleasure is not only a function of physical stimulation but also heavily influenced by emotional connection and trust between partners.

Techniques for Internal Stimulation

When exploring internal stimulation, the following techniques can enhance pleasure:

- **Gentle Curvature:** When inserting the hand, a gentle curve can help target sensitive areas like the G-spot or prostate. A slight upward angle during insertion can maximize contact with these areas.

- **Rhythmic Movement:** Establishing a rhythm can create a pleasurable wave of sensations. Varying the speed and depth of thrusting can help maintain excitement and prevent discomfort.

- **Pressure Play:** Experimenting with different levels of pressure can yield varying sensations. Some may enjoy firm pressure against the G-spot or prostate, while others may prefer a lighter touch.

- **Exploration of Surrounding Areas:** Engaging with the surrounding tissues, such as the vaginal or anal walls, can enhance overall pleasure. This can include massaging the perineum or the outer labia during internal stimulation.

Psychological Aspects of Pleasure

The experience of pleasure during internal stimulation is deeply intertwined with psychological factors. The mind plays a pivotal role in sexual arousal and satisfaction. Factors such as body image, emotional safety, and the context of the encounter can significantly influence the experience.

- **Mindfulness and Presence:** Being present in the moment can enhance the experience of pleasure. Mindfulness techniques, such as focusing on breath or bodily sensations, can help individuals connect more deeply with their sensations.

- **Fantasy and Imagination:** Engaging in fantasy can amplify arousal and pleasure. Discussing fantasies with a partner before fisting can create a more exciting and fulfilling experience.

- **Overcoming Psychological Barriers:** Many individuals may experience anxiety or fear surrounding fisting and internal stimulation. Open communication about concerns and setting boundaries can alleviate these feelings and foster a more enjoyable experience.

Common Challenges and Solutions

While exploring internal stimulation can be pleasurable, it may also present challenges. Here are some common issues and potential solutions:

- **Discomfort or Pain:** If discomfort arises, it is crucial to communicate immediately. Adjusting technique, using more lubrication, or taking breaks can help alleviate pain.

- **Difficulty Reaching Orgasm:** Some may find it challenging to reach orgasm through internal stimulation alone. Incorporating external stimulation or focusing on the clitoris or other erogenous zones can enhance pleasure.

- **Emotional Responses:** Internal stimulation can evoke strong emotional reactions. Providing aftercare and discussing feelings post-session can help partners process these emotions and build intimacy.

Conclusion

Exploring internal stimulation through fisting can be a deeply satisfying experience when approached with care, consent, and open communication. By understanding anatomy, employing effective techniques, and addressing psychological factors, partners can enhance their pleasure and intimacy. Always prioritize safety and comfort, and remember that every body is unique—what works for one may not work for another. The journey of exploration is as significant as the destination, fostering deeper connections and understanding between partners.

Understanding the Importance of Patience and Communication

In the realm of fisting, the significance of patience and communication cannot be overstated. Engaging in this intimate and complex form of sexual expression requires a foundation of trust, understanding, and a commitment to the well-being of all parties involved. This section will delve into the theoretical underpinnings of patience and communication, the potential challenges that may arise, and practical strategies to enhance these crucial elements in fisting practice.

Theoretical Foundations

At the core of effective communication is the concept of *active listening*, which involves fully concentrating on what is being said rather than just passively hearing the message. According to Carl Rogers' person-centered approach, active listening fosters an environment of empathy and understanding, allowing partners to express their desires, boundaries, and concerns freely. This is particularly important in fisting, where physical and emotional vulnerabilities are heightened.

Patience, on the other hand, can be understood through the lens of *self-regulation theory*, which posits that the ability to manage one's emotions, thoughts, and behaviors in the face of challenges is crucial for successful interpersonal interactions. In the context of fisting, patience allows partners to navigate the intricacies of physical sensations and emotional responses, ensuring a more fulfilling and safe experience.

Challenges in Communication and Patience

Despite the importance of patience and communication, several challenges may arise during fisting:

- **Miscommunication:** Partners may misinterpret verbal and non-verbal cues, leading to misunderstandings about comfort levels and desires.

- **Anxiety and Pressure:** The desire to please or meet certain expectations can create anxiety, making it difficult for individuals to communicate their needs effectively.

- **Physical Discomfort:** As fisting can involve intense sensations, partners may struggle to articulate their feelings, especially if they experience discomfort or pain.

- **Emotional Vulnerability:** The intimate nature of fisting may evoke strong emotions, which can complicate communication and lead to misunderstandings.

Strategies for Enhancing Patience and Communication

To foster an environment conducive to open communication and patience, consider the following strategies:

1. **Establish Clear Communication Channels:** Before engaging in fisting, discuss preferred communication styles. Determine whether verbal cues, safe words, or hand signals will be used to indicate comfort levels and boundaries. For example, using a safe word like "red" to indicate a need to stop can provide clarity and reassurance.

2. **Practice Active Listening:** Encourage each partner to practice active listening by summarizing what they heard and asking clarifying questions. This not only enhances understanding but also demonstrates respect for each other's feelings and boundaries.

3. **Engage in Ongoing Check-Ins:** During the fisting experience, implement regular check-ins to assess comfort levels. Simple questions like "How does that feel?" or "Are you okay?" can provide opportunities for partners to express their needs and adjust accordingly.

4. **Cultivate a Non-Judgmental Space:** Create an environment where partners feel safe to express their thoughts and feelings without fear of judgment. This can be achieved by affirming each other's experiences and validating emotions.

5. **Be Patient with the Process:** Recognize that fisting is a journey that requires time and practice. Allow for gradual exploration of sensations, and be prepared for moments of discomfort or uncertainty. Emphasize that it is acceptable to pause or slow down if needed.

6. **Reflect After the Experience:** Aftercare is a vital component of the fisting experience. Take time to discuss what worked well and what could be improved. This reflection can deepen understanding and strengthen the bond between partners.

Practical Examples

Consider the following scenarios that illustrate the importance of patience and communication in fisting:

- **Scenario 1:** During a fisting session, one partner begins to feel discomfort but is hesitant to speak up. By implementing regular check-ins, the other partner notices the change in body language and prompts, "How are you feeling right now?" This question creates a safe space for the first partner to express their discomfort and adjust the pace accordingly.

- **Scenario 2:** A couple is exploring fisting for the first time. They establish a safe word and agree to pause if either partner feels overwhelmed. During the session, one partner experiences a sudden wave of anxiety. By using the safe word, they communicate their need to stop, allowing both partners to regroup and discuss their feelings before continuing.

- **Scenario 3:** After a fisting session, partners engage in aftercare, discussing their experiences. One partner shares that they felt a deep emotional release during the session. The other partner listens actively, expressing gratitude for the vulnerability shared, which strengthens their emotional connection and fosters trust for future exploration.

Conclusion

In conclusion, patience and communication are foundational elements in the practice of fisting. By understanding their theoretical underpinnings, recognizing potential challenges, and implementing practical strategies, partners can enhance their experiences and foster a deeper sense of intimacy and trust. Ultimately, the journey of fisting is not solely about the physical act but also about the emotional connection and mutual respect that underpin it. Embracing patience and communication transforms fisting from a mere physical exploration into a profound expression of love, trust, and shared vulnerability.

Incorporating Toys and Accessories

In the exploration of fisting, the incorporation of toys and accessories can enhance pleasure, facilitate safety, and broaden the range of sensations experienced. This section delves into the various types of toys and accessories that can be utilized during fisting, their benefits, and considerations for safe use.

Types of Toys and Accessories

1. **Fisting Gloves:** Fisting gloves are designed to provide a barrier between partners, enhancing hygiene and reducing the risk of infection. They can be made from latex, nitrile, or vinyl. When selecting gloves, consider the following:

- **Material Sensitivity:** Some individuals may have allergies to latex; in such cases, nitrile gloves are a suitable alternative.
- **Fit and Comfort:** Gloves should fit snugly without being too tight, allowing for dexterity during play.

2. **Lubricants:** The importance of lubrication cannot be overstated in fisting. A good lubricant reduces friction, enhances comfort, and allows for smoother insertion. Consider the following types:

- **Water-Based Lubricants:** These are easy to clean and safe to use with most toys. However, they may require reapplication during extended sessions.
- **Silicone-Based Lubricants:** Longer-lasting and ideal for fisting, silicone lubricants are not compatible with silicone toys but are excellent for skin-on-skin contact.
- **Oil-Based Lubricants:** While providing excellent glide, oil-based lubricants can degrade latex condoms and gloves, so caution is advised.

3. **Fisting Toys:** Various toys can be employed to enhance the fisting experience, including:

- **Fisting Dildos:** These are specifically designed for fisting, often featuring a wider girth and a flared base for safety. Materials can vary from silicone to glass.
- **Anal Beads:** These can be used to warm up the anal area before fisting, providing varying sensations as they are inserted or removed.

THE ART OF FISTING: TECHNIQUES AND POSITIONS

- **Butt Plugs:** A butt plug can help relax the anal sphincter and prepare the body for fisting. Choose a size that is comfortable and gradually increase the size as comfort allows.

4. **Sensory Accessories:** Incorporating sensory accessories can enhance the overall experience. Consider:

- **Blindfolds and Restraints:** These can heighten anticipation and focus on sensations, allowing individuals to explore their bodies and their partner's bodies more deeply.

- **Warming or Cooling Gels:** These products can create unique sensations on the skin and enhance arousal.

Benefits of Incorporating Toys and Accessories

Incorporating toys and accessories into fisting play offers several benefits:

- **Enhanced Pleasure:** Toys can provide stimulation in ways that manual fisting cannot, allowing for a wider range of sensations.

- **Safety:** Utilizing gloves and appropriate lubricants can mitigate risks associated with fisting, such as tearing or infection.

- **Exploration:** Toys can facilitate exploration of different sensations and fantasies, enriching the overall experience.

Considerations for Safe Use

When incorporating toys and accessories into fisting, it is essential to keep safety in mind:

- **Hygiene:** Always clean toys before and after use. Use soap and water or a suitable toy cleaner. For shared toys, consider using condoms over the toy to ensure cleanliness.

- **Communication:** Discuss preferences and boundaries with your partner before introducing new toys. Ensure that both partners are comfortable and enthusiastic about the inclusion of accessories.

- **Gradual Introduction:** If using toys for the first time, start with smaller sizes and gradually work up to larger ones. This approach helps the body adjust and minimizes discomfort.

Example Scenario

Consider a couple, Alex and Jamie, who are exploring fisting for the first time. They decide to incorporate a silicone fisting dildo and a water-based lubricant into their play. Before beginning, they communicate openly about their boundaries and establish a safe word.

As they start, Jamie uses the dildo to warm up, allowing Alex to adjust to the sensation before introducing fingers. They take their time, focusing on comfort and pleasure, ensuring that they are both enjoying the experience. The use of toys not only enhances the physical sensations but also deepens their emotional connection, allowing them to explore vulnerability and trust.

Conclusion

Incorporating toys and accessories into fisting can significantly enhance the experience, providing added pleasure, safety, and opportunities for exploration. By choosing the right tools and maintaining open communication, partners can create a fulfilling and enjoyable fisting journey. Always prioritize safety, hygiene, and consent, ensuring that the experience is positive for all involved.

Advanced Techniques and Positions

As you delve deeper into the art of fisting, exploring advanced techniques and positions can significantly enhance the experience for both the giver and receiver. This section covers various strategies, anatomical considerations, and positions that allow for deeper exploration while prioritizing safety and pleasure.

Understanding Advanced Techniques

Advanced fisting techniques build upon the fundamental principles of fisting, emphasizing communication, body awareness, and adaptability. Key elements to consider include:

- **Body Mechanics:** Understanding the biomechanics of your body and your partner's body is crucial. This includes knowing how to position your arm and hand for maximum comfort and access while minimizing strain.

- **Breath Control:** Utilizing breath as a tool can enhance relaxation and pleasure. Deep, rhythmic breathing can help the receiver relax their pelvic floor, making the experience smoother and more enjoyable.

THE ART OF FISTING: TECHNIQUES AND POSITIONS 113

- **Gradual Progression:** Advanced techniques often involve gradually increasing depth and intensity. Begin with gentle movements and slowly build to more intense sensations, always checking in with your partner.

Common Advanced Positions

Several positions can facilitate deeper penetration and enhance pleasure during fisting. Here are some examples:

1. **The Modified Missionary:** In this position, the receiver lies on their back with their legs raised and supported by their partner's shoulders. This allows for deep access while maintaining eye contact and intimacy. The giver can use their free hand to stimulate other erogenous zones, enhancing the experience.

2. **Side-Lying Spooning:** Both partners lie on their sides, with the receiver's back against the giver's front. This position allows for a gentle, intimate connection and makes it easier for the giver to maintain control over depth and angle. The receiver can also adjust their body to find their optimal pleasure point.

3. **Kneeling Entry:** The receiver kneels on all fours, while the giver kneels behind them. This position allows for deeper penetration and the ability to adjust the angle for maximum pleasure. The giver can also use their free hand to explore the receiver's body or apply pressure to the lower back for added support.

4. **The Chair Position:** The receiver sits on the edge of a sturdy chair, with their legs spread. The giver stands or kneels in front, allowing for a unique angle of entry that can stimulate different areas. This position can also facilitate eye contact and emotional connection.

5. **The Cross-Legged Position:** The receiver sits cross-legged on the floor or a soft surface, allowing the giver to sit behind them. This position encourages relaxation and can create a sense of safety, making it easier for the receiver to let go and enjoy the experience. The giver can also use their body to support the receiver's back.

Incorporating Advanced Techniques

Beyond positions, advanced fisting also involves a variety of techniques that can enhance pleasure and safety:

- **Varying Speed and Rhythm:** Experimenting with different speeds and rhythms can create a dynamic experience. Alternating between slow, deep thrusts and faster, shallower movements can heighten arousal and lead to more intense orgasms.

- **Using the Whole Hand:** While many may start with just fingers, using the entire hand can create a fuller sensation. As comfort levels increase, the giver can explore different hand shapes and angles, such as cupping or curling the fingers, to stimulate the internal walls.

- **Pressure Points:** Learning to identify and stimulate specific pressure points within the vagina or anus can enhance pleasure. For instance, applying pressure to the anterior vaginal wall can stimulate the G-spot, while focusing on the rectal wall can create a unique sensation.

- **Incorporating Toys:** Advanced fisters often use toys to enhance the experience. Vibrating toys can provide additional stimulation, while anal beads can create a unique sensation during withdrawal. Ensure all toys are body-safe, properly cleaned, and used with ample lubricant.

Addressing Potential Challenges

As with any advanced sexual practice, challenges may arise. Here are some common issues and solutions:

- **Discomfort or Pain:** If the receiver experiences discomfort or pain, it is crucial to stop immediately. Communicate openly about what feels good and what does not. Adjusting the angle, depth, or speed can often alleviate discomfort.

- **Lack of Lubrication:** Adequate lubrication is essential for a pleasurable fisting experience. If the lubricant begins to dry out, pause and reapply. Silicone-based lubricants often last longer than water-based options, making them a preferred choice for fisting.

- **Fatigue:** Fisting can be physically demanding for both partners. If either partner feels fatigued, take breaks as needed. Using a supportive cushion or pillow can help alleviate strain on the giver's arm and back.

- **Communication Barriers:** Establishing clear communication is vital. Use safe words and signals to indicate comfort levels and boundaries. Regularly check in with your partner to ensure they are enjoying the experience.

Conclusion

Advanced techniques and positions in fisting open up a world of exploration and intimacy. By focusing on communication, body awareness, and adaptability, partners can create a safe and pleasurable environment that enhances their connection. Remember that every body is different; what works for one may not work for another. The key to a fulfilling fisting experience lies in mutual respect, consent, and a willingness to explore together.

$$P = \int_a^b f(x)\,dx \tag{15}$$

where P represents the pleasure derived from fisting, and $f(x)$ is the function of techniques and positions explored over the range $[a, b]$ of experiences shared.

Safety and Risk Management

Safety and Risk Management

Safety and Risk Management

In the realm of fisting, safety and risk management are paramount. Engaging in this intimate act carries inherent risks that can range from physical injuries to emotional distress. Understanding these risks, along with proactive measures to mitigate them, is essential for ensuring a safe and pleasurable experience for all involved parties.

Understanding the Risks of Fisting

Fisting, while often pleasurable, can lead to various physical and emotional risks. Recognizing these risks is the first step in effective risk management.

- **Potential Physical Injuries and Damage:** Fisting involves the insertion of the hand into the vagina or anus, which can lead to injuries if not performed with care. Common injuries include tears in the vaginal or anal tissues, which can cause pain and bleeding.

- **Internal Bleeding and Bruising:** The internal structure of the body can be sensitive. Excessive force or improper technique may lead to internal bleeding or bruising, which can be serious and require medical attention.

- **Nerve Damage and Sensation Loss:** Overzealous fisting can potentially damage nerves, leading to temporary or permanent loss of sensation in the affected area. Participants should be aware of their limits and communicate openly about any discomfort.

- **Infection and Hygiene Concerns:** The risk of infection is significant in fisting, particularly if proper hygiene is not maintained. Bacterial infections can arise from the introduction of bacteria into the body during the act.

- **Emotional and Psychological Risks:** Fisting can evoke strong emotional responses. Participants may experience feelings of vulnerability, fear, or anxiety, particularly if they are new to the practice. It is essential to address these emotional aspects before engaging in fisting.

Practicing Harm Reduction Strategies

To minimize the risks associated with fisting, practitioners should adopt harm reduction strategies. These strategies are designed to promote safety and well-being for all participants.

- **Education and Communication:** Prior to engaging in fisting, partners should educate themselves about the anatomy involved, potential risks, and safe practices. Open communication about desires, fears, and boundaries is crucial.

- **Establishing Safe Words and Signals:** Safe words and signals are vital for ensuring that all parties can communicate their comfort levels during the act. A commonly used safe word is "red" to indicate an immediate stop, while "yellow" can suggest slowing down or checking in.

- **Gradual Progression:** Beginners should start slowly, gradually increasing the depth and intensity of fisting. This allows the body to adapt and reduces the risk of injury.

- **Using Adequate Lubrication:** Lubrication is essential in fisting to reduce friction and facilitate smoother insertion. Water-based or silicone-based lubricants are recommended, ensuring that they are safe for use with gloves and any toys.

- **Hand Hygiene and Nail Care:** Maintaining proper hygiene is crucial. Hands should be thoroughly washed, and nails should be trimmed and smooth to prevent cuts or tears during insertion. Wearing gloves can further minimize the risk of infection.

- **Monitoring Physical and Emotional Responses:** Partners should regularly check in with each other during the act, both physically and emotionally. This can help identify any discomfort or pain early on, allowing for adjustments to be made.

Recognizing and Addressing Trauma

It is essential to recognize that some individuals may have past trauma related to their bodies or sexual experiences. Fisting can trigger these memories or feelings, making it critical to approach the act with sensitivity.

- **Pre-Engagement Discussions:** Before engaging in fisting, partners should discuss any past trauma and how it may affect their experience. This conversation can help establish trust and understanding.

- **Creating a Safe Space:** Establishing an emotionally safe environment is key. This can involve setting the mood, ensuring privacy, and removing distractions that may cause anxiety.

- **Post-Scene Debriefing:** Aftercare is an integral part of fisting. Partners should take time to discuss their experiences, feelings, and any discomfort that may have arisen during the act. This practice fosters emotional connection and healing.

Conclusion

In summary, safety and risk management are critical components of fisting. By understanding the risks, practicing harm reduction strategies, and fostering open communication, participants can engage in this intimate act safely and enjoyably. The combination of physical safety and emotional awareness creates a fulfilling experience that honors the trust and connection between partners. Through education and practice, fisting can be a deeply rewarding exploration of intimacy and pleasure.

Understanding the Risks of Fisting

Potential Physical Injuries and Damage

Fisting, while an intimate and pleasurable experience for many, carries inherent risks that participants must understand and manage. Awareness of potential physical injuries and damage is crucial for ensuring safety and enhancing the experience. This section delves into various types of injuries that can occur during fisting, the mechanisms behind them, and strategies for prevention.

Types of Injuries

Fisting can lead to several types of injuries, including but not limited to:

- **Tissue Damage:** The insertion of a hand into the vagina or anus can cause stretching and tearing of the delicate tissues. This is particularly true if adequate lubrication is not used or if the insertion is too forceful. Tearing can lead to immediate pain and long-term complications, such as scarring or infection.

- **Internal Bruising:** The force applied during fisting can result in bruising of internal structures. This can manifest as pain and discomfort in the pelvic region, and in severe cases, may require medical attention. Bruising is often a result of excessive force or rapid movements that exceed the body's capacity for safe stretching.

- **Nerve Damage:** Excessive pressure on nerves, particularly in the anal region, can lead to temporary or permanent nerve damage. Symptoms may include numbness, tingling, or loss of sensation in the area. Understanding the anatomy of the pelvic floor and surrounding nerves is essential to avoid this risk.

- **Infection:** Introducing foreign objects or hands into the body can increase the risk of infection, especially if hygiene practices are not followed. Bacterial infections can occur, leading to conditions such as bacterial vaginosis or urinary tract infections (UTIs). It is vital to maintain strict hygiene protocols to minimize this risk.

- **Internal Bleeding:** In rare cases, fisting can cause internal bleeding, particularly if there is significant trauma to the vaginal or anal walls. Symptoms may include severe pain, swelling, or unusual discharge. If any of these symptoms occur, it is crucial to seek medical assistance immediately.

Mechanisms of Injury

Understanding the mechanisms behind these injuries can aid in prevention. The following factors contribute to the likelihood of injury during fisting:

- **Lack of Preparation:** Fisting requires both physical and emotional preparation. Failing to warm up the body and gradually increase the size of the insertion can lead to injuries. Engaging in activities such as vaginal or anal dilation prior to fisting can help prepare the body.

- **Inadequate Lubrication:** Proper lubrication is critical in reducing friction and allowing for smoother insertion. Insufficient lubrication can lead to tearing and discomfort. It is recommended to use a high-quality, body-safe lubricant that is compatible with the body and any toys being used.

- **Poor Communication:** Effective communication between partners is essential. Failing to discuss comfort levels, boundaries, and safe words can lead to misunderstandings and unintentional harm. Establishing clear communication channels before and during the act can help mitigate risks.

- **Excessive Force or Speed:** Rushing the process or applying too much force can lead to immediate injuries. Participants should prioritize a slow and gentle approach, allowing the receiving partner to adjust and respond to sensations.

Prevention Strategies

To minimize the risk of injuries during fisting, consider the following strategies:

- **Education and Research:** Engaging in thorough research on fisting techniques, anatomy, and safety protocols can empower individuals to make informed decisions. Understanding the body's limits and responses is crucial for safe exploration.

- **Gradual Progression:** Start with smaller insertions and gradually increase size and depth as comfort allows. This approach helps the body adapt and reduces the likelihood of tearing or bruising.

- **Regular Health Check-Ups:** Maintaining regular health check-ups, including STI screenings and pelvic health assessments, can help identify any underlying issues that may predispose individuals to injury.

- **Hygiene Practices:** Prioritize hygiene by washing hands and using gloves if necessary. Ensure that any toys or accessories are thoroughly cleaned and sanitized before use.

- **Listening to Your Body:** Pay attention to your body's signals. If pain or discomfort arises, communicate with your partner and consider stopping or adjusting the activity. Recognizing the difference between pleasurable sensations and pain is crucial for safety.

Conclusion

Understanding the potential physical injuries and damage associated with fisting is essential for safe exploration. By prioritizing communication, preparation, and hygiene, individuals can significantly reduce the risks involved. Remember, safety and consent should always be at the forefront of any intimate experience. Engaging in fisting can be a fulfilling and pleasurable journey when approached with care and respect for one's body and boundaries.

Internal Bleeding and Bruising

Internal bleeding and bruising are critical considerations when exploring fisting, as they can result from excessive force, improper technique, or lack of preparation. Understanding the anatomy involved, the potential risks, and the signs to watch for is essential for ensuring safety and enjoyment during this intimate practice.

Understanding Internal Bleeding

Internal bleeding occurs when blood vessels are damaged, leading to blood leaking into surrounding tissues or body cavities. In the context of fisting, this can happen if excessive pressure is applied to delicate structures, such as the vaginal or anal walls. The potential for internal bleeding can be influenced by several factors, including:

- **Anatomical Variability:** Individuals have different anatomical structures, which can affect how their bodies respond to fisting. For instance, the thickness and elasticity of the rectal or vaginal walls can vary significantly among individuals.

- **Technique:** The manner in which fisting is performed plays a crucial role in minimizing the risk of injury. Rushing the process or using excessive force can lead to trauma.

- **Prior Conditions:** Pre-existing medical conditions, such as blood clotting disorders or vascular fragility, can increase susceptibility to internal bleeding.

Bruising: A Common Outcome

Bruising, or contusions, occur when small blood vessels break due to trauma, causing blood to leak into the surrounding tissue, resulting in discoloration. While bruising is often superficial, in the context of fisting, it can indicate more serious underlying issues. The severity of bruising can depend on:

- **Force Applied:** Higher levels of force can lead to more extensive bruising. It is crucial to communicate with partners about the intensity of pressure being applied.
- **Duration of Pressure:** Prolonged pressure on a specific area can exacerbate bruising. Regularly checking in with partners can help gauge comfort levels.
- **Body Positioning:** Certain positions may place additional strain on specific areas of the body, increasing the likelihood of bruising.

Signs and Symptoms of Internal Bleeding

Recognizing the signs and symptoms of internal bleeding is vital for timely intervention. Symptoms may include:

- **Pain:** Sudden or severe pain in the abdominal or pelvic area can indicate internal bleeding. This pain may be accompanied by tenderness upon palpation.
- **Swelling:** The affected area may appear swollen or distended, signaling fluid accumulation.
- **Changes in Bowel or Urinary Habits:** If bleeding occurs in the rectal area, individuals may experience changes in bowel habits, such as diarrhea or constipation. In cases involving the urinary tract, blood in urine may be present.
- **Dizziness or Weakness:** Systemic symptoms such as dizziness, fainting, or weakness may indicate significant internal bleeding and require immediate medical attention.

Preventive Measures

To minimize the risk of internal bleeding and bruising during fisting, consider the following preventive measures:

- **Warm-Up:** Engaging in adequate warm-up activities can help prepare the body for deeper penetration. This may include external stimulation, relaxation techniques, and gradual insertion of fingers or toys.

- **Communication:** Establishing open lines of communication with partners is essential. Discuss boundaries, comfort levels, and safe words before engaging in fisting.

- **Technique:** Focus on gentle and gradual insertion, maintaining awareness of the partner's comfort levels. It is advisable to start with smaller fingers or toys and progressively increase size and depth as comfort allows.

- **Lubrication:** Adequate lubrication is crucial for reducing friction and preventing tears. Use high-quality, body-safe lubricants that are compatible with the body and any toys used.

- **Regular Breaks:** Taking breaks during the session allows partners to assess their comfort levels and adjust techniques as necessary.

When to Seek Medical Attention

In the event of suspected internal bleeding or significant bruising, it is important to seek medical attention. Indicators that warrant immediate medical evaluation include:

- Severe or persistent pain that does not improve with rest or over-the-counter pain relief.

- Noticeable swelling or changes in skin color in the abdominal or pelvic area.

- Any signs of shock, including rapid heartbeat, shallow breathing, or confusion.

- Presence of blood in stool or urine, as this may indicate a more serious injury.

Conclusion

Internal bleeding and bruising are serious considerations in the practice of fisting. By understanding the risks, recognizing the signs, and implementing preventive measures, individuals can engage in this intimate act safely and enjoyably. Always prioritize communication, consent, and the well-being of all partners involved to foster a positive and fulfilling fisting experience.

Nerve Damage and Sensation Loss

When exploring the intimate act of fisting, it is essential to understand the potential risks involved, particularly concerning nerve damage and sensation loss. The human body is a complex network of nerves that play a critical role in sensation, movement, and overall bodily function. Understanding how fisting can impact these nerves is crucial for both safety and pleasure.

Understanding Nerve Anatomy

The human nervous system can be divided into two main components: the central nervous system (CNS), which comprises the brain and spinal cord, and the peripheral nervous system (PNS), which includes all the nerves that branch out from the CNS to the rest of the body. The PNS is responsible for transmitting sensory information to the CNS and relaying motor commands from the CNS to the muscles.

Nerves can be classified into three types:

- **Sensory Nerves:** These nerves transmit sensory information from the body to the brain, including touch, temperature, and pain.
- **Motor Nerves:** These nerves carry signals from the brain to the muscles, facilitating movement.
- **Autonomic Nerves:** These nerves control involuntary functions, such as heart rate and digestion.

During fisting, the hands and fingers exert significant pressure on the internal structures of the body, which may lead to potential nerve compression or damage, particularly in the pelvic region.

Potential Causes of Nerve Damage

Nerve damage during fisting can occur due to several factors:

- **Excessive Force:** Applying too much pressure during insertion can compress nerves, leading to temporary or permanent damage.
- **Improper Technique:** Lack of knowledge regarding safe fisting techniques can result in awkward angles or movements that may strain nerves.
- **Lack of Lubrication:** Insufficient lubrication can increase friction and resistance, leading to excessive force and potential injury.

- **Duration of Activity:** Prolonged fisting sessions without breaks can lead to nerve fatigue and damage.
- **Pre-existing Conditions:** Individuals with pre-existing nerve conditions, such as neuropathy or diabetes, may be at greater risk for nerve damage during fisting.

Symptoms of Nerve Damage

Recognizing the symptoms of nerve damage is vital for addressing issues promptly. Common symptoms may include:

- **Numbness or Tingling:** A loss of sensation or a tingling feeling in the fingers, hands, or pelvic region may indicate nerve compression.
- **Weakness:** Difficulty in moving the fingers or pelvic muscles can signal nerve impairment.
- **Pain:** Sharp or shooting pains in the hands or pelvic area may suggest nerve damage.
- **Sensitivity Changes:** Heightened sensitivity to touch or pressure can occur if nerves are irritated or compressed.

Preventing Nerve Damage

To minimize the risk of nerve damage during fisting, consider the following safety measures:

- **Educate Yourself:** Familiarize yourself with proper fisting techniques and anatomy to ensure a safe experience.
- **Communicate with Your Partner:** Open dialogue about comfort levels, boundaries, and sensations can help prevent injury.
- **Use Plenty of Lubrication:** Ensure adequate lubrication to reduce friction and ease insertion.
- **Start Slow:** Gradually increase intensity and depth, allowing the body to adjust to the sensations.
- **Take Breaks:** Allow for rest periods during prolonged sessions to prevent nerve fatigue.

- **Listen to Your Body:** Pay attention to any signs of discomfort or pain and adjust accordingly.

Addressing Sensation Loss

If sensation loss occurs, it is essential to take immediate action:

- **Stop the Activity:** Cease any further fisting until the symptoms resolve.
- **Rest and Recover:** Allow time for the body to heal; this may take hours or days, depending on the severity of the nerve compression.
- **Consult a Medical Professional:** If symptoms persist, seek medical advice to rule out serious injury or underlying conditions.

Conclusion

Understanding the risks of nerve damage and sensation loss is crucial for anyone exploring fisting. By prioritizing safety, communication, and education, individuals can engage in this intimate act while minimizing the potential for injury. Remember, the goal of fisting is to enhance pleasure and intimacy, not to cause harm. Always listen to your body and prioritize your well-being and that of your partner.

Infection and Hygiene Concerns

Engaging in fisting, while potentially pleasurable and intimate, does come with significant considerations regarding infection and hygiene. Understanding these concerns is crucial for ensuring a safe and enjoyable experience.

The Importance of Hygiene

Hygiene plays a pivotal role in preventing infections during fisting. The human body hosts a variety of bacteria, some of which can lead to infections if they enter the bloodstream or other vulnerable areas. Thus, maintaining cleanliness before, during, and after fisting activities is essential.

Common Types of Infections

Fisting can lead to several types of infections, including:

- **Bacterial Infections:** These can arise from the introduction of bacteria from the hands or the anal/vaginal area into the body. Common bacteria include *Escherichia coli* (E. coli) and *Staphylococcus aureus*.

- **Viral Infections:** The risk of transmitting viruses such as Human Immunodeficiency Virus (HIV), Herpes Simplex Virus (HSV), and Human Papillomavirus (HPV) can increase with fisting, especially if there are cuts or abrasions on the hands or in the receiving partner's body.

- **Fungal Infections:** Yeast infections can occur, particularly in individuals with vulvas, if the vaginal flora is disrupted during fisting.

- **Parasitic Infections:** Though less common, parasites such as *Giardia* can potentially be transmitted through fecal matter, emphasizing the need for thorough hygiene practices.

Preventative Measures

To mitigate the risk of infections, several preventative measures should be taken:

1. **Hand Hygiene:** Before engaging in fisting, it is crucial to thoroughly wash hands with soap and water. This includes cleaning under the nails and between fingers. Hand sanitizers can be used as an additional precaution, but they should not replace thorough washing.

2. **Nail Care:** Keeping nails trimmed and smooth is essential to prevent cuts or abrasions. Jagged or long nails can easily cause micro-tears in the anal or vaginal lining, increasing the risk of infection.

3. **Use of Gloves:** Wearing disposable latex or nitrile gloves can significantly reduce the risk of transmitting bacteria and viruses. Gloves should be changed if they become soiled or if switching between different areas of the body (e.g., from anal to vaginal).

4. **Lubrication:** Using a generous amount of water-based or silicone-based lubricant can help reduce friction and prevent tearing of sensitive tissues. Avoid oil-based lubricants if using latex gloves, as they can degrade the material.

5. **Environment Preparation:** Ensure that the environment is clean and sanitary. This includes using clean sheets or towels, and having disinfectant

wipes or sprays available for surfaces that may come into contact with bodily fluids.

6. **Post-Activity Hygiene:** After fisting, both partners should clean their hands and any areas that may have come into contact with bodily fluids. Showering and changing into clean clothes can further reduce the risk of infection.

7. **Regular Health Check-Ups:** Engaging in regular STI testing and health check-ups can help catch any potential infections early. Open communication with partners about sexual health is essential.

Recognizing Symptoms of Infection

Awareness of the symptoms of infection is critical for early detection and treatment. Common signs include:

- **Unusual Discharge:** Any change in the color, consistency, or smell of vaginal or anal discharge may indicate an infection.

- **Pain or Discomfort:** Persistent pain during or after fisting, especially if accompanied by swelling or redness, should be evaluated by a healthcare professional.

- **Fever or Chills:** Systemic symptoms such as fever can indicate a more serious infection that requires immediate medical attention.

- **Itching or Irritation:** Unexplained itching or irritation in the anal or vaginal area may suggest a yeast infection or other types of irritation.

Conclusion

In conclusion, while fisting can be a fulfilling and intimate experience, it is imperative to prioritize hygiene and infection prevention. By implementing thorough hygiene practices, recognizing potential risks, and maintaining open communication with partners, individuals can significantly reduce the likelihood of infections and enhance their overall experience. Remember, safety and pleasure can coexist through informed and responsible practices.

Emotional and Psychological Risks

Engaging in fisting can evoke a range of emotional and psychological responses, both positive and negative. Understanding these risks is crucial for anyone considering this intimate act, as it involves deep trust and vulnerability. This section explores the potential emotional and psychological risks associated with fisting, drawing on relevant theories and providing examples to illustrate these concepts.

Understanding Emotional Responses

The act of fisting can elicit intense emotional reactions due to its intimate nature. For some individuals, the experience may lead to feelings of euphoria, connection, and empowerment. However, for others, it may trigger anxiety, fear, or past trauma. The emotional responses can be influenced by various factors, including personal history, relationship dynamics, and individual psychological makeup.

Attachment Theory Attachment theory posits that early relationships with caregivers shape our expectations and behaviors in adult relationships [?]. Individuals with secure attachment styles may find fisting to be a positive experience that enhances intimacy and trust. Conversely, those with anxious or avoidant attachment styles might struggle with feelings of insecurity or vulnerability during the act. For instance, an individual with an avoidant attachment style may feel overwhelmed by the level of intimacy involved in fisting, leading to emotional withdrawal or discomfort.

Triggers and Trauma Responses

Fisting can be a profound experience, but it may also trigger unresolved trauma for some individuals. Past experiences of sexual abuse, assault, or other forms of trauma can resurface during fisting, leading to panic attacks, dissociation, or emotional distress. It is essential for participants to engage in open communication about their histories and any potential triggers before exploring fisting.

Example of Triggering Situations Consider a scenario where a person who has experienced sexual trauma engages in fisting without adequately discussing their past with their partner. During the experience, they may suddenly feel a sense of helplessness or fear, reminiscent of their previous trauma. This reaction can lead to a breakdown in communication and trust, making it imperative to establish a safe space for dialogue beforehand.

Managing Emotional Risks

To mitigate emotional and psychological risks, it is vital to prioritize communication and consent. Establishing clear boundaries and safe words can help participants navigate their emotional landscapes during fisting. Additionally, engaging in pre-scene discussions about desires, fears, and boundaries can foster a sense of safety and trust.

The Role of Aftercare Aftercare is a crucial component of any BDSM or kink-related activity, including fisting. It involves providing emotional support and reassurance to partners after an intense experience. This practice can help individuals process their feelings, address any discomfort, and reinforce the emotional connection between partners. For example, aftercare may include cuddling, discussing the experience, or engaging in activities that promote relaxation and comfort.

Potential for Emotional Growth

While fisting carries emotional risks, it also offers opportunities for personal growth and emotional resilience. Engaging in this act can foster deeper intimacy and trust between partners, allowing them to explore their boundaries and desires in a safe environment. For some, the experience may lead to a greater understanding of their bodies and emotional landscapes, ultimately enhancing their sexual and relational satisfaction.

Example of Positive Outcomes An individual who has previously felt shame about their body may find empowerment through fisting. By engaging in this act with a trusted partner, they may learn to embrace their body and sexuality, leading to improved self-esteem and body positivity. This transformative experience can be a powerful testament to the potential for emotional healing and growth within the context of consensual kink.

Conclusion

In conclusion, while fisting can be a deeply fulfilling and intimate experience, it is essential to acknowledge and address the emotional and psychological risks involved. By fostering open communication, establishing boundaries, and prioritizing aftercare, participants can navigate these risks effectively. Ultimately, the journey of exploring fisting can lead to profound emotional connections and personal growth when approached with care and consideration.

Recognizing and Addressing Trauma

Trauma is a complex and multifaceted experience that can significantly impact an individual's emotional, psychological, and physical well-being. Understanding how trauma intersects with fisting, and more broadly with sexual practices, is essential for creating a safe and supportive environment for exploration.

The Nature of Trauma

Trauma can be defined as an emotional response to a distressing event or series of events that overwhelm an individual's ability to cope. This may include experiences such as sexual assault, physical abuse, emotional neglect, or witnessing violence. The impact of trauma can manifest in various ways, including anxiety, depression, dissociation, and an altered sense of self-worth.

Types of Trauma

Trauma can be categorized into several types, including:

- **Acute Trauma:** Resulting from a single distressing event.

- **Chronic Trauma:** Resulting from repeated and prolonged exposure to distressing events, such as ongoing domestic violence or childhood abuse.

- **Complex Trauma:** Referring to exposure to multiple traumatic events, often of an invasive and interpersonal nature, such as repeated abuse or neglect.

Recognizing Trauma Responses

Individuals may exhibit various responses to trauma, which can include:

- **Hyperarousal:** Increased anxiety, irritability, or heightened startle response.

- **Avoidance:** Steering clear of reminders of the trauma, including certain sexual practices or situations.

- **Dissociation:** Feelings of detachment from oneself or the surrounding environment, which can affect intimacy and connection during sexual activities.

- **Intrusive Thoughts:** Recurrent memories or flashbacks of the traumatic event that can surface unexpectedly.

Recognizing these responses in oneself or a partner is crucial for fostering a safe space for fisting or any intimate exploration.

Addressing Trauma in Fisting Practices

When engaging in fisting, it is vital to prioritize emotional safety alongside physical safety. Here are some strategies to recognize and address trauma effectively:

Open Communication Establishing an open line of communication with partners about past traumas can help create a foundation of trust. Discussing boundaries, triggers, and safe words is essential. For instance, a partner may disclose that certain hand movements remind them of a past trauma, prompting a discussion on how to adjust techniques to ensure comfort.

Establishing Safe Words Safe words serve as a critical tool for managing consent and comfort levels during fisting. A safe word allows individuals to pause or stop the activity if they begin to feel uncomfortable or triggered. The use of a safe word can help mitigate the risk of re-traumatization.

Gradual Exposure For individuals with a history of trauma, a gradual approach to fisting can be beneficial. This may involve starting with less invasive forms of intimacy and slowly progressing to more intense experiences as comfort and trust build.

Aftercare Aftercare is an essential practice following any intense sexual activity, especially for those with trauma histories. Aftercare can include physical comfort, emotional support, and open dialogue about the experience. It allows individuals to process their feelings and reinforces the bond between partners.

Professional Support For those struggling to navigate their trauma, seeking professional support from a therapist trained in trauma-informed care can be invaluable. Therapists can provide tools and techniques to help individuals process their trauma, develop coping strategies, and enhance their sexual health.

The Role of Trauma-Informed Care

Trauma-informed care is an approach that recognizes the impact of trauma on individuals and emphasizes safety, empowerment, and collaboration. It involves:

- **Safety:** Ensuring a physically and emotionally safe environment.

- **Trustworthiness:** Building trust through consistent and transparent communication.

- **Peer Support:** Encouraging support networks that foster shared experiences and understanding.

- **Empowerment:** Fostering a sense of agency and control over one's body and experiences.

Incorporating these principles into fisting practices can create a more inclusive and supportive atmosphere for individuals who have experienced trauma.

Conclusion

Recognizing and addressing trauma is a vital aspect of engaging in fisting and other intimate practices. By fostering open communication, establishing safe words, practicing gradual exposure, and prioritizing aftercare, individuals can navigate their experiences with greater safety and awareness. Ultimately, creating a trauma-informed approach to fisting not only enhances the experience but also nurtures deeper intimacy and connection between partners.

Through understanding and compassion, we can transform the experience of fisting into one of empowerment and healing, allowing individuals to reclaim their bodies and their pleasure.

Understanding Risk Factors and Vulnerabilities

Fisting, while an intimate and pleasurable act for many, carries inherent risks that can be exacerbated by individual vulnerabilities and situational factors. Understanding these risks is crucial for ensuring a safe and enjoyable experience.

Physical Vulnerabilities

Individuals may have varying physical vulnerabilities based on their anatomy, health conditions, and prior experiences. For instance, those with a history of pelvic floor dysfunction or injuries may be at a higher risk for pain or injury during fisting.

Pelvic Floor Dysfunction Pelvic floor dysfunction can manifest as tightness, weakness, or coordination issues in the pelvic muscles. Individuals with such conditions may experience discomfort or pain during fisting due to an inability to relax adequately. It is essential to engage in pelvic floor exercises, such as Kegel exercises or relaxation techniques, to enhance muscle control and comfort.

Medical Conditions

Certain medical conditions may increase the likelihood of complications during fisting. For example, individuals with conditions such as Crohn's disease, ulcerative colitis, or hemorrhoids may be more susceptible to injury or exacerbation of their symptoms. It is advisable for individuals with such conditions to consult with a healthcare provider before engaging in fisting.

Medication Effects Medications can also play a role in vulnerability. For instance, blood thinners can increase the risk of bleeding, while certain antidepressants may affect sensation and lubrication. Understanding the potential effects of medications on sexual health is critical for safe fisting practices.

Emotional and Psychological Vulnerabilities

Emotional and psychological factors can significantly influence an individual's experience with fisting. Past trauma, anxiety, and body image issues can all create barriers to fully engaging in the act.

Trauma and Trust Individuals with a history of sexual trauma may find fisting to be triggering or overwhelming. Establishing a strong foundation of trust and communication with partners is essential in these cases. Engaging in pre-scene discussions about boundaries, triggers, and aftercare can help mitigate emotional risks.

Anxiety and Performance Pressure Performance anxiety can also impact the experience. The pressure to achieve certain outcomes, whether they be related to pleasure or technique, can lead to tension and discomfort. Practicing mindfulness and focusing on the sensations of the moment rather than expectations can help alleviate this pressure.

Social and Cultural Vulnerabilities

Societal attitudes towards fisting can create additional layers of vulnerability. Stigma and discrimination may lead individuals to feel shame or fear about their desires, which can hinder open communication with partners and affect overall enjoyment.

Navigating Stigma Addressing societal stigma involves fostering open discussions about sexual desires and practices within relationships. Creating a non-judgmental space allows partners to explore their interests without fear of shame or rejection.

Situational Factors

The environment in which fisting occurs can also influence risk levels. Factors such as privacy, comfort, and the availability of necessary supplies (like lubricant and gloves) play a critical role in ensuring safety.

Creating a Safe Environment Establishing a safe and comfortable environment is paramount. This includes ensuring that the space is clean, private, and equipped with all necessary supplies. Engaging in pre-scene rituals, such as setting the mood with lighting and music, can enhance relaxation and comfort.

Risk Awareness and Harm Reduction

Understanding risk factors and vulnerabilities is a vital component of harm reduction strategies. Practicing informed consent, establishing clear communication channels, and engaging in continuous education about fisting can empower individuals to navigate their desires safely.

Continuous Education Engaging in ongoing education about fisting techniques, safety protocols, and personal health can help individuals make informed decisions. Participating in workshops, reading literature, and joining supportive communities can provide valuable insights and resources.

Self-Reflection and Assessment Regular self-reflection and assessment of one's physical and emotional state can help individuals identify vulnerabilities before engaging in fisting. Keeping a journal or engaging in discussions with trusted partners can facilitate this process.

In conclusion, understanding the risk factors and vulnerabilities associated with fisting is essential for fostering a safe and enjoyable experience. By recognizing individual physical, emotional, and situational factors, individuals can take proactive steps to mitigate risks and enhance their fisting journey.

Practicing Harm Reduction Strategies

Harm reduction strategies are essential in ensuring that fisting, like any other intimate practice, is approached with safety, respect, and care. These strategies focus on minimizing the risks associated with fisting while promoting a positive and empowering experience for all participants.

Understanding Harm Reduction

Harm reduction is an approach that acknowledges the reality of risky behaviors while aiming to reduce their negative consequences. In the context of fisting, this means recognizing the potential physical and emotional risks involved and proactively implementing strategies to mitigate those risks.

Key Components of Harm Reduction Strategies

1. **Education and Awareness**: Understanding the anatomy involved in fisting, as well as the techniques that promote safety, is crucial. Educating oneself about the risks of internal injuries, nerve damage, and infection can empower individuals to make informed choices. Resources such as workshops, literature, and community discussions can provide valuable information.

2. **Open Communication**: Clear and honest communication between partners is vital. Discussing boundaries, desires, and concerns before engaging in fisting can help establish trust and ensure that all parties feel comfortable. Utilizing safe words and signals can further enhance communication during the act.

3. **Gradual Progression**: When exploring fisting, it is important to start slowly and gradually increase intensity. This can involve beginning with smaller objects or fingers before progressing to the whole hand. Gradual progression allows the body to adapt and reduces the risk of injury.

4. **Proper Preparation**: Preparing the body and environment is essential. This includes: - **Hygiene**: Ensuring that both the fister and the recipient practice good hygiene by washing hands and using gloves can significantly reduce the risk of infection. Additionally, using safe and appropriate lubricants can facilitate smoother insertion and reduce friction. - **Warm-Up**: Engaging in foreplay and other forms of stimulation can help relax the pelvic floor muscles and enhance comfort during fisting.

5. **Listening to the Body**: Paying attention to physical sensations is crucial. Partners should be attuned to each other's comfort levels and be willing to stop or slow down if any discomfort or pain is experienced. Pain should never be ignored, as it can be an indicator of potential injury.

6. **Aftercare**: Aftercare is an essential component of any intimate experience, particularly after fisting. It involves providing emotional and physical support to one another post-scene. This can include cuddling, discussing the experience, and checking in on each other's emotional state. Aftercare helps reinforce trust and connection between partners.

Examples of Harm Reduction Strategies

- **Using Gloves**: Wearing gloves during fisting can protect against the transmission of infections and reduce the risk of cuts or abrasions on the hands.

- **Choosing the Right Lubricant**: Using a high-quality, body-safe lubricant can minimize friction and enhance comfort. Water-based or silicone-based lubricants are often recommended for this purpose.

- **Establishing a Safe Word**: Agreeing on a safe word that either partner can use if they feel uncomfortable can help ensure that both parties feel safe and respected throughout the experience.

- **Regular Health Check-Ups**: Engaging in regular STI testing and health check-ups can provide peace of mind and help partners make informed decisions about their sexual health.

Conclusion

Practicing harm reduction strategies is crucial for anyone exploring fisting. By prioritizing education, communication, and safety, individuals can create a positive and fulfilling experience that respects the boundaries and well-being of all involved. Embracing these strategies not only enhances the physical safety of fisting but also fosters emotional intimacy and trust between partners.

In summary, harm reduction is not just about minimizing risks; it is about enhancing the overall experience of fisting, turning what may be perceived as a taboo into a journey of exploration, connection, and empowerment.

Seeking Professional Help and Support

Engaging in fisting can be an intense and transformative experience, but it can also bring up a range of emotions and psychological complexities. It is crucial to acknowledge when professional help is needed to navigate these feelings safely and effectively. This section will explore the importance of seeking professional support, the types of professionals who can assist, and how to approach these resources.

The Importance of Professional Support

When exploring practices that push personal boundaries, such as fisting, individuals may encounter emotional challenges, trauma triggers, or feelings of shame and anxiety. Seeking professional help can provide a safe space to process these experiences and emotions. Professionals can offer guidance on:

- **Understanding Emotional Responses:** Engaging in fisting may elicit unexpected emotional reactions, including joy, fear, or vulnerability. A trained therapist can help individuals understand these responses and develop coping strategies.

- **Addressing Trauma:** For some, fisting may trigger past traumas. Therapy can assist in processing these triggers, ensuring that the experience remains consensual and pleasurable.

- **Improving Communication Skills:** Professional support can enhance communication skills, which are essential for discussing boundaries, desires, and consent with partners.

- **Building Self-Esteem:** Engaging in fisting can sometimes lead to body image issues or feelings of inadequacy. Therapists can help individuals cultivate a positive self-image and embrace their bodies.

Types of Professionals to Consider

When seeking help, it is vital to find professionals who are knowledgeable about sexual health, kink, and the specific dynamics of fisting. Here are some types of professionals to consider:

- **Sex Therapists:** These professionals specialize in sexual issues and can provide insights into healthy sexual practices, including fisting. They can help clients explore their desires and address any psychological barriers.

- **Counselors and Psychologists:** General mental health professionals can offer support for emotional and psychological challenges. It is essential to find someone who is open-minded and knowledgeable about alternative sexual practices.

- **Sexual Health Educators:** These educators can provide information about safe practices, consent, and communication strategies. They may also facilitate workshops that focus on fisting and related topics.

- **Support Groups:** Peer-led support groups can offer a sense of community and shared experiences. They can be particularly beneficial for individuals navigating feelings of shame or stigma.

How to Approach Seeking Help

When considering professional help, the following steps can facilitate the process:

1. **Identify Your Needs:** Reflect on what specific issues you wish to address. Are you struggling with emotional responses, communication with partners, or past trauma? Understanding your needs will guide you in selecting the right professional.

2. **Research Professionals:** Look for therapists or educators who specialize in sexual health, kink, or trauma-informed care. Online directories, community recommendations, and local LGBTQ+ organizations can be valuable resources.

3. **Prepare for the First Session:** Consider writing down your thoughts and feelings about fisting, as well as any specific questions or concerns. This preparation can help you articulate your needs during the session.

4. **Establish Boundaries:** Before beginning therapy, communicate your boundaries and expectations with the professional. This can create a safe environment for exploration and discussion.

5. **Be Open to the Process:** Therapy is a journey, and it may take time to uncover and address underlying issues. Be patient with yourself and the process.

Examples of Professional Support Scenarios

To illustrate the importance of seeking professional help, consider the following scenarios:

- **Scenario 1: Overcoming Trauma:** Jamie has a history of trauma associated with intimacy. After discussing their interest in fisting with a partner, they find themselves experiencing anxiety and flashbacks. By working with a trauma-informed therapist, Jamie learns grounding techniques and communication skills, allowing them to engage in fisting safely while addressing their emotional responses.

- **Scenario 2: Improving Communication:** Alex and Taylor are exploring fisting but struggle to communicate their desires and boundaries effectively. They seek the guidance of a sex therapist who facilitates discussions about consent and helps them develop a shared language for their experiences. This support enhances their intimacy and trust during fisting play.

- **Scenario 3: Building Self-Esteem:** Jordan feels self-conscious about their body and worries that it will affect their fisting experiences. They attend therapy sessions focused on body positivity and self-acceptance. Through this process, Jordan learns to embrace their body and feel empowered in their sexual experiences.

Conclusion

Seeking professional help and support is a valuable step in ensuring a safe and fulfilling fisting experience. By addressing emotional challenges, improving communication skills, and fostering self-acceptance, individuals can navigate their fisting journeys with confidence and resilience. Remember, it is perfectly normal to seek help, and doing so can enhance both personal growth and the quality of intimate relationships.

Consensual Non-Consent and Risk Awareness

Consensual non-consent (CNC) is a complex and nuanced aspect of sexual exploration, particularly in the context of fisting. It involves the negotiation of scenarios where one or more participants agree to engage in activities that mimic non-consensual acts. This can include role-play scenarios where power dynamics are explored, often with the intent of pushing boundaries and exploring deeper emotional and psychological territories. However, it is crucial to approach CNC with a profound understanding of the inherent risks and the necessity of clear communication and consent.

Understanding Consensual Non-Consent

CNC is predicated on the foundation of informed consent. Participants must engage in thorough discussions prior to any activity to establish boundaries, safe words, and aftercare protocols. The essence of CNC lies in the paradox of consent: while the act may appear non-consensual, it is rooted in mutual agreement and understanding. This requires an elevated level of trust between partners, as well as an acute awareness of each other's emotional and physical states throughout the experience.

Theoretical Framework

The theoretical framework surrounding CNC can be informed by several key concepts:

- **Power Exchange Dynamics:** Understanding the dynamics of power in sexual relationships is crucial. CNC often involves a dominant and a submissive role, where the dominant partner may take control while the submissive partner surrenders agency within the agreed-upon limits.

- **Psychological Safety:** Engaging in CNC requires a high level of psychological safety. Participants must feel secure in expressing their limits and desires without fear of judgment or violation of trust.

- **Risk Awareness:** Understanding and acknowledging the potential risks involved in CNC scenarios is paramount. This includes both physical risks associated with fisting and emotional risks tied to vulnerability and trust.

Potential Problems and Considerations

While CNC can be a fulfilling aspect of sexual exploration, it is not without its challenges and potential pitfalls:

- **Miscommunication:** The ambiguity surrounding consent in CNC scenarios can lead to misunderstandings. It is essential to have explicit discussions about what is and isn't acceptable, and to revisit these conversations regularly.

- **Emotional Aftermath:** Participants may experience unexpected emotional responses post-scene. It is vital to incorporate aftercare practices to help partners process their experiences and feelings.

- **Boundary Overstepping:** Even in CNC scenarios, boundaries must be respected. Participants should have a clear understanding of what constitutes a violation of consent, even in a role-play context.
- **Social Stigma:** Engaging in CNC can carry societal stigma, leading individuals to feel shame or guilt about their desires. It is essential to cultivate a supportive community that understands and respects the complexities of CNC.

Examples of Consensual Non-Consent in Fisting

To illustrate CNC in the context of fisting, consider the following scenarios:

- **Role-Play Scenario:** A couple agrees to enact a scenario where one partner pretends to resist while the other partner fists them. Prior to the scene, they establish a safe word that, when spoken, will immediately halt all activities. This allows the submissive partner to explore feelings of vulnerability while maintaining control over the situation.
- **Exploring Limits:** A participant may express a desire to push their limits during fisting. They may agree to a scene where they are "forced" to take more than they typically would, but with a pre-established understanding that they can withdraw at any moment. This requires a high level of trust and communication to ensure safety.
- **Fantasy Exploration:** In a safe and consensual environment, partners may explore fantasies of non-consent through fisting, where one partner takes on a more dominant role. This can be a way to explore deeper desires while ensuring that both parties are aware of and agree to the boundaries set forth.

Best Practices for Engaging in CNC

To engage in consensual non-consent safely, consider the following best practices:

- **Comprehensive Negotiation:** Before engaging in any CNC activities, partners should engage in extensive discussions to outline desires, limits, and safe words. This negotiation should be revisited regularly to ensure ongoing consent.
- **Establish Safe Words:** Safe words are critical in CNC scenarios. They provide an immediate way to communicate discomfort or the need to stop, ensuring that participants can maintain control over their boundaries.

- **Aftercare:** Aftercare is essential in CNC scenarios, particularly after intense experiences. This may include physical comfort, emotional support, and time to discuss the experience. Aftercare helps partners reconnect and process their feelings.

- **Continuous Check-Ins:** During the scene, partners should engage in continuous check-ins, either verbally or through non-verbal cues, to gauge comfort levels and ensure that both parties are still consenting to the activities.

- **Education and Resources:** Engaging in CNC requires a solid understanding of both the physical and emotional aspects of the activities involved. Participants should seek out educational resources and communities that focus on safe practices in CNC and fisting.

Conclusion

Consensual non-consent can be an enriching aspect of sexual exploration when approached with care, communication, and respect. Understanding the complexities of CNC within the context of fisting not only enhances the experience but also fosters deeper connections and trust between partners. By prioritizing risk awareness and maintaining open lines of communication, participants can navigate the exhilarating yet intricate world of CNC safely and consensually.

Hygiene and Cleanliness

Cleaning and Preparing the Environment

Creating a safe and hygienic environment is a fundamental aspect of fisting. The physical act of fisting involves significant bodily engagement, and thus, ensuring a clean space is paramount to minimize health risks and enhance the overall experience. This section outlines essential practices for cleaning and preparing the environment before engaging in fisting.

Understanding the Importance of a Clean Environment

A clean environment reduces the risk of infections, injuries, and other complications associated with fisting. Bacteria and pathogens can thrive in unclean spaces, potentially leading to urinary tract infections (UTIs), sexually transmitted infections (STIs), or other health issues. Additionally, a well-prepared space

HYGIENE AND CLEANLINESS

contributes to emotional comfort and psychological safety, allowing participants to focus on pleasure and connection.

Steps for Cleaning the Environment

1. **Choose the Right Space:** Select a location that is private, comfortable, and free from distractions. Consider using a room that can be easily cleaned, such as a bathroom or bedroom.

2. **Declutter the Area:** Remove any unnecessary items from the space. This not only prevents accidents but also creates a calming atmosphere. Ensure that all tools and supplies are organized and within reach.

3. **Surface Cleaning:** Use disinfectant wipes or sprays to clean all surfaces that may come into contact with bodily fluids. Pay special attention to:

    - Bedsheets and blankets
    - Tables or surfaces where activities may occur
    - Any toys or accessories that will be used

   Ensure that the cleaning products used are safe for the materials being cleaned and do not leave harmful residues.

4. **Floor Cleaning:** Vacuum or sweep the floor to remove dust and debris. If engaging in activities that may lead to spills, consider laying down a protective covering such as a tarp or old sheet that can be easily washed afterward.

5. **Air Quality:** Ensure proper ventilation in the room. Open windows or use an air purifier to maintain good air quality. This can help reduce any odors and create a more pleasant atmosphere.

6. **Personal Hygiene Stations:** Set up a personal hygiene station equipped with:

    - Antibacterial soap
    - Clean towels
    - Hand sanitizer
    - Disposable gloves
    - Lubricants (preferably water-based or silicone-based, depending on the materials used)

This station should be easily accessible to all participants.

7. **Post-Cleaning Check:** Before beginning, conduct a final check of the environment to ensure that everything is clean, organized, and ready for use. This includes confirming that all necessary supplies are in place.

Potential Problems and Solutions

While preparing the environment, several potential problems may arise. Here are common issues and their solutions:

- **Inadequate Cleaning:** If surfaces are not properly disinfected, there is a risk of infection. Always use appropriate cleaning agents and verify that they are effective against a broad spectrum of pathogens. For example, using a bleach solution (1:10 ratio of bleach to water) can effectively disinfect surfaces.

- **Allergic Reactions:** Some individuals may have allergies to certain cleaning products. It is advisable to use hypoallergenic and fragrance-free cleaning supplies. Always communicate with partners about any known allergies before cleaning.

- **Discomfort Due to Temperature:** An environment that is too hot or too cold can detract from the experience. Adjust the temperature of the space to ensure comfort. Consider using blankets or space heaters if the environment is too cold, or fans if it is too warm.

- **Lack of Privacy:** Noise or interruptions can disrupt the experience. Ensure that the chosen space is private and, if necessary, use soundproofing methods such as thick curtains or rugs to dampen noise.

Examples of Effective Cleaning Practices

To illustrate effective cleaning practices, consider the following examples:

- **Using Natural Cleaners:** For those who prefer eco-friendly options, vinegar and baking soda can be effective natural cleaners. A mixture of vinegar and water can be used to wipe down surfaces, while baking soda can be sprinkled on carpets or upholstery to eliminate odors.

- **Creating a Cleaning Checklist:** Develop a checklist for cleaning and preparing the environment. This can include tasks such as:

- Disinfect surfaces
- Organize toys and supplies
- Set up personal hygiene stations
- Check for privacy and comfort

A checklist can ensure that no steps are overlooked and can be particularly useful for individuals new to fisting.

- **Utilizing Protective Covers:** For added protection, use disposable or washable covers on surfaces where activities will occur. This not only protects the surfaces but also simplifies cleanup after the session.

In conclusion, cleaning and preparing the environment is a crucial step in ensuring a safe and enjoyable fisting experience. By following these guidelines, participants can create a space that is not only hygienic but also conducive to intimacy and pleasure. Taking the time to prepare the environment thoughtfully reflects a commitment to safety and mutual respect, laying the foundation for a fulfilling exploration of fisting.

Personal Hygiene Practices

Maintaining personal hygiene is crucial for anyone engaging in fisting, as it significantly impacts both safety and pleasure. Personal hygiene encompasses a variety of practices that help prevent infections, promote comfort, and enhance the overall experience. In this section, we will explore essential hygiene practices, common challenges, and practical examples to ensure a safe and enjoyable fisting experience.

Importance of Personal Hygiene

Personal hygiene is essential in fisting for several reasons:

- **Infection Prevention:** The introduction of hands into the body can potentially transfer bacteria, viruses, or other pathogens. Good hygiene practices significantly reduce the risk of infections such as bacterial vaginosis, yeast infections, or sexually transmitted infections (STIs).

- **Comfort:** Maintaining cleanliness can enhance comfort levels during play. Participants are more likely to relax and enjoy the experience when they feel clean and fresh.

- **Respect for Partners:** Practicing good hygiene demonstrates care and respect for partners, fostering trust and intimacy.
- **Psychological Well-being:** Feeling clean can enhance self-esteem and body image, contributing to a more positive sexual experience.

Key Hygiene Practices

1. Hand Hygiene

Before engaging in fisting, it is vital to wash hands thoroughly. The Centers for Disease Control and Prevention (CDC) recommends the following steps for effective handwashing:

1. Wet hands with clean, running water (warm or cold).
2. Apply soap and lather by rubbing hands together, ensuring to scrub all surfaces, including between fingers, under nails, and the backs of hands.
3. Scrub hands for at least 20 seconds. A helpful tip is to sing the "Happy Birthday" song twice.
4. Rinse hands under clean, running water.
5. Dry hands using a clean towel or air dry.

2. Nail Care

Long or unkempt nails can harbor bacteria and cause injury during fisting. It is essential to:

- Keep nails short and well-trimmed.
- Smooth any rough edges with a nail file to prevent scratches or tears.
- Avoid nail polish or artificial nails, as they can chip and create sharp edges.

3. Personal Grooming

While personal grooming preferences vary, some individuals may choose to trim or shave pubic hair. This can enhance hygiene by reducing the risk of bacterial growth and making cleaning easier. If grooming is performed, it should be done carefully to avoid cuts or irritation.

4. Body Cleansing

HYGIENE AND CLEANLINESS

A thorough shower before engaging in fisting is recommended. Use a gentle, unscented soap to cleanse the body, focusing on the genital area and hands. Avoid harsh chemicals or fragrances that may irritate sensitive skin.

5. Lubrication Considerations

Using appropriate lubricants is crucial for a safe fisting experience. Water-based or silicone-based lubricants are recommended, as they are less likely to cause irritation or infection. Avoid oil-based lubricants, as they can break down latex gloves or condoms and may lead to infections.

Challenges and Solutions

While maintaining personal hygiene is essential, some challenges may arise:

- **Time Constraints:** In a spontaneous setting, individuals may feel rushed. It is essential to prioritize hygiene, even if it means taking a few extra minutes to wash hands and bodies.

- **Body Image Issues:** Some individuals may feel self-conscious about their bodies. Open communication with partners about hygiene practices can alleviate anxiety and foster a supportive environment.

- **Access to Facilities:** In situations where access to a shower or bathroom is limited, consider using antibacterial wipes or hand sanitizers as a temporary solution. However, these should not replace proper handwashing when possible.

Examples of Personal Hygiene Practices

Example 1: Pre-Fisting Routine

Before engaging in fisting, a couple may establish a routine that includes:

- Showering together to enhance intimacy while ensuring cleanliness.

- Taking turns washing each other's hands and bodies, which can be a sensual experience.

- Discussing any preferences for grooming and hygiene practices to ensure both partners feel comfortable.

Example 2: Hygiene During Fisting

During fisting, participants should:

- Use gloves to maintain hygiene and prevent the transfer of bacteria.

- Change gloves if there is a need to touch other body parts, such as transitioning from anal to vaginal play.

- Keep lubricant easily accessible to avoid friction, which can lead to irritation or injury.

Conclusion

In conclusion, personal hygiene practices are a fundamental aspect of safe and pleasurable fisting experiences. By prioritizing cleanliness, individuals can reduce the risk of infections, enhance comfort, and foster intimacy with their partners. Open communication about hygiene preferences and practices can further strengthen connections and ensure a positive experience for all involved. Remember, a little preparation goes a long way in creating a safe and enjoyable environment for exploration.

Bibliography

[1] Centers for Disease Control and Prevention. (2021). *Handwashing: Clean Hands Save Lives.* Retrieved from https://www.cdc.gov/handwashing/index.html

[2] World Health Organization. (2020). *WHO Guidelines on Hand Hygiene in Health Care.* Retrieved from https://www.who.int/publications/i/item/9789241597906

Proper Hand Hygiene and Nail Care

Ensuring proper hand hygiene and nail care is critical in the practice of fisting, as it not only promotes safety but also enhances the overall experience for all participants. This section will outline the theoretical underpinnings of hand hygiene, the importance of nail care, common problems that can arise, and practical examples to illustrate best practices.

The Importance of Hand Hygiene

Hand hygiene is a vital component in preventing the transmission of infections. The Centers for Disease Control and Prevention (CDC) emphasizes that proper handwashing can reduce the risk of infections significantly. According to the CDC, hand hygiene can reduce the risk of respiratory infections by 21% and gastrointestinal infections by 31% [?].

The skin, particularly on the hands, can harbor various pathogens, including bacteria, viruses, and fungi. When engaging in intimate activities such as fisting, these pathogens can be transferred to the receiving partner, potentially leading to infections. Therefore, maintaining clean hands is essential to ensure both partners' health and safety.

Handwashing Techniques

To achieve effective hand hygiene, follow these steps:

1. Wet your hands with clean, running water (warm or cold).

2. Apply soap and lather by rubbing your hands together. Be sure to lather the backs of your hands, between your fingers, and under your nails.

3. Scrub your hands for at least 20 seconds. Need a timer? Hum the "Happy Birthday" song twice.

4. Rinse your hands well under clean, running water.

5. Dry your hands using a clean towel or air dry them.

It is crucial to wash your hands before and after engaging in fisting to minimize the risk of infection.

Nail Care: A Critical Component

Proper nail care is equally important as it can be a source of injury or infection. Long or unkempt nails can harbor bacteria and can also cause abrasions or tears during fisting. The following guidelines should be adhered to:

- **Keep nails trimmed:** Regularly trim your nails to a short length. The American Academy of Dermatology recommends keeping fingernails no longer than the tips of your fingers.

- **File edges:** Smooth out the edges of your nails with a nail file to prevent sharp edges that could cause cuts or scratches.

- **Avoid artificial nails:** While they may look appealing, artificial nails can harbor bacteria and may break off during play, leading to potential injury.

- **Regular cleaning:** Clean under your nails regularly to remove dirt and debris, as these can introduce pathogens into the receiving partner's body.

Common Problems and Solutions

Despite best practices, common issues can arise related to hand hygiene and nail care. Here are a few potential problems and their solutions:

- **Dry or cracked skin:** Frequent handwashing can lead to dry skin, which may crack and bleed. To combat this, use a gentle, moisturizing soap and apply hand cream after washing your hands.

- **Nail infections:** Ingrown nails or fungal infections can occur, especially if nails are not properly cared for. If you notice redness, swelling, or pus, seek medical attention promptly.

- **Bacterial transmission:** If you or your partner have any cuts or abrasions on your hands, it is crucial to avoid fisting until they have healed to prevent introducing bacteria into the body.

Practical Examples

To illustrate the importance of proper hand hygiene and nail care, consider the following scenarios:

- **Scenario 1:** A couple decides to engage in fisting after a long day. They wash their hands thoroughly but neglect to trim their nails. During the act, one partner experiences discomfort due to a jagged nail edge, leading to a minor cut. This could have been avoided with proper nail care.

- **Scenario 2:** Before a fisting session, one partner has a small cut on their hand but does not inform their partner. During the act, bacteria from the cut enter the receiving partner's body, resulting in an infection. Open communication about any injuries is vital for safety.

Conclusion

In conclusion, proper hand hygiene and nail care are essential components of safe fisting practices. By adhering to the guidelines outlined in this section, individuals can significantly reduce the risk of infections and enhance their intimate experiences. Remember, a little preparation goes a long way in ensuring a safe and pleasurable journey into the world of fisting.

Choosing Safe and Appropriate Lubricants

When it comes to fisting, selecting the right lubricant is crucial for both safety and pleasure. Lubricants reduce friction, enhance sensation, and help prevent injuries, making them an essential component of the experience. However, not all lubricants are created equal, and understanding their properties, compatibility, and safety is vital.

Types of Lubricants

Lubricants can be categorized into three main types: water-based, silicone-based, and oil-based. Each type has its own advantages and disadvantages, which can affect your choice depending on the specific context of your fisting experience.

- **Water-Based Lubricants:** Water-based lubes are versatile and easy to clean up. They are safe to use with condoms and sex toys, making them a popular choice for many. However, they can dry out quickly, requiring reapplication, especially during extended sessions. Common ingredients include glycerin and aloe vera, which can provide additional soothing properties. It's important to choose a water-based lubricant that is free from irritating additives, such as parabens or fragrances.

- **Silicone-Based Lubricants:** Silicone-based lubes offer a longer-lasting glide than water-based options, making them ideal for fisting. They are also safe to use with latex condoms but may not be compatible with certain silicone sex toys. Silicone lubricants can provide a silky feel and are less likely to dry out, allowing for extended play without frequent reapplication. However, they can be more challenging to clean off surfaces and may require soap and water for complete removal.

- **Oil-Based Lubricants:** Oil-based lubes, such as coconut oil or almond oil, provide excellent lubrication and a luxurious feel. They are not safe to use with latex condoms, as they can cause them to break. However, they can be compatible with certain polyurethane or polyisoprene condoms. Oil-based lubricants can be more difficult to clean up and may stain fabrics. Additionally, some individuals may experience irritation or allergic reactions to specific oils, so it's important to patch-test before use.

Safety Considerations

When selecting a lubricant for fisting, safety should always be a priority. Here are key considerations to keep in mind:

- **Compatibility with Condoms and Toys:** Always check the compatibility of the lubricant with any condoms or toys you plan to use. Water-based lubes are generally the safest option for all types of condoms and toys. Silicone lubes can be used with latex condoms but may not be suitable for silicone toys. Oil-based lubes should be avoided with latex condoms altogether.

- **Irritation and Allergies:** Some lubricants contain ingredients that can cause irritation or allergic reactions. Always read the ingredient list and avoid products with parabens, glycerin (if you are sensitive), and synthetic fragrances. Consider using hypoallergenic options or those specifically designed for sensitive skin.

- **pH Balance:** The vaginal and anal areas have a specific pH balance that can be disrupted by certain lubricants. Using a pH-balanced lubricant can help maintain the natural flora and prevent infections. Look for products labeled as pH-balanced for intimate use.

- **Testing for Sensitivity:** Before using a new lubricant, conduct a patch test on a small area of skin to check for any adverse reactions. Apply a small amount and wait 24 hours to see if any irritation occurs.

Recommended Products

Here are a few recommended lubricants known for their safety and effectiveness:

- **Water-Based:**
    - *Sliquid H2O* - A vegan-friendly, glycerin-free water-based lubricant that is gentle on the skin.
    - *Aloe Cadabra* - An organic aloe vera-based lubricant that is soothing and pH-balanced.

- **Silicone-Based:**
    - *Pjur Original* - A high-quality silicone lubricant that lasts longer and provides a silky feel.

- *Wet Platinum* - A silicone lubricant that is long-lasting and safe for use with latex condoms.

+ **Oil-Based:**

  - *Coconut Oil* - A natural option that is moisturizing and has antifungal properties.
  - *Boy Butter* - A hybrid lubricant that combines coconut oil and silicone for enhanced performance.

Conclusion

Choosing the right lubricant for fisting is essential for ensuring a safe and pleasurable experience. By understanding the different types of lubricants, their compatibility, and safety considerations, you can make an informed decision that enhances your exploration. Always prioritize your comfort and safety, and don't hesitate to experiment with different products to find what works best for you and your partner(s). Remember, the right lubricant can transform your fisting journey, allowing for deeper connection, pleasure, and exploration.

Sterilizing and Cleaning Toys and Accessories

The importance of proper sterilization and cleaning of toys and accessories cannot be overstated in the context of fisting and other intimate activities. Ensuring that all items used are clean and safe significantly reduces the risk of infections and other complications, thereby enhancing the overall experience.

Understanding the Need for Sterilization

Fisting often involves the use of various toys and accessories, which can come into contact with bodily fluids and mucous membranes. This makes them potential vectors for pathogens, including bacteria, viruses, and fungi. The primary goal of sterilization is to eliminate these microorganisms, ensuring that the items are safe for use.

Types of Contaminants

Contaminants can be categorized into three main types:

+ **Biological Contaminants:** These include bacteria, viruses, and fungi that can cause infections.

- **Chemical Contaminants:** Residues from lubricants, soaps, or other substances that can cause irritation or allergic reactions.
- **Physical Contaminants:** Dust, dirt, or other physical debris that may accumulate on toys and accessories.

Cleaning vs. Sterilizing

It is essential to understand the difference between cleaning and sterilizing:

- **Cleaning:** This process involves removing visible dirt and contaminants from surfaces using soap and water. It is the first step before sterilization.
- **Sterilizing:** This process goes a step further by using methods that kill all microorganisms, including spores. Common methods include boiling, using chemical disinfectants, or employing autoclaving techniques.

Recommended Cleaning Procedures

To ensure that your toys and accessories are safe for use, follow these recommended cleaning procedures:

1. **Initial Rinse:** After use, rinse the toy or accessory under warm running water to remove any bodily fluids or lubricant residues.
2. **Soap and Water Cleaning:** Use a mild, unscented antibacterial soap to wash the item thoroughly. Pay special attention to any crevices or textured areas where contaminants may hide.
3. **Rinse Again:** Rinse the item thoroughly under warm water to remove any soap residue.
4. **Drying:** Allow the item to air dry completely on a clean towel or drying rack. Avoid using shared towels to prevent cross-contamination.

Sterilization Techniques

Once the item is cleaned, you can proceed with sterilization. Here are some effective methods:

- **Boiling:** Submerge the item in boiling water for at least 10 minutes. This method is effective for most non-electronic toys made of materials like silicone, glass, or stainless steel.

- **Chemical Disinfectants:** Use a solution of 70% isopropyl alcohol or a specialized toy cleaner. Ensure that the product is safe for the material of the toy. Follow the manufacturer's instructions for contact time.

- **Dishwasher:** If the toy is dishwasher safe, placing it on the top rack and running a hot cycle can effectively clean and sterilize it. Avoid using detergent with fragrances or additives.

- **UV Sterilizers:** Some modern toys come with UV sterilization features. Alternatively, you can use a UV sterilizer specifically designed for sex toys.

Material Considerations

Different materials require different cleaning and sterilization methods:

- **Silicone:** Generally safe for boiling and chemical disinfectants. Avoid using oil-based lubricants that can degrade silicone.

- **Glass and Stainless Steel:** These materials can withstand high temperatures and are safe for boiling and dishwashers.

- **Rubber and PVC:** These materials may not withstand boiling and should be cleaned with soap and water, followed by a chemical disinfectant.

- **Electronics:** Always refer to the manufacturer's guidelines. Most electronic toys should not be submerged in water.

Storage and Maintenance

Proper storage is equally important for maintaining the cleanliness of toys and accessories. Consider the following tips:

- **Use a Dedicated Storage Bag or Box:** Store toys in a clean, dry, and dedicated space to prevent contamination from dust or other items.

- **Keep Toys Separate:** Avoid storing different materials together, as they can react with one another and degrade.

- **Regular Inspections:** Periodically check your toys for any signs of wear, damage, or degradation. Discard any items that show signs of deterioration.

Conclusion

Maintaining a rigorous cleaning and sterilization routine for your toys and accessories is essential for safe and pleasurable fisting experiences. By understanding the differences between cleaning and sterilizing, utilizing appropriate techniques, and considering material-specific needs, you can significantly reduce the risk of infections and enhance your intimate experiences. Remember that safety is paramount, and taking these precautions will allow you to explore your fantasies with confidence and care.

Understanding the Importance of Gloves

In the realm of fisting, the use of gloves is not merely a suggestion; it is a critical component of safety and hygiene. The importance of gloves can be understood through several lenses: health considerations, risk management, and the enhancement of the overall experience.

Health Considerations

First and foremost, gloves serve as a barrier to prevent the transmission of pathogens. When engaging in intimate activities such as fisting, the risk of exposure to sexually transmitted infections (STIs) increases. According to the Centers for Disease Control and Prevention (CDC), many STIs can be transmitted through skin-to-skin contact, making it essential to minimize direct contact with bodily fluids.

$$P(T) = 1 - (1-p)^n \qquad (16)$$

Where:

- $P(T)$ = Probability of transmission
- p = Probability of transmission per contact
- n = Number of contacts

This equation illustrates that as the number of contacts increases, so does the probability of transmission, emphasizing the need for protective measures such as gloves.

Risk Management

Using gloves can significantly reduce the risk of physical injuries during fisting. The vaginal and anal tissues are delicate and can be easily damaged. Abrasions or tears can occur, creating openings for bacteria and viruses to enter the body. Gloves provide a smooth surface that can help prevent friction-related injuries.

In addition to protecting the receiving partner, gloves also safeguard the inserting partner from potential exposure to blood, fecal matter, or other bodily fluids that may carry infections. This mutual protection fosters a sense of safety and trust between partners, which is essential for a positive fisting experience.

Enhancing the Experience

Beyond health and safety, gloves can enhance the sensory experience of fisting. The choice of glove material can impact the level of sensation felt by both partners. For instance, latex gloves are thin and provide a high level of sensitivity, allowing for a more intimate connection. However, some individuals may have latex allergies; in such cases, nitrile gloves are an excellent alternative, offering both safety and sensitivity.

The texture of the gloves can also play a role in the experience. Textured gloves may provide additional stimulation, while smooth gloves can facilitate easier insertion. Experimenting with different types of gloves can add an exciting element to the fisting experience.

Choosing the Right Gloves

When selecting gloves for fisting, consider the following factors:

- **Material:** Choose between latex, nitrile, or vinyl based on personal preferences and any allergies.

- **Size:** Ensure the gloves fit well. Gloves that are too tight can restrict movement, while those that are too loose may slip off during play.

- **Texture:** Decide whether a smooth or textured surface is preferred for enhanced sensation.

- **Thickness:** Thinner gloves may provide more sensitivity, while thicker gloves offer added protection.

Proper Glove Use

To maximize the benefits of gloves during fisting, follow these guidelines:

1. **Wash Hands:** Always wash your hands thoroughly before putting on gloves to minimize contamination.

2. **Inspect Gloves:** Check for any tears or defects before use. Discard any damaged gloves immediately.

3. **Change Gloves:** Change gloves between different activities or partners to prevent cross-contamination.

4. **Dispose Properly:** After use, dispose of gloves in a sanitary manner. Do not flush them down the toilet.

Conclusion

In conclusion, the use of gloves during fisting is a fundamental practice that enhances safety, reduces health risks, and can even improve the overall experience. By understanding the importance of gloves, individuals can engage in fisting with confidence, knowing they are taking necessary precautions to protect themselves and their partners. Embracing this practice not only promotes a healthier sexual experience but also fosters a deeper sense of trust and intimacy between partners.

Bibliography

[1] Centers for Disease Control and Prevention. (n.d.). *Sexually Transmitted Diseases (STDs)*. Retrieved from `https://www.cdc.gov/std/default.htm`

Maintaining a Clean and Sanitary Space

Creating a clean and sanitary environment is paramount when engaging in fisting, as it significantly reduces the risk of infections and promotes a more enjoyable experience. This section will delve into the necessary steps and considerations for maintaining cleanliness and hygiene in your fisting practice.

The Importance of a Sanitary Space

A clean environment not only safeguards physical health but also enhances emotional well-being. Engaging in fisting can evoke vulnerability and intimacy; thus, knowing that the space is hygienic allows participants to relax and fully engage in the experience. A sanitary space can also foster a sense of trust and care between partners, reinforcing the emotional connection that is vital in such intimate activities.

Cleaning and Preparing the Environment

Before any intimate activity, it is essential to prepare the space. Here are key steps to ensure cleanliness:

- **Surface Cleaning:** Use disinfectant wipes or sprays to clean all surfaces that may come into contact with bodily fluids. Focus on areas like beds, couches, or any surfaces where fisting will occur. Ensure that the cleaning agents used are safe for the materials of the surfaces.

- **Floor Hygiene:** Vacuum or mop the floor to remove any dust or debris. If the floor is carpeted, consider placing a clean, washable blanket or towel over the area where the activity will occur.

- **Ventilation:** Ensure the space is well-ventilated to promote air circulation. This can help reduce the presence of any lingering odors and create a more comfortable atmosphere.

Personal Hygiene Practices

Maintaining personal hygiene is equally important for both participants. Here are some recommendations:

- **Showering Beforehand:** Both partners should shower before engaging in fisting. This includes washing hands, arms, and any areas of the body that may come into contact during the activity. Use mild soap to avoid irritation.

- **Nail Care:** Ensure that nails are trimmed and filed to prevent any accidental scratches or tears. Long or jagged nails can cause significant discomfort and injury, so it is advisable to keep them short and smooth.

- **Gloves:** Wearing disposable gloves is highly recommended. Gloves act as a barrier against bacteria and viruses, providing an additional layer of protection. Always use new gloves for each session and dispose of them properly afterward.

Proper Hand Hygiene and Nail Care

Hand hygiene is crucial in preventing the transfer of pathogens. The following practices should be observed:

- **Handwashing:** Wash hands thoroughly with soap and water for at least 20 seconds before and after the activity. Pay special attention to the areas between fingers and under nails.

- **Use of Hand Sanitizer:** If soap and water are not readily available, an alcohol-based hand sanitizer with at least 60% alcohol can be used as an alternative. However, it should not replace thorough handwashing.

- **Nail Maintenance:** Regularly inspect nails for any signs of damage or dirt. Keeping nails clean and well-maintained is essential to ensure safety during fisting.

Choosing Safe and Appropriate Lubricants

Lubrication is critical in fisting to minimize friction and enhance comfort. However, the choice of lubricant can impact hygiene:

- **Types of Lubricants:** Water-based lubricants are generally recommended as they are easy to clean and less likely to cause irritation. Silicone-based lubricants can also be effective but may require more effort to clean up.

- **Avoiding Oil-Based Products:** Oil-based lubricants can degrade latex gloves and condoms, increasing the risk of breakage and infection. Always check the compatibility of the lubricant with the materials being used.

- **Storage:** Store lubricants in a cool, dry place, and ensure they are tightly sealed to prevent contamination.

Sterilizing and Cleaning Toys and Accessories

If incorporating toys or accessories into fisting, proper cleaning and sterilization are essential:

- **Material Considerations:** Different materials require different cleaning methods. For example, silicone and glass toys can typically be boiled or washed with soap and water, while porous materials may require specific cleaning solutions.

- **Post-Use Cleaning:** Clean all toys immediately after use to prevent the growth of bacteria. Use warm water and soap, or follow the manufacturer's cleaning instructions.

- **Storage:** Store toys in a clean, dry place, preferably in a dedicated storage bag or container to prevent contamination.

Establishing Hygiene Protocols with Partners

Creating hygiene protocols with partners can enhance safety and comfort. Consider the following:

- **Pre-Session Discussions:** Discuss hygiene practices with your partner before engaging in fisting. Agree on what measures will be taken to ensure cleanliness.

- **Regular Health Check-Ups:** Encourage regular STI testing and health check-ups among partners. Open discussions about sexual health can help build trust and ensure a safer experience.

- **Post-Session Care:** Aftercare is important not only for emotional support but also for hygiene. Ensure that both partners clean up properly after the session and discuss any concerns that may arise.

Managing and Preventing Infections

Awareness and proactive measures can help prevent infections related to fisting:

- **Recognizing Symptoms:** Be vigilant for any signs of infection, such as redness, swelling, or unusual discharge. If any symptoms arise, seek medical attention promptly.

- **Educating Yourself:** Stay informed about common infections associated with fisting and how to prevent them. Understanding the risks can help in making informed decisions.

- **Consulting Professionals:** If you have concerns about hygiene or health related to fisting, do not hesitate to consult a healthcare professional for personalized advice and guidance.

In conclusion, maintaining a clean and sanitary space is a fundamental aspect of safe fisting practices. By prioritizing hygiene, individuals can enhance their experiences while minimizing risks. Remember that cleanliness is not just about physical health; it also plays a significant role in fostering trust, intimacy, and emotional safety in the exploration of fisting.

Establishing Hygiene Protocols with Partners

Establishing hygiene protocols with partners is a crucial aspect of ensuring safe and enjoyable fisting experiences. This section outlines the necessary steps to promote cleanliness, prevent infections, and foster open communication regarding hygiene practices. The importance of hygiene cannot be overstated, as it not only protects physical health but also enhances emotional safety and trust between partners.

The Importance of Hygiene in Fisting

Fisting involves significant physical intimacy and can introduce various health risks if proper hygiene practices are not followed. The following points highlight the importance of hygiene in fisting:

- **Infection Prevention:** The rectum and vagina are home to various bacteria that can lead to infections if introduced to other areas of the body. Proper hygiene reduces the risk of bacterial infections, sexually transmitted infections (STIs), and other complications.

- **Physical Comfort:** Cleanliness enhances the overall experience by minimizing unpleasant odors and discomfort, allowing partners to focus on pleasure and connection.

- **Emotional Safety:** Open discussions about hygiene foster trust and respect in the relationship, making partners feel valued and cared for.

Creating a Hygiene Protocol

To establish effective hygiene protocols, partners should engage in open dialogue and agree on specific practices before engaging in fisting. The following steps can serve as a guideline:

1. **Discuss Hygiene Expectations:** Partners should openly discuss their hygiene expectations and preferences. This includes preferences for showering before play, the use of gloves, and the types of lubricants that will be used.

2. **Set Up a Pre-Play Routine:** Establish a routine that includes washing hands, cleaning the body, and preparing the play area. For example, both partners can agree to shower together before engaging in fisting, using mild soap and water to clean the relevant areas.

3. **Use Protection:** The use of gloves can significantly reduce the risk of transmitting bacteria and infections. Partners should agree on whether to use gloves during fisting and ensure that they are properly fitted and made of a suitable material (e.g., latex, nitrile).

4. **Choose Appropriate Lubricants:** Selecting the right lubricant is essential for comfort and safety. Partners should agree on using water-based or silicone-based lubricants, avoiding oil-based products that can degrade latex gloves.

5. **Establish Cleaning Protocols for Toys:** If using toys during fisting, it is vital to establish cleaning protocols. Toys should be cleaned with soap and water or a suitable toy cleaner before and after use. Partners should discuss the types of toys they plan to incorporate and how they will be maintained.

6. **Post-Play Hygiene:** After engaging in fisting, partners should clean themselves and the play area. This may include washing hands, showering, and sanitizing any surfaces or toys used during play.

7. **Regular Health Check-Ups:** Partners should agree to undergo regular STI testing and health check-ups to ensure both parties are aware of their sexual health status. This promotes transparency and trust in the relationship.

Addressing Potential Problems

While establishing hygiene protocols is beneficial, partners may encounter challenges. Some common issues include:

- **Discomfort Discussing Hygiene:** Some individuals may feel embarrassed or uncomfortable discussing hygiene practices. It is essential to create a non-judgmental space where both partners feel safe to express their concerns and preferences.

- **Differences in Hygiene Standards:** Partners may have differing hygiene standards or practices. Open communication and compromise are vital to finding a middle ground that satisfies both parties.

- **Forgetting Protocols:** In the heat of the moment, partners may forget to follow established hygiene protocols. It is helpful to create a checklist or reminder to ensure that all necessary steps are followed before engaging in fisting.

Examples of Hygiene Protocols in Action

To illustrate the establishment of hygiene protocols, consider the following scenarios:

- **Scenario 1: Pre-Play Agreement** - Two partners, Alex and Jamie, decide to engage in fisting for the first time. They agree to shower together beforehand, use nitrile gloves during play, and clean any toys with soap and water. After their session, they both wash their hands and clean the play area together, reinforcing their commitment to hygiene.

- **Scenario 2: Addressing Discomfort** - During a discussion about hygiene, Taylor expresses discomfort with the idea of using gloves. Their partner, Morgan, listens empathetically and suggests trying gloves during their next session to see how they feel. This approach fosters open communication and respect for each other's boundaries.
- **Scenario 3: Post-Play Reflection** - After a fisting session, Sam and Jordan take time to discuss their experience. They reflect on their hygiene practices and agree to add a step to clean the play area more thoroughly next time. This ongoing dialogue helps them improve their hygiene protocols over time.

Conclusion

Establishing hygiene protocols with partners is an essential component of safe and pleasurable fisting experiences. By engaging in open communication, setting clear expectations, and addressing potential challenges, partners can create a supportive environment that prioritizes health and emotional safety. Remember, effective hygiene practices not only enhance physical well-being but also deepen the connection and trust between partners, allowing for more fulfilling intimate experiences.

Managing and Preventing Infections

In the context of fisting, managing and preventing infections is paramount to ensure a safe and pleasurable experience. The intimate nature of fisting, which involves the insertion of a hand into the body, can pose various health risks, including the transmission of sexually transmitted infections (STIs) and other pathogens. This section will explore the theoretical foundations of infection management, common problems associated with fisting, and practical examples to illustrate effective prevention strategies.

Theoretical Foundations of Infection Control

Infection control in fisting practices hinges on understanding the transmission pathways of pathogens. Pathogens can enter the body through:

- **Mucosal Surfaces:** The vagina, anus, and urethra are mucosal surfaces that can facilitate the entry of bacteria and viruses.
- **Open Wounds or Cuts:** Any abrasions or cuts on the hand or body can serve as entry points for pathogens.

- **Fecal Contamination:** The anus is home to a variety of bacteria, and improper hygiene can lead to infections.

To prevent infections, it is essential to adopt a multifaceted approach that includes personal hygiene, environmental cleanliness, and the use of protective barriers.

Common Problems Associated with Fisting

Several issues can arise during fisting that may increase the risk of infection:

- **Inadequate Hygiene:** Failure to wash hands, use gloves, or clean toys can introduce bacteria into the body.

- **Improper Lubrication:** Insufficient lubrication can lead to tears in the mucosal lining, increasing the risk of infection.

- **Delayed Medical Attention:** Ignoring signs of infection, such as unusual discharge, pain, or swelling, can lead to severe complications.

Practical Strategies for Infection Prevention

To effectively manage and prevent infections during fisting, the following strategies should be implemented:

1. Personal Hygiene Practices

- **Handwashing:** Before and after engaging in fisting, thoroughly wash hands with soap and water for at least 20 seconds. Pay special attention to the nails and cuticles, where bacteria can accumulate.

- **Nail Care:** Keep nails short and smooth to prevent cuts and tears in the mucosal lining. Avoid artificial nails, as they can harbor bacteria.

- **Skin Preparation:** Clean the skin around the anal and vaginal areas with mild soap and water before fisting. This reduces the risk of introducing bacteria into the body.

2. Use of Protective Barriers

- **Gloves:** Wearing latex or nitrile gloves during fisting is highly recommended. Gloves provide a barrier against pathogens and can be changed easily if they become torn or contaminated.

- **Lubricants:** Use high-quality, body-safe lubricants to minimize friction and reduce the risk of tears. Avoid oil-based lubricants if using latex gloves, as they can degrade the material.

3. Environmental Cleanliness

- **Sanitizing Surfaces:** Ensure that all surfaces in the fisting area are clean and sanitized. Use disinfectant wipes or sprays on surfaces that may come into contact with bodily fluids.

- **Toys and Accessories:** If using any toys or accessories, clean them thoroughly before and after use according to the manufacturer's instructions. Consider using toys made from non-porous materials that can be easily sanitized.

4. Recognizing Signs of Infection

It is crucial to be aware of the signs of potential infections, which may include:

- Unusual discharge from the vagina or anus
- Persistent pain or discomfort during or after fisting
- Swelling, redness, or warmth around the insertion site
- Fever or chills, which may indicate a systemic infection

If any of these symptoms arise, it is essential to seek medical attention promptly to address potential infections.

Case Study: Effective Infection Management

Consider a scenario where a couple engages in fisting for the first time. They discuss their boundaries and establish consent, but they overlook hygiene practices. After the session, one partner develops symptoms of an infection. This situation highlights the importance of implementing infection prevention strategies:

- **Before the Session:** The couple should have washed their hands and used gloves, ensuring that the environment was clean and that toys were sanitized.

- **During the Session:** They should have used sufficient lubricant to prevent tearing and communicated openly about comfort levels.

- **After the Session:** They should have monitored for any signs of infection and sought medical advice if symptoms arose.

This case illustrates that proactive infection management can significantly reduce the risk of complications and enhance the overall experience.

Conclusion

Managing and preventing infections during fisting requires a comprehensive understanding of hygiene practices, the use of protective barriers, and awareness of potential risks. By prioritizing cleanliness and communication, individuals can engage in fisting safely while minimizing the likelihood of infections. Emphasizing these practices not only enhances physical safety but also fosters a deeper sense of trust and intimacy between partners, allowing for a more fulfilling exploration of this intimate act.

Regular Health Check-Ups and STI Testing

Engaging in fisting, like any other sexual activity, necessitates a commitment to health and safety. Regular health check-ups and STI testing are crucial components of a responsible sexual health regimen, particularly for individuals who participate in high-risk sexual practices. This section will explore the importance of these practices, the recommended testing intervals, and the implications of results.

The Importance of Regular Health Check-Ups

Regular health check-ups serve as a proactive measure to maintain overall health and well-being. These check-ups typically include a comprehensive review of an individual's medical history, physical examinations, and screenings for various health conditions. For individuals engaging in fisting, these check-ups are vital for several reasons:

- **Early Detection of Health Issues:** Regular visits to a healthcare provider can facilitate the early detection of potential health issues, including sexually transmitted infections (STIs), which can often be asymptomatic in their early stages.

- **Monitoring of Sexual Health:** Healthcare professionals can provide tailored advice regarding sexual health, including safe practices and potential risks associated with fisting.

- **Building a Relationship with Healthcare Providers:** Establishing a rapport with healthcare providers can lead to more open discussions about sexual health, reducing stigma and promoting a supportive environment for discussing sensitive topics.

STI Testing: Frequency and Recommendations

STI testing is a critical aspect of sexual health, especially for individuals who engage in practices like fisting that may involve higher risk factors. The Centers for Disease Control and Prevention (CDC) recommends the following guidelines for STI testing:

- **Annual Testing:** Individuals who are sexually active should undergo STI testing at least once a year. This includes testing for common STIs such as chlamydia, gonorrhea, syphilis, and HIV.

- **Increased Frequency for High-Risk Individuals:** Those who have multiple sexual partners, engage in non-monogamous relationships, or participate in high-risk sexual behaviors should consider more frequent testing, ideally every 3 to 6 months.

- **Testing After New Partners:** It is advisable to get tested after engaging in sexual activities with a new partner, particularly if fisting or other high-risk behaviors are involved.

Understanding STI Testing Results

Understanding the results of STI tests is crucial for informed decision-making regarding sexual health. The following outlines how to interpret common STI test results:

- **Negative Results:** A negative result typically indicates that no infection is present at the time of testing. However, it is essential to consider the window period for each STI, as infections may not be detectable immediately after exposure.

- **Positive Results:** A positive result indicates the presence of an STI. It is vital to consult with a healthcare provider to discuss treatment options, potential implications for partners, and strategies for preventing transmission.

- **Follow-Up Testing:** In some cases, follow-up testing may be necessary to confirm results or to monitor the effectiveness of treatment.

Addressing Stigma and Barriers to Testing

Despite the importance of regular health check-ups and STI testing, many individuals face barriers that prevent them from seeking care. These barriers may include:

- **Stigma:** The stigma associated with STIs and sexual health can deter individuals from seeking testing. Education and open discussions about sexual health can help reduce this stigma.

- **Access to Healthcare:** Limited access to healthcare services, including financial constraints and lack of insurance, can hinder regular testing. Seeking out community health centers or clinics that offer sliding scale fees can provide affordable options.

- **Fear of Judgment:** Many individuals fear being judged by healthcare providers when discussing sexual practices. Finding a healthcare provider who is knowledgeable and non-judgmental can create a safe space for open dialogue.

Conclusion

In conclusion, regular health check-ups and STI testing are essential components of a responsible sexual health regimen for individuals engaging in fisting and other high-risk sexual practices. By prioritizing these health measures, individuals can not only protect themselves but also contribute to the overall health of their partners and communities. Open communication with healthcare providers, along with a commitment to regular testing, can foster a healthier and more informed approach to sexual well-being.

$$\text{Health Check-Up Frequency} = \begin{cases} \text{Every year} & \text{for sexually active individuals} \\ \text{Every 3-6 months} & \text{for high-risk individuals} \end{cases}$$

(17)

By integrating these practices into one's sexual health routine, individuals can navigate their fisting journey with confidence and care, ensuring a safer and more fulfilling experience.

Consent, Boundaries, and Communication

Establishing Clear Consent Guidelines

Consent is the cornerstone of any intimate interaction, particularly in practices that challenge societal norms, such as fisting. Establishing clear consent guidelines not only safeguards physical and emotional well-being but also fosters an environment of trust, respect, and mutual enjoyment. This section will delve into the theoretical frameworks of consent, practical strategies for establishing consent, potential problems that may arise, and illustrative examples.

Theoretical Framework of Consent

Consent is often defined as a mutual agreement between participants to engage in a specific activity. It is essential to understand that consent must be:

- **Informed:** All parties should have a comprehensive understanding of the activity, including potential risks and benefits.

- **Voluntary:** Consent must be given freely, without coercion, manipulation, or undue pressure.

- **Reversible:** Individuals retain the right to withdraw consent at any point, regardless of prior agreements.

- **Enthusiastic:** Consent should be expressed actively and enthusiastically, rather than assumed or coerced.

These principles align with the broader concept of affirmative consent, which emphasizes the importance of active participation and clear communication in the consent process.

Practical Strategies for Establishing Consent

To establish clear consent guidelines, participants should engage in open and honest communication before, during, and after the fisting experience. Here are some practical strategies:

1. **Pre-Engagement Conversations:** Prior to any intimate activity, partners should discuss their desires, boundaries, and limits. This conversation should include topics such as:

    - Personal comfort levels with fisting.
    - Specific techniques or positions that are preferred or off-limits.
    - Any medical concerns or physical limitations.

2. **Establishing Safe Words:** Safe words are pre-agreed terms that signal the need to slow down, stop, or check in. It is crucial to choose a safe word that is easy to remember and unlikely to be confused with normal conversation. Common examples include "red" for stop and "yellow" for slow down or check in.

3. **Ongoing Consent:** Consent is not a one-time agreement. Partners should check in with each other regularly throughout the experience, ensuring that both parties feel comfortable and safe. Phrases such as "How are you feeling?" or "Is this okay?" can facilitate ongoing communication.

4. **Post-Engagement Debriefing:** After the fisting session, partners should engage in a debriefing conversation to discuss their experiences, feelings, and any physical discomfort. This practice not only reinforces trust but also helps to identify areas for improvement in future encounters.

Potential Problems and Challenges

Despite the best intentions, issues may arise in the consent process. Some common challenges include:

- **Miscommunication:** Differences in understanding or interpreting consent can lead to misunderstandings. It is vital to ensure that all parties are on the same page regarding what consent entails.

- **Assumptions:** Partners may assume that consent is implied based on prior experiences or relationships. Clear, explicit communication is essential to avoid these pitfalls.

- **Power Dynamics:** In relationships with unequal power dynamics, such as those involving dominant and submissive roles, it is crucial to navigate consent carefully. The dominant partner must ensure that the submissive partner's consent is given freely and without coercion.

- **Emotional Vulnerability:** Engaging in fisting can evoke strong emotions. Partners should be prepared for the possibility that one or both individuals may experience emotional reactions during or after the act, and they should have strategies in place to address these feelings.

Examples of Clear Consent Guidelines in Practice

To illustrate the importance of establishing clear consent guidelines, consider the following scenarios:

- **Scenario 1: The Enthusiastic Agreement** - Before engaging in fisting, Alex and Jamie have a thorough discussion about their desires and limits. Alex expresses a strong interest in exploring fisting, while Jamie is initially hesitant. They agree to start slowly, using safe words to communicate comfort levels. As they proceed, Jamie feels empowered to voice any discomfort, leading to a positive experience for both.

- **Scenario 2: The Miscommunication** - During a fisting session, Sam assumes that their partner, Taylor, is comfortable with deeper penetration based on previous experiences. However, Taylor had not communicated a change in their boundaries. When Taylor begins to feel discomfort but is unsure how to express it, the situation escalates. This highlights the need for ongoing consent and check-ins.

- **Scenario 3: The Power Dynamic** - In a BDSM context, the dominant partner, Casey, establishes clear consent guidelines with their submissive partner, Morgan. They discuss boundaries and safe words before engaging in fisting. During the act, Casey remains vigilant for any signs of distress in Morgan, ensuring that consent is respected at all times.

Conclusion

Establishing clear consent guidelines is essential for creating a safe and enjoyable fisting experience. By prioritizing informed, voluntary, reversible, and enthusiastic consent, partners can navigate the complexities of this intimate practice with confidence and care. Open communication, ongoing check-ins, and a commitment to mutual respect will lay the foundation for a fulfilling exploration of fisting that honors the desires and boundaries of all involved.

Understanding the Dynamics of Power and Control

The exploration of fisting, like many forms of sexual expression, often intersects with the dynamics of power and control. Understanding these dynamics is crucial for creating a safe and consensual environment, where all parties feel empowered and respected. This section delves into the theoretical frameworks surrounding power dynamics, the potential issues that may arise, and practical examples that illustrate these concepts in the context of fisting.

Theoretical Frameworks

Power dynamics in sexual relationships can be analyzed through various theoretical lenses, including social exchange theory, feminist theory, and psychoanalytic theory.

Social Exchange Theory posits that relationships are formed based on the perceived rewards and costs associated with them. In the context of fisting, individuals may weigh the physical pleasure and emotional intimacy gained against the risks and potential discomfort involved. This balancing act can influence how power is negotiated within the relationship. For instance, one partner may feel more empowered to explore fisting if they perceive the experience as rewarding and consensual, whereas the other may feel vulnerable if they are uncertain about their partner's intentions or the safety of the act.

Feminist Theory provides a critical lens through which to examine power dynamics, particularly in heterosexual relationships. It emphasizes the importance of consent and mutual respect in sexual encounters. In fisting, the dynamics of power can become complex, as traditional gender roles may influence how partners communicate their desires and boundaries. For example, a male partner might feel societal pressure to assert dominance, while a female partner may feel expected to submit. Acknowledging these societal influences is essential for fostering a more equitable power dynamic.

Psychoanalytic Theory explores the unconscious motivations behind sexual behavior, including the desire for control or submission. Fisting may evoke deep-seated feelings of vulnerability or empowerment, depending on the individual's psychological makeup and past experiences. Understanding these motivations can help partners navigate their desires and establish a consensual framework for their exploration.

Potential Issues in Power Dynamics

While exploring power dynamics can enhance intimacy, it can also lead to potential issues if not navigated carefully.

Miscommunication is a common problem that can arise when partners have different expectations regarding power dynamics. For instance, one partner may interpret the act of fisting as a dominant expression, while the other views it as a shared experience. This discrepancy can lead to feelings of discomfort or betrayal if not addressed openly.

Coercion is another critical concern. Even in consensual BDSM contexts, the line between persuasion and coercion can be blurred. A partner may feel pressured to engage in fisting despite reservations, leading to potential emotional harm. Establishing clear communication and consent protocols, including safe words, can help mitigate this risk.

Internalized Shame can also impact power dynamics. Individuals may struggle with feelings of shame related to their desires, which can lead to power imbalances in the relationship. For instance, a partner may feel unworthy of pleasure and therefore acquiesce to their partner's desires without voicing their own. Encouraging open dialogue about desires and boundaries can help combat this internalized shame.

Examples of Power Dynamics in Fisting

To illustrate the complexities of power dynamics in fisting, consider the following examples:

Example 1: Negotiation of Boundaries In a scenario where one partner expresses interest in fisting, the other partner may initially feel apprehensive. Through open communication, they establish boundaries and safe words, ensuring that both partners feel comfortable. This negotiation empowers both individuals, allowing them to explore their desires within a consensual framework.

Example 2: Role Reversal In a BDSM context, a couple may engage in role play where traditional power dynamics are inverted. The submissive partner may take on a dominant role during fisting, challenging societal norms and allowing both partners to explore their desires in a safe environment. This role reversal can foster deeper intimacy and trust, as both partners navigate the complexities of power together.

Example 3: Addressing Past Trauma A partner with a history of trauma may approach fisting with trepidation. Open discussions about their past experiences and establishing clear boundaries can help create a safe space for exploration. By acknowledging the impact of past trauma on their current desires, both partners can work together to build trust and intimacy.

Conclusion

Understanding the dynamics of power and control in fisting is essential for fostering a consensual and empowering experience. By recognizing the theoretical frameworks that inform these dynamics, addressing potential issues, and engaging in open communication, partners can navigate their desires safely and respectfully. Ultimately, the goal is to cultivate a shared experience that honors the autonomy and agency of all involved, allowing for deeper intimacy and connection.

$$\text{Empowerment} = \frac{\text{Trust} + \text{Communication}}{\text{Fear} + \text{Coercion}} \qquad (18)$$

This equation illustrates that empowerment in sexual dynamics is achieved when trust and communication outweigh fear and coercion. By prioritizing these elements, partners can create a fulfilling and safe environment for exploring their desires, including fisting.

Handling Boundaries, Limits, and Red Flags

When exploring the intimate practice of fisting, it is crucial to approach the experience with a clear understanding of boundaries, limits, and the identification of red flags. This section aims to provide insight into how to effectively manage these aspects to ensure a safe and consensual experience for all parties involved.

Understanding Boundaries and Limits

Boundaries are the personal limits that individuals set to protect their emotional and physical well-being. They define what is acceptable and what is not in any intimate interaction. Limits, on the other hand, refer to the extent to which one is willing to go within those boundaries. Establishing clear boundaries and limits is essential in any sexual activity, particularly in practices that may involve vulnerability, such as fisting.

Types of Boundaries   Boundaries can be categorized into several types:

- **Physical Boundaries:** These pertain to personal space and physical touch. For example, a participant may set a boundary regarding how much pressure they are comfortable with during fisting.

- **Emotional Boundaries:** These involve protecting one's emotional state. Participants should communicate their emotional triggers and ensure that they feel safe expressing their feelings.

- **Time Boundaries:** These refer to the duration of the activity. Setting a time limit can help participants manage their energy and emotional state.

- **Sexual Boundaries:** These define what sexual activities are acceptable. For instance, a participant might be comfortable with fisting but not with any additional sexual acts during the same session.

Communicating Boundaries and Limits

Effective communication is vital when establishing boundaries and limits. Participants should engage in open dialogues before, during, and after the fisting experience. Here are some strategies for effective communication:

- **Pre-Scene Negotiation:** Discuss boundaries and limits before engaging in fisting. This conversation should include what each participant is comfortable with, any specific triggers, and safe words or signals.

- **Active Listening:** Ensure that all parties feel heard and understood. This involves not only verbal communication but also paying attention to non-verbal cues.

- **Check-Ins During Play:** Regularly check in with each other during the experience to ensure comfort levels remain consistent. Questions like "How are you feeling?" or "Is this okay?" can help maintain a safe environment.

- **Post-Scene Debriefing:** After the experience, discuss what worked well and what could be improved. This helps build trust and enhances future interactions.

Recognizing Red Flags

Red flags are warning signs that indicate a potential issue in the dynamic between partners. Recognizing these signs early can prevent harm and ensure a positive experience. Some common red flags include:

- **Disregard for Boundaries**: If a partner consistently pushes past established boundaries, this is a significant red flag. For example, if a participant has communicated a limit on depth and their partner disregards it, this indicates a lack of respect for their comfort.

- **Inconsistent Communication**: If one partner seems uncertain or evasive about their feelings or limits, it may signal discomfort or unease.

- **Unwillingness to Discuss Safety**: A partner who avoids conversations about safety, hygiene, or consent should be approached with caution. Open discussions about these topics are essential for a healthy dynamic.

- **Physical Signs of Distress**: Pay attention to body language. If a partner appears tense, withdrawn, or uncomfortable, it is crucial to address these signs immediately.

- **Manipulation or Coercion**: Any form of pressure to engage in activities that one partner is not comfortable with is unacceptable. This includes guilt-tripping or emotional manipulation.

Responding to Red Flags

If a red flag is identified, it is important to respond appropriately:

- **Pause the Activity**: If any discomfort arises, it is essential to stop the activity immediately. Safety should always be the priority.

- **Communicate Openly**: Address the red flag directly. Use "I" statements to express feelings without placing blame. For instance, "I feel uncomfortable when…" can open a productive dialogue.

- **Reassess Boundaries**: After addressing the red flag, take time to reassess boundaries and limits together. This may involve redefining what is acceptable moving forward.

- **Seek Support**: If the situation escalates or if there are unresolved issues, consider seeking guidance from a trusted friend or a professional in the community.

The Importance of Trust and Respect

Ultimately, the foundation of any intimate experience, including fisting, is built on trust and respect. Both partners should feel safe to express their desires, boundaries, and concerns. Establishing a culture of respect allows for a more fulfilling and enjoyable experience.

Building Trust   Building trust takes time and requires consistent effort. Here are some ways to foster trust in the relationship:

- **Consistency:** Be reliable in communication and actions. Follow through on commitments made during negotiations.
- **Vulnerability:** Share personal experiences and feelings to deepen the emotional connection. This openness can enhance intimacy.
- **Respect for Autonomy:** Recognize and honor each other's autonomy. Each partner should feel empowered to make choices about their bodies and experiences.

In conclusion, handling boundaries, limits, and red flags in fisting requires thoughtful communication, awareness, and mutual respect. By prioritizing these elements, participants can create a safe and pleasurable environment that enhances their intimate experiences. Remember that consent is an ongoing process, and it is essential to remain attentive and responsive to each other's needs throughout the journey.

Active Listening and Effective Communication

Effective communication is the cornerstone of any intimate relationship, particularly in the context of exploring fisting. When partners engage in this intimate act, the need for clear, open, and honest dialogue becomes paramount. This section will delve into the principles of active listening and effective communication, exploring their significance in fostering trust, consent, and safety during fisting experiences.

The Importance of Active Listening

Active listening is more than just hearing words; it involves fully engaging with the speaker and demonstrating understanding and empathy. This practice is essential in intimate relationships, especially when discussing sensitive topics like fisting. According to [?], active listening can significantly enhance emotional intimacy and connection between partners.

Key Components of Active Listening

The process of active listening comprises several key components:

- **Attention:** Giving your full focus to the speaker, minimizing distractions, and demonstrating that you are present in the moment.

- **Reflection:** Paraphrasing or summarizing what the speaker has said to confirm understanding and validate their feelings.

- **Empathy:** Acknowledging the speaker's emotions and experiences without judgment, allowing them to feel heard and understood.

- **Clarification:** Asking open-ended questions to encourage deeper dialogue and to clarify any points of confusion.

Barriers to Effective Communication

Despite the importance of active listening, several barriers can hinder effective communication in intimate settings:

- **Assumptions:** Making assumptions about what a partner feels or thinks can lead to misunderstandings. For example, assuming that a partner is comfortable with a certain level of intensity in fisting without explicitly discussing it can lead to discomfort or even trauma.

- **Defensiveness:** Responding defensively to feedback can shut down communication. If a partner expresses discomfort with a technique or approach, a defensive response may prevent further dialogue.

- **Emotional Triggers:** Past experiences can create emotional triggers that affect how partners communicate. Recognizing these triggers can help partners navigate sensitive conversations more effectively.

- **Distractions:** External distractions, such as noise or interruptions, can detract from the quality of communication. Creating a safe and quiet environment can enhance the effectiveness of conversations.

Examples of Effective Communication in Fisting

To illustrate the principles of active listening and effective communication, consider the following scenarios:

> **Example**
>
> **Scenario 1: Discussing Boundaries**
> Partner A expresses a desire to explore fisting but is unsure about their limits. Partner B practices active listening by maintaining eye contact, nodding, and summarizing Partner A's feelings. They say, "It sounds like you're excited but also a bit nervous about how far you want to go. Let's talk about what feels good for you."

In this scenario, Partner B demonstrates active listening by validating Partner A's feelings and inviting further discussion about boundaries.

> **Example**
>
> **Scenario 2: Addressing Discomfort**
> During a fisting session, Partner A suddenly feels discomfort and wants to stop. Partner B, having established a safe word, pauses and checks in: "I noticed you tensed up. Are you okay? Do you want to use our safe word?" This approach shows that Partner B is attentive to Partner A's needs and is willing to prioritize their comfort.

In this example, Partner B's proactive communication helps ensure that both partners feel safe and respected throughout the experience.

Techniques for Enhancing Communication

To foster effective communication, partners can implement several techniques:

- **Establishing Safe Words:** Safe words are crucial in any intimate exploration, especially in fisting. They provide a clear and unambiguous way for partners to communicate discomfort or the need to stop. Using a safe word allows for immediate cessation of activity without fear of judgment or misunderstanding.

- **Regular Check-Ins:** Partners can agree to check in with each other periodically during a session. Simple questions like, "How are you feeling?"

or "Is this okay for you?" can reinforce trust and ensure both partners are comfortable.

- **Post-Session Debriefing:** Aftercare is an essential part of any intimate experience. Taking time to discuss what worked well, what could be improved, and how each partner felt during the session fosters ongoing communication and growth in the relationship.

Conclusion

Active listening and effective communication are vital components of exploring fisting safely and consensually. By cultivating these skills, partners can create a nurturing environment that promotes trust, intimacy, and mutual satisfaction. As with any intimate practice, the journey of fisting is enhanced through open dialogue, empathy, and a commitment to understanding one another's needs and boundaries.

Honoring and Respecting Changing Consent

Consent is not a static agreement; it is a dynamic process that evolves throughout any intimate experience, including fisting. This section explores the importance of recognizing and respecting the fluid nature of consent, addressing the theoretical underpinnings, potential challenges, and practical examples to enhance understanding and application.

Theoretical Framework

Consent can be understood through the lens of several theories, including the **Social Exchange Theory**, which posits that interpersonal interactions are based on the perceived benefits and costs. In the context of fisting, participants must continually assess their comfort levels and desires, which may shift during the act.

Furthermore, the **Transactional Model of Stress and Coping** suggests that individuals evaluate situations based on their ability to cope with stressors. When engaging in fisting, if one partner feels overwhelmed or uncomfortable, their ability to consent may change, necessitating a reevaluation of boundaries.

Recognizing Changes in Consent

It is critical to understand that consent can change for various reasons, including physical discomfort, emotional triggers, or shifts in mood. Recognizing these changes requires active communication and attentiveness. Partners should engage in continuous dialogue, checking in with each other regularly.

Examples of verbal check-ins include:

- "How are you feeling right now?"
- "Is this still good for you?"
- "Do you want to try something different?"

Non-verbal cues also play a significant role in understanding changing consent. Body language, facial expressions, and even breathing patterns can indicate discomfort or hesitation. It is essential for partners to be attuned to these signals and respond appropriately.

Practical Strategies for Honoring Changing Consent

1. **Establish Safe Words:** Before engaging in fisting, partners should establish clear safe words or signals that can be used to pause or stop the activity. This provides a straightforward way to communicate discomfort without the need for lengthy explanations in the moment.

2. **Practice Active Listening:** Partners should practice active listening, which involves fully concentrating on what the other person is saying. This includes acknowledging verbal cues and responding empathetically to concerns or changes in comfort levels.

3. **Encourage Openness:** Create an environment where both partners feel safe to express their feelings about the experience. This can be reinforced by discussing the importance of changing consent before engaging in any intimate activity.

4. **Conduct Post-Scene Debriefing:** Aftercare is vital in any intimate interaction, especially in the context of fisting. Partners should take time to discuss what felt good, what didn't, and how consent may have shifted throughout the experience. This reflection can enhance future encounters and strengthen trust.

Addressing Challenges

Despite best efforts, challenges may arise when navigating changing consent. Some common problems include:

- **Fear of Hurting Feelings:** Partners may hesitate to express discomfort out of fear of disappointing the other. It is crucial to emphasize that prioritizing one's own comfort is not only acceptable but necessary for a healthy interaction.

- **Power Dynamics:** In relationships with inherent power imbalances, such as those found in BDSM dynamics, one partner may feel pressured to continue despite discomfort. Continuous dialogue about consent can help mitigate this issue.

- **Miscommunication:** Misunderstandings can occur if partners do not clearly articulate their feelings. Utilizing established safe words and regular check-ins can minimize these risks.

Case Study Example

Consider a couple, Alex and Jordan, exploring fisting for the first time. They have established a safe word, "red," to indicate a need to stop. During the experience, Jordan begins to feel overwhelmed and uncertain about continuing but hesitates to speak up. Noticing Jordan's tense body language, Alex initiates a check-in:

"Hey, I notice you seem a bit tense. How are you feeling?"

Jordan expresses discomfort, saying, "I'm not sure if I want to continue." Alex respects this change in consent, using the safe word to pause the activity. They then engage in a discussion about what led to this feeling, which not only honors Jordan's consent but also strengthens their emotional connection.

Conclusion

Honoring and respecting changing consent is essential in any intimate relationship, particularly in the context of fisting. By fostering open communication, recognizing non-verbal cues, and employing strategies to address challenges, partners can create a safe and fulfilling environment that respects the dynamic nature of consent. This commitment to ongoing consent not only enhances the physical experience but also deepens emotional intimacy and trust, ultimately enriching the relationship as a whole.

Navigating Consent in Non-Monogamous Relationships

In the realm of non-monogamous relationships, the dynamics of consent can become complex due to the involvement of multiple partners, each with their own

CONSENT, BOUNDARIES, AND COMMUNICATION

boundaries, desires, and emotional needs. Navigating consent in these contexts requires intentional communication, clear agreements, and a profound understanding of the nuances of each relationship.

Understanding the Framework of Non-Monogamy

Non-monogamous relationships can take various forms, including polyamory, swinging, and open relationships. Each form presents unique challenges and opportunities for consent. At the core, non-monogamy emphasizes the importance of autonomy and the ability to engage with multiple partners consensually.

$$C = \{P_1, P_2, P_3, \ldots, P_n\} \qquad (19)$$

Where C represents the consent framework and P denotes individual partners involved in the relationship. Each partner must feel empowered to express their needs and boundaries, fostering a culture of respect and understanding.

The Importance of Communication

Effective communication is the cornerstone of navigating consent in non-monogamous relationships. Partners must engage in ongoing conversations about their desires, limits, and expectations. This can involve:

- **Regular Check-Ins**: Establishing a routine for discussing relationship dynamics can help partners stay aligned and address any emerging concerns.

- **Open Dialogue**: Encouraging a non-judgmental space where partners can express their feelings and fears promotes emotional safety.

- **Utilizing Tools**: Some couples find it helpful to use tools such as consent contracts or communication apps to outline agreements and revisit them as needed.

Establishing Boundaries

Boundaries in non-monogamous relationships can be fluid and may change over time. It is crucial for partners to articulate their boundaries clearly and to respect those of others. This process involves:

$$B_i = \{b_1, b_2, b_3, \ldots, b_m\} \qquad (20)$$

Where B_i represents the boundaries of partner i and b denotes individual boundary elements. Some common boundaries include:

- **Sexual Boundaries**: Defining what sexual activities are acceptable with other partners.
- **Emotional Boundaries**: Discussing the level of emotional involvement allowed with others.
- **Time Boundaries**: Outlining how much time can be spent with other partners versus primary partners.

Consent Models in Non-Monogamous Contexts

Different models of consent can be applied in non-monogamous relationships. The following frameworks can guide discussions around consent:

- **Enthusiastic Consent**: All parties actively express their desire to engage in specific activities, ensuring that consent is not only given but also desired.
- **Ongoing Consent**: Consent is not a one-time agreement but an ongoing conversation. Partners should feel free to withdraw consent at any point.
- **Informed Consent**: All parties must have a clear understanding of the dynamics at play, including the potential risks and emotional implications of non-monogamous engagements.

Addressing Common Challenges

Navigating consent in non-monogamous relationships can present several challenges, including:

- **Jealousy and Insecurity**: These feelings can arise when partners perceive threats to their connection. Addressing these emotions openly can help mitigate their impact.
- **Differing Levels of Comfort**: Partners may have varying degrees of comfort with non-monogamy. It is essential to respect individual limits and negotiate compromises.
- **Miscommunication**: Assumptions can lead to misunderstandings. Regular, honest communication is necessary to ensure everyone is on the same page.

Practical Examples

Consider a scenario where two partners, Alex and Jamie, are in a polyamorous relationship and wish to explore fisting with other partners. They might approach the conversation like this:

- **Initial Discussion**: Alex expresses interest in fisting with another partner. They discuss what that would mean for their relationship, exploring feelings of excitement and potential jealousy.

- **Setting Boundaries**: They agree that Alex can explore fisting but will check in with Jamie before any new partner is involved. Jamie expresses a need to know details about who Alex is seeing.

- **Ongoing Communication**: After Alex engages in fisting with another partner, they have a debriefing session to discuss feelings, experiences, and any discomfort that may have arisen.

Conclusion

Navigating consent in non-monogamous relationships is an evolving process that requires dedication to communication, respect for boundaries, and the ability to address challenges as they arise. By fostering an environment of trust and openness, partners can explore the rich landscape of non-monogamy while ensuring that consent remains a foundational element of their connections.

In summary, the principles of consent in non-monogamous relationships can be distilled into the following key takeaways:

- Prioritize communication and regular check-ins.

- Clearly articulate and respect boundaries.

- Embrace various models of consent, adapting them to fit the unique dynamics of each relationship.

- Address challenges collaboratively, creating a supportive space for emotional exploration.

Balancing Power Dynamics in Fisting Play

In the realm of fisting, power dynamics play a crucial role in shaping the experiences of all participants. Understanding how to balance these dynamics is essential for fostering a safe, consensual, and pleasurable environment. This section explores the theoretical frameworks surrounding power dynamics, the potential challenges that can arise, and practical strategies for maintaining balance during fisting play.

Theoretical Frameworks of Power Dynamics

Power dynamics in sexual relationships can be understood through various theoretical lenses, including:

- **Feminist Theory:** This framework emphasizes the importance of consent and the negotiation of power in sexual encounters. It advocates for equitable power distribution, challenging traditional gender roles that often place one partner in a dominant position.

- **BDSM Frameworks:** BDSM practices often involve explicit negotiations of power dynamics. The concepts of Dominance and Submission (D/s) are central to understanding how power can be consensually exchanged and managed. The principles of Risk-Aware Consensual Kink (RACK) are particularly relevant, as they encourage participants to be aware of the risks involved and to establish clear boundaries.

- **Transactional Analysis:** This psychological theory posits that individuals operate from different ego states—Parent, Adult, and Child. Understanding which ego state a partner is operating from can help in navigating power dynamics, ensuring that interactions remain consensual and respectful.

Potential Challenges in Balancing Power Dynamics

While power dynamics can enhance the experience of fisting, they also present challenges that must be addressed:

- **Miscommunication:** A lack of clear communication can lead to misunderstandings about consent and boundaries. For example, one partner may assume that a certain level of intensity is acceptable, while the other may not feel comfortable with it.

- **Assumed Roles:** Participants may enter a scene with preconceived notions about their roles based on societal norms or past experiences. This can result in one partner feeling pressured to conform to a dominant or submissive role, even if it does not align with their desires.

- **Power Imbalance:** Existing power imbalances in a relationship, such as those stemming from socioeconomic status or emotional dependency, can complicate the dynamics of fisting play. A partner may feel coerced into participating in ways that do not genuinely reflect their desires.

Strategies for Balancing Power Dynamics

To navigate and balance power dynamics effectively, consider the following strategies:

- **Open Communication:** Prior to engaging in fisting, partners should have an open dialogue about their desires, limits, and concerns. Establishing a safe word or signal can provide a means for either partner to pause or stop the activity if they feel uncomfortable.

- **Role Negotiation:** Discuss and negotiate the roles that each partner wishes to embody during the scene. This should include an exploration of what being dominant or submissive means to each individual and how they can express those roles authentically.

- **Regular Check-Ins:** During the fisting experience, it is important to check in with each other. Simple questions like "How does this feel?" or "Are you okay?" can help maintain awareness of each other's comfort levels and reinforce consent.

- **Aftercare:** Aftercare is essential for processing the emotional and physical experiences of fisting. It provides an opportunity to reconnect, discuss what worked, and address any feelings that may have arisen during the scene. This can help reinforce trust and balance in the relationship.

- **Education and Training:** Engaging in workshops or reading materials about power dynamics, consent, and fisting techniques can enhance understanding and skill. Knowledge empowers partners to navigate their experiences with confidence and clarity.

Examples of Power Dynamics in Fisting Play

To illustrate how power dynamics can manifest in fisting play, consider the following scenarios:

- **Scenario 1: Dominance and Submission** - In a consensual D/s relationship, one partner may take on a dominant role during fisting. They may enjoy guiding their submissive partner through the experience, using verbal cues and physical direction. The submissive partner, in turn, may find pleasure in surrendering control, trusting their dominant partner to prioritize their safety and pleasure.

- **Scenario 2: Equal Partners** - Two partners who view themselves as equals may negotiate the dynamics of fisting based on mutual exploration. They might take turns being the one who fists and the one receiving, emphasizing communication and shared pleasure. This scenario highlights the importance of collaboration in balancing power.

- **Scenario 3: Role Reversal** - A couple may typically engage in traditional gender roles, with one partner often taking a dominant position. However, they may decide to experiment with role reversal during a fisting session. This can be an enlightening experience, allowing both partners to explore different aspects of their sexuality and challenge preconceived notions about power and pleasure.

Conclusion

Balancing power dynamics in fisting play requires intentional communication, negotiation, and mutual respect. By understanding the theoretical frameworks of power, recognizing potential challenges, and implementing effective strategies, partners can create a fulfilling and safe fisting experience. Ultimately, the goal is to foster an environment where both participants feel empowered and connected, enhancing the physical and emotional aspects of their intimate exploration.

Handling Post-Scene Debriefing and Care

Post-scene debriefing is an essential aspect of any intimate experience, particularly in the context of fisting, where the physical and emotional stakes can be high. This process allows participants to reflect on their experience, address any concerns, and reinforce the trust and connection established during the scene. The following sections outline the importance of post-scene debriefing, the key components to include, and practical strategies to ensure that both partners feel safe and supported.

Importance of Post-Scene Debriefing

Debriefing serves multiple purposes:

- **Emotional Processing:** Engaging in a debrief allows both partners to articulate their feelings about the experience. This can include discussing moments of pleasure, discomfort, or surprise. Articulating these feelings is crucial for emotional processing and can help mitigate any feelings of shame or confusion that may arise post-scene.

- **Reinforcing Consent:** A debriefing session provides an opportunity to reaffirm consent and discuss any boundaries that may have been tested during the scene. This reinforces the notion that consent is an ongoing process rather than a one-time agreement.

- **Identifying Areas for Improvement:** Participants can discuss what worked well and what could be improved in future sessions. This constructive feedback can enhance future experiences and help partners grow together.

- **Building Trust:** Sharing thoughts and feelings post-scene can deepen intimacy and trust between partners. It shows a commitment to each other's well-being and an understanding of the emotional complexities involved in kink.

- **Aftercare:** This is often an integral part of debriefing, as it focuses on the physical and emotional care needed following intense scenes. Aftercare can include physical comfort, such as cuddling or providing water, as well as emotional support through conversation.

Key Components of a Post-Scene Debrief

A thorough debriefing should include the following components:

1. **Check-in:** Start with a simple check-in to gauge how each partner is feeling. Questions like "How are you feeling right now?" or "What was your favorite part of the scene?" can open the dialogue.

2. **Discussing Boundaries:** Review any boundaries that were established before the scene and discuss whether they were respected. If any boundaries were crossed, it is important to address this openly and honestly.

3. **Sharing Experiences:** Encourage each partner to share their perspective on the scene. This can include discussing sensations experienced, emotional responses, and any unexpected reactions.

4. **Addressing Concerns:** If any physical discomfort or emotional distress was experienced, it is crucial to address these concerns openly. This discussion can help identify if any injuries occurred and how to care for them.

5. **Aftercare Needs:** Discuss what aftercare each partner needs. This may include physical comforts such as blankets, water, or snacks, as well as emotional support like reassurance or quiet time together.

6. **Future Planning:** Talk about what both partners would like to explore in future scenes. This can include new techniques, different dynamics, or adjusting boundaries based on the current experience.

Practical Strategies for Effective Debriefing

To facilitate a successful debriefing session, consider the following strategies:

- **Create a Safe Space:** Ensure that the environment is comfortable and private, allowing both partners to express themselves freely without fear of judgment.

- **Use Open-Ended Questions:** Encourage discussion by asking open-ended questions that invite deeper reflection. For example, instead of asking, "Did you enjoy it?" try "What did you enjoy most about the experience?"

- **Practice Active Listening:** Show that you are engaged in the conversation by practicing active listening. This includes nodding, maintaining eye contact, and summarizing what your partner has shared to demonstrate understanding.

- **Be Mindful of Tone:** The tone of the conversation should be compassionate and non-judgmental. Acknowledge any negative feelings without dismissing them, and validate your partner's experiences.

- **Allow for Silence:** Silence can be a powerful tool in debriefing. Give your partner time to process their thoughts and feelings before responding.

- **Follow Up:** After the debriefing session, check in with your partner in the days following the scene. This ongoing communication reinforces care and support.

Example Scenario

Consider a scenario where two partners engage in a fisting scene. After the scene, they sit together to debrief.

> Partner A: "I felt really nervous at first, but once we started, I was surprised by how much I enjoyed it. What about you?"
>
> Partner B: "I loved the intimacy, but I was worried when you seemed to tense up. I want to make sure we communicate better next time."
>
> Partner A: "Yes, I noticed that too. I think I need to work on relaxing more. I'd like to try some breathing exercises next time to help."
>
> Partner B: "That sounds great! And I'll make sure to check in more often during the scene."

In this exchange, both partners express their feelings, acknowledge concerns, and collaboratively plan for future experiences. This kind of dialogue fosters trust and enhances the overall dynamic of their relationship.

Conclusion

Post-scene debriefing is a vital practice in the realm of fisting and other intimate experiences. It not only serves to process the physical and emotional aspects of the scene but also strengthens the bonds of trust and communication between partners. By prioritizing this practice, individuals can enhance their experiences and ensure that both partners feel valued, safe, and understood. Remember, the journey of exploration in intimacy is ongoing, and the lessons learned in debriefing can lead to deeper connections and more fulfilling experiences in the future.

Handling Consent Violations and Conflict Resolution

Consent is the cornerstone of any intimate interaction, particularly in practices like fisting, where trust and communication are paramount. However, despite best intentions, consent violations can occur. This section explores how to recognize, address, and resolve these violations effectively, fostering a culture of safety and respect.

Understanding Consent Violations

Consent violations occur when an individual engages in sexual activity without the explicit agreement of all parties involved. These can range from subtle breaches, such as ignoring established boundaries, to overt acts of coercion or assault. Understanding the nature of consent is crucial:

- **Informed Consent:** All parties must have a clear understanding of the activity, its risks, and their own limits.

- **Revocable Consent:** Consent can be withdrawn at any time. It is a dynamic process that requires ongoing communication.

- **Enthusiastic Consent:** Consent should be given freely, enthusiastically, and without pressure. It is not merely the absence of a "no" but the presence of a "yes."

Identifying Consent Violations

Recognizing a consent violation can be challenging, as the signs may not always be overt. Common indicators include:

- **Non-verbal cues:** Body language, facial expressions, or withdrawal can indicate discomfort or reluctance.

- **Verbal cues:** Statements like "I'm not sure," "I don't want to," or silence can signal a lack of consent.

- **Changes in behavior:** Sudden shifts in enthusiasm or engagement can indicate that a partner is feeling unsafe or uncomfortable.

Immediate Steps to Take

When a consent violation is suspected or recognized, immediate action is crucial:

1. **Pause the Activity:** Stop all activities immediately. This allows space for communication and assessment of the situation.

2. **Check In:** Ask the affected partner how they feel. Use open-ended questions to encourage dialogue, such as "What's going on for you right now?" or "Can you share what you're feeling?"

CONSENT, BOUNDARIES, AND COMMUNICATION

3. **Acknowledge Feelings:** Validate their feelings without judgment. A simple acknowledgment like, "I understand you feel uncomfortable," can go a long way.

Conflict Resolution Strategies

Once the immediate situation is addressed, it is vital to engage in conflict resolution. Here are some effective strategies:

- **Open Dialogue:** Encourage honest communication about what went wrong. Discuss boundaries, expectations, and feelings without blame.

- **Active Listening:** Practice active listening techniques, such as reflecting back what you hear, to ensure understanding and show empathy.

- **Apologize When Necessary:** If a violation occurred due to a misunderstanding or oversight, a sincere apology can help rebuild trust. Use "I" statements to express remorse, e.g., "I'm sorry for not respecting your limits."

Rebuilding Trust

Rebuilding trust after a consent violation is essential for the continuation of the relationship. Here are steps to consider:

- **Establish New Boundaries:** Work together to redefine boundaries and establish clear consent protocols moving forward.

- **Engage in Aftercare:** Aftercare is crucial in the aftermath of intense experiences, particularly following a conflict. Provide emotional support and reassurance to each other.

- **Seek Professional Help:** In cases where trust has been significantly damaged, consider seeking the help of a therapist or counselor who specializes in sexual health and relationships.

Education and Prevention

Preventing consent violations requires ongoing education and awareness. Here are some practices to incorporate:

- **Workshops and Training:** Participate in workshops focused on consent, communication, and healthy sexual practices.
- **Community Discussions:** Engage in discussions within your community about consent and boundaries, sharing experiences and strategies for improvement.
- **Personal Reflection:** Regularly reflect on your own boundaries, desires, and communication styles to ensure alignment with your partners.

Conclusion

Handling consent violations is a delicate process that requires compassion, understanding, and a commitment to ongoing dialogue. By recognizing the signs of consent violations, taking immediate action, and engaging in effective conflict resolution, individuals can foster healthier, more respectful intimate relationships. Ultimately, the goal is to create an environment where all parties feel safe, respected, and empowered to express their desires and boundaries openly.

$$\text{Trust} = \frac{\text{Communication} + \text{Respect}}{\text{Violations}} \quad \text{(The Trust Equation)} \tag{21}$$

Consent in Public and Private Play Spaces

In the realm of intimate exploration, the concept of consent serves as the cornerstone of ethical engagement, particularly within both public and private play spaces. Understanding the nuances of consent in these varying contexts is essential for fostering a safe and respectful environment for all participants.

Understanding Consent

Consent is defined as the voluntary agreement to engage in a specific activity, which must be informed, enthusiastic, and revocable at any time. In the context of fisting and other intimate practices, consent becomes even more critical due to the physical and emotional vulnerabilities involved.

$$C = V + I + E + R \tag{22}$$

Where:

- C = Consent

CONSENT, BOUNDARIES, AND COMMUNICATION

- V = Voluntary
- I = Informed
- E = Enthusiastic
- R = Revocable

This equation illustrates the multifaceted nature of consent, emphasizing that all components must be present for consent to be valid.

Public Play Spaces

Public play spaces, such as BDSM clubs, workshops, or community events, often have specific guidelines and protocols regarding consent. These environments can foster a sense of community and shared understanding, but they also present unique challenges.

Challenges in Public Spaces   1. **Crowd Dynamics**: The presence of others can complicate consent. Participants may feel pressure to engage in activities due to social dynamics or the fear of judgment. It is crucial to establish clear boundaries and safe words before entering such spaces.
   2. **Visibility and Privacy**: In public settings, the visibility of acts can lead to misunderstandings or unwanted attention. It is essential to communicate openly with partners about what is acceptable in the presence of others and to respect the privacy of all participants.
   3. **Consent Culture**: Many public spaces promote a culture of consent, often requiring explicit verbal consent before any physical contact. This can help mitigate misunderstandings but may also feel daunting for newcomers.

Private Play Spaces

Private play spaces, such as a home or a secluded area, often allow for a more intimate setting where participants can explore their desires without the distractions of an audience. However, consent remains equally important in these contexts.

Challenges in Private Spaces   1.   **Assumptions of Consent**: In private settings, there can be a tendency to assume consent based on prior engagements or relationships. This assumption can lead to violations of boundaries. It is vital to check in regularly with partners, even if consent has been established previously.

2. **Emotional Vulnerability**: The intimacy of private spaces can heighten emotional vulnerabilities. Participants may feel pressured to engage in activities they are uncomfortable with due to the closeness of the relationship. Open communication about feelings and boundaries is essential.

3. **Aftercare and Debriefing**: Aftercare is a critical component of intimate play, particularly in private settings. Discussing experiences, feelings, and any discomforts post-play can help reinforce trust and ensure that all parties feel respected and valued.

Practical Strategies for Ensuring Consent

To navigate consent effectively in both public and private play spaces, consider implementing the following strategies:

- **Pre-Play Discussions**: Engage in open conversations about desires, boundaries, and safe words before any activities begin. This ensures that all participants are on the same page.

- **Use of Safe Words**: Establish clear safe words that can be used to halt any activity immediately. This is especially important in public spaces where distractions may occur.

- **Check-Ins During Play**: Regularly check in with partners during play to ensure comfort levels are maintained. Simple questions like "Are you okay?" or "Do you want to continue?" can facilitate ongoing consent.

- **Post-Play Debriefing**: After engaging in intimate activities, take the time to discuss what went well, what could be improved, and any feelings that arose during the experience. This reinforces trust and helps address any potential issues.

- **Education and Training**: Encourage participation in workshops or training sessions focused on consent and communication. Educating oneself and partners on these topics can enhance the overall experience and foster a culture of respect.

Conclusion

In conclusion, navigating consent in both public and private play spaces requires intentionality, communication, and a shared commitment to safety and respect. By understanding the dynamics of consent and implementing practical strategies, individuals can create enriching and consensual experiences that honor the desires and boundaries of all participants. Consent is not merely a checkbox; it is an ongoing dialogue that enriches the intimate landscape of exploration.

Physical and Emotional Safety

Understanding Your Physical Limits and Capacities

Understanding your physical limits and capacities is crucial for a safe and enjoyable fisting experience. This section will explore the anatomy involved, the importance of self-awareness, and how to recognize and respect your body's signals.

Anatomy and Physiology of Fisting

Fisting involves the insertion of a hand into the vagina or anus, which requires an understanding of the relevant anatomy. The primary structures involved include:

- **Vagina:** The vagina is a muscular canal that connects the external genitals to the uterus. It is elastic and can stretch significantly, but it is important to recognize its limits to avoid injury.

- **Anus:** The anus is surrounded by sphincter muscles that control its opening. It is less elastic than the vagina and requires careful preparation and relaxation to accommodate larger objects safely.

- **Pelvic Floor Muscles:** These muscles support the pelvic organs and play a crucial role in sexual function. Understanding how to relax and engage these muscles can enhance the fisting experience.

Recognizing Your Limits

Every individual has unique physical limits, influenced by factors such as anatomy, experience, and comfort levels. It is essential to engage in self-reflection and communication with your partner to establish these limits. Here are some key considerations:

- **Pain Threshold:** Each person's pain threshold varies. It is vital to differentiate between pleasurable sensations and pain that indicates potential injury. A common approach is to use a scale from 1 to 10 to communicate discomfort levels, where 1 is minimal discomfort and 10 is extreme pain.

- **Physical Health:** Pre-existing medical conditions, such as pelvic floor dysfunction, previous injuries, or surgeries, can impact your ability to engage in fisting. Consulting with a healthcare provider can help assess your physical readiness.

- **Experience Level:** Newcomers to fisting should start slowly and gradually increase the intensity and depth of penetration as they become more comfortable and aware of their limits.

Listening to Your Body

Being attuned to your body is essential for a safe fisting experience. Here are some strategies to enhance body awareness:

- **Mindfulness Practices:** Engaging in mindfulness techniques, such as deep breathing and body scans, can help you tune into your physical sensations and emotional responses during fisting.

- **Warm-Up Exercises:** Prior to fisting, consider engaging in warm-up exercises that promote relaxation and increase blood flow to the pelvic area. This can include gentle stretching, kegel exercises, or using fingers for gradual insertion.

- **Feedback Mechanisms:** Establish a clear communication system with your partner, including safe words and gestures, to indicate when you need to slow down, stop, or adjust the technique.

Common Problems and Solutions

Despite careful preparation, individuals may encounter challenges during fisting. Here are some common issues and how to address them:

- **Discomfort or Pain:** If you experience discomfort or pain, it is crucial to stop immediately. Communicate with your partner and assess the situation. Consider using more lubrication or adjusting the angle or depth of penetration.

- **Inadequate Lubrication:** Insufficient lubrication can lead to friction and discomfort. Always use a generous amount of high-quality lubricant suitable for anal or vaginal use. Reapply as necessary throughout the experience.

- **Tension in the Pelvic Floor:** If you notice tension in your pelvic floor muscles, take a moment to breathe deeply and consciously relax these muscles. Engaging in pelvic floor relaxation techniques can help alleviate this tension.

Empowerment Through Knowledge

Understanding your physical limits and capacities is not only about safety; it is also an empowering aspect of sexual exploration. By educating yourself about your body, you can embrace your desires with confidence and clarity. Engaging in fisting can be a profound expression of trust, intimacy, and self-discovery when approached with awareness and care.

In summary, recognizing your physical limits and capacities involves understanding your anatomy, being aware of your pain threshold, and actively listening to your body. By fostering open communication with your partner and engaging in practices that enhance body awareness, you can create a safe and pleasurable fisting experience.

Recognizing and Managing Pain Levels

Pain is a complex and subjective experience that can vary significantly between individuals, especially in the context of fisting. Understanding how to recognize and manage pain levels is crucial for ensuring a safe and pleasurable experience. This section will explore the nature of pain, the different types of pain that may be experienced during fisting, and strategies for effectively managing pain levels.

Understanding Pain

Pain can be categorized into two primary types: acute pain and chronic pain. Acute pain is typically a direct response to an injury or a specific stimulus, while chronic pain persists beyond the expected period of healing and can be influenced by psychological factors. In the context of fisting, individuals may experience acute pain due to the physical nature of the activity, but it is essential to differentiate between pain that signals injury and pain that may be part of the experience.

Recognizing Pain Levels

Recognizing pain levels involves developing an awareness of one's body and its responses during fisting. The following scale can be used to help individuals articulate their pain levels:

- **0: No Pain** - No sensation of discomfort.

- **1-3: Mild Pain** - A slight discomfort that is manageable and does not detract from the experience.

- **4-6: Moderate Pain** - Noticeable discomfort that may require adjustments in technique or position to alleviate.

- **7-9: Severe Pain** - Intense discomfort that is difficult to tolerate and may indicate potential injury.

- **10: Unbearable Pain** - Extreme pain that necessitates immediate cessation of the activity.

It is essential for participants to communicate openly about their pain levels using this scale, ensuring that both partners are aware of each other's comfort and limits.

The Role of Pain in Fisting

While pain is often viewed negatively, it can also play a role in the experience of fisting. Some individuals may find pleasure in the sensation of pain, especially when it is consensual and part of a broader context of trust and intimacy. The relationship between pain and pleasure is complex and can be influenced by various factors, including psychological state, emotional connection, and individual preferences.

Managing Pain Levels

Effective pain management during fisting involves several strategies:

1. **Communication:** Establishing open lines of communication with your partner is essential. Use safe words and signals to indicate when pain levels become uncomfortable. For instance, a simple phrase like "red" can signal the need to stop, while "yellow" can indicate the need to slow down or adjust.

2. **Mindfulness:** Practicing mindfulness techniques can help individuals stay attuned to their bodies and recognize pain levels as they fluctuate. Focusing on breath and sensation can enhance awareness and facilitate better communication about discomfort.

3. **Gradual Progression:** Start slowly and gradually increase intensity and depth. This approach allows the body to adapt and helps minimize the risk of injury. For example, begin with gentle insertion and slowly progress to deeper penetration as comfort levels increase.

4. **Positioning:** Experimenting with different positions can significantly affect pain levels. Certain angles may reduce discomfort and enhance pleasure. For instance, adjusting the angle of penetration or the position of the receiving partner can create a more comfortable experience.

5. **Lubrication:** Adequate lubrication is essential for minimizing friction and reducing the risk of pain. Use a high-quality lubricant specifically designed for anal or vaginal play to ensure comfort and safety.

6. **Physical Preparation:** Engaging in warm-up exercises, such as gentle stretching or the use of smaller toys, can help prepare the body for fisting. This practice can relax the muscles and enhance overall comfort during the experience.

7. **Aftercare:** Aftercare is crucial for emotional and physical recovery. Engaging in soothing activities, such as cuddling, gentle massage, or discussing the experience, can help partners reconnect and process any sensations or emotions that arose during play.

Conclusion

Recognizing and managing pain levels is an integral part of a safe and enjoyable fisting experience. By fostering open communication, practicing mindfulness, and employing effective pain management strategies, partners can navigate the complexities of pain and pleasure. Remember that every body is different, and what may be pleasurable for one person could be painful for another. Always prioritize consent, comfort, and safety to create a fulfilling and intimate experience.

$$\text{Pain Level} = \frac{\text{Intensity of Pain}}{\text{Duration of Pain}} \qquad (23)$$

This equation highlights the importance of both the intensity and duration of pain in determining the overall pain experience. By being mindful of these factors, individuals can better manage their pain levels and enhance their fisting journey.

Using Pain as an Indicator of Potential Injury

Pain is a complex and subjective experience that serves as a crucial indicator of our body's state and potential injury. In the context of fisting, understanding pain and its implications is essential for maintaining safety and enhancing pleasure. This section explores the theoretical framework surrounding pain perception, the types of pain one may experience during fisting, and how to distinguish between acceptable sensations and those that signal potential harm.

Theoretical Framework of Pain Perception

Pain is often classified into two primary types: acute and chronic. Acute pain is a direct response to injury or harm, serving as a warning signal that prompts protective behaviors. Chronic pain, on the other hand, persists beyond the typical healing time and may not have a clear physical cause.

The *Gate Control Theory of Pain*, proposed by Melzack and Wall in 1965, posits that pain perception is not solely determined by the physical injury but is also influenced by psychological factors and the nervous system's modulation. According to this theory, non-painful stimuli can close the "gates" to painful input, thus preventing the sensation of pain from reaching the brain. This theory underscores the importance of psychological and emotional states in pain perception, particularly in a sexual context where arousal and anticipation may alter pain experiences.

Types of Pain Experienced During Fisting

During fisting, individuals may experience a range of sensations, some of which may be perceived as pain. Understanding these sensations is crucial for differentiating between pleasurable discomfort and harmful pain.

- **Pleasurable Discomfort:** This type of sensation is often described as a deep pressure or stretching feeling. It may accompany the initial stages of fisting as the body adjusts to the intrusion. This discomfort can be pleasurable when approached with patience and proper technique.

- **Sharp or Stinging Pain:** This sensation often indicates that something is wrong. Sharp pain may arise from improper technique, lack of lubrication, or anatomical issues such as tightness or tension in the pelvic floor muscles. It is crucial to listen to these signals and reassess the situation.

PHYSICAL AND EMOTIONAL SAFETY

- **Throbbing or Aching Pain:** This type of pain may occur after prolonged fisting sessions or if the body is not adequately warmed up. It can indicate overexertion or strain on the muscles and tissues involved.

Distinguishing Between Acceptable Sensations and Warning Signs

Recognizing the difference between pleasurable sensations and warning signs of potential injury is vital for safe fisting practices. Here are some guidelines to help distinguish between the two:

1. **Listen to Your Body:** Pay attention to the sensations you are experiencing. If the sensation shifts from pleasurable to painful, it is essential to stop and reassess.

2. **Communicate with Your Partner:** Open communication with your partner is crucial. Establishing a safe word or signal can help ensure that both partners feel comfortable expressing discomfort or pain.

3. **Use the Pain Scale:** Consider using a subjective pain scale (0-10) to rate your pain during the experience. A rating of 0 indicates no pain, while 10 represents unbearable pain. Ideally, pleasurable sensations should remain below a 5 on this scale.

4. **Check for Physical Signs:** Look for physical indicators of distress, such as excessive redness, swelling, or bleeding. If these signs are present, it is essential to stop immediately and assess the situation.

Example Scenarios

To illustrate the importance of using pain as an indicator of potential injury, consider the following scenarios:

- **Scenario 1: Warming Up Properly** A couple begins their fisting journey without sufficient foreplay or warm-up. One partner experiences sharp pain upon insertion. This pain indicates that the body is not adequately prepared for the experience, suggesting a need for more extensive warm-up and relaxation techniques.

- **Scenario 2: Communication Breakdown** During a fisting session, one partner feels a throbbing pain but does not communicate this to their partner. The session continues, leading to significant discomfort and potential injury. This scenario highlights the critical importance of communication and listening to one's body.

- **Scenario 3: Recognizing Limits** A participant in a fisting workshop pushes themselves to try advanced techniques without proper preparation. They experience a sharp pain that signals a potential injury. Recognizing this pain allows them to stop and seek guidance, preventing further harm.

Conclusion

Understanding and interpreting pain during fisting is essential for safe and pleasurable experiences. By recognizing the different types of pain, communicating openly with partners, and listening to one's body, individuals can navigate the complexities of fisting while minimizing the risk of injury. Remember, pain is not just a sensation; it is a vital signal that can guide you toward a more fulfilling and safe exploration of your desires.

Key Takeaway: Always prioritize communication, consent, and body awareness. Pain should never be ignored or dismissed, as it serves as a critical indicator of your body's well-being.

Knowing When to Stop or Slow Down

In the context of fisting, understanding when to stop or slow down is crucial for ensuring both physical safety and emotional well-being. The act of fisting can bring about intense sensations, both pleasurable and painful, which necessitates a heightened awareness of one's own body and the dynamics at play between partners. This section will explore the indicators for pausing or ceasing activity, the importance of communication, and strategies to facilitate a safe and enjoyable experience.

Physical Indicators

Recognizing physical signs that signal the need to stop or slow down is paramount. Some common indicators include:

- **Pain Levels:** Pain is a natural part of many sexual experiences, but it is essential to differentiate between pleasurable discomfort and pain that signals injury. A common guideline is the *10-point pain scale*, where 0 indicates no pain and 10 indicates extreme pain. Ideally, the pain level should remain at or below a 3 during fisting.

$$\text{Pain Level} = \frac{\text{Current Pain}}{\text{Maximum Pain}} \times 10$$

If the pain level exceeds 3, it may be time to slow down or stop altogether.

- **Physical Responses:** The body may exhibit signs of distress such as excessive sweating, changes in breathing patterns, or involuntary muscle tension. These responses can indicate that the body is reaching its limits and may require a pause.

- **Discomfort or Tightness:** If the receiving partner feels an unusual tightness or discomfort in their pelvic area, it may signal that they are not adequately relaxed or that the insertion is too forceful. This is an important moment to communicate and reassess the approach.

Emotional Indicators

Emotional safety is equally important as physical safety. Partners should be attuned to each other's emotional states, which can be indicated by:

- **Verbal Cues:** Partners should use clear language to express their feelings. Phrases such as "I need a break" or "That's too much" should be respected without hesitation. Establishing safe words or signals prior to engaging in fisting can facilitate easier communication during the act.

- **Non-Verbal Signals:** Body language can reveal discomfort or distress. If a partner's body becomes tense, they may be signaling a need to stop. Observing facial expressions and posture can provide important context to the emotional state of the partner.

- **Emotional Triggers:** Fisting can elicit a range of emotions, including vulnerability, fear, or anxiety. If either partner begins to feel overwhelmed, it is critical to take a step back and assess the situation. Engaging in a conversation about feelings and experiences can help navigate these emotional landscapes.

Communication Strategies

Effective communication is the cornerstone of safe fisting practices. Here are some strategies to enhance communication between partners:

- **Establishing Safe Words:** Safe words should be predetermined and easy to remember. Common choices include "red" for stop and "yellow" for slow down. This creates a clear and immediate way to communicate discomfort without ambiguity.

- **Regular Check-Ins:** During the experience, partners should check in with each other at regular intervals. Simple questions like "How are you feeling?" or "Do you want to continue?" can help ensure that both partners remain comfortable and engaged.

- **Post-Scene Debriefing:** Aftercare is an essential component of any intimate experience, especially in activities that involve vulnerability. Taking time to discuss what felt good, what was challenging, and how both partners felt about the experience can foster a deeper connection and understanding.

The Importance of Trust and Comfort

The ability to stop or slow down during fisting is deeply rooted in the levels of trust and comfort established between partners. When both individuals feel safe and respected, they are more likely to express their needs openly. Building this trust can be achieved through:

- **Prior Discussions:** Before engaging in fisting, partners should have thorough discussions about boundaries, desires, and fears. This not only sets the stage for a safer experience but also reinforces the emotional bond between partners.

- **Gradual Exploration:** Starting with less intense forms of play can help build confidence and comfort. Gradually increasing intensity allows partners to assess their limits and communicate effectively.

- **Being Attentive:** Actively listening and responding to each other's needs during the act is vital. This attentiveness can help partners navigate the experience together, ensuring that both feel heard and respected.

Conclusion

In conclusion, knowing when to stop or slow down during fisting is a multifaceted process that involves recognizing physical sensations, emotional cues, and maintaining open lines of communication. By fostering an environment of trust and respect, partners can engage in this intimate act safely and enjoyably.

Remember, the goal of fisting is not only physical pleasure but also emotional connection and mutual satisfaction. Prioritizing safety and communication will enhance the experience and deepen the bond between partners.

Emotional Safety and Support Systems

Emotional safety in the context of fisting and other intimate practices is paramount for both participants. It encompasses the ability to express feelings, boundaries, and vulnerabilities without fear of judgment, rejection, or harm. Establishing emotional safety not only enhances the experience but also fosters trust and connection between partners.

Understanding Emotional Safety

Emotional safety can be defined as a state in which individuals feel secure enough to express their thoughts and feelings openly. This involves:

- **Open Communication:** Partners should feel free to discuss their desires, fears, and boundaries without fear of negative repercussions.

- **Active Listening:** Each partner must engage in active listening, which involves fully concentrating on what the other is saying, understanding it, responding thoughtfully, and remembering the information later.

- **Validation:** Acknowledging and validating each other's feelings and experiences is crucial for emotional safety. This can be as simple as saying, "I understand that you're feeling anxious about this."

The Role of Support Systems

Support systems play a critical role in maintaining emotional safety. They can include friends, community groups, or professionals who provide encouragement, understanding, and guidance. Having a robust support system can help individuals navigate their feelings and experiences related to fisting, especially if they encounter challenges or emotional triggers.

Identifying Emotional Triggers

Understanding personal emotional triggers is vital for fostering emotional safety. Triggers may arise from past experiences or societal stigma surrounding fisting. For instance, someone may feel anxious about being judged for their interest in fisting, which could inhibit their ability to engage fully. Recognizing these triggers allows partners to:

- **Discuss Triggers Openly:** Partners should talk about their triggers before engaging in fisting to avoid unexpected emotional responses during the experience.
- **Develop Coping Strategies:** Creating strategies to manage triggers, such as taking breaks or using safe words, can help maintain emotional safety.

Creating a Supportive Environment

To foster emotional safety, it is essential to create a supportive environment. This includes:

- **Setting the Scene:** A comfortable and private space can help individuals feel more secure. Consider factors such as lighting, temperature, and privacy.
- **Establishing Rituals:** Rituals, such as a pre-scene check-in or post-scene debriefing, can enhance emotional safety. These rituals provide structure and reassurance that both partners are cared for and respected.

Aftercare as Emotional Support

Aftercare is a vital component of emotional safety in fisting. It involves the care and attention given to each partner after an intimate experience. This can include:

- **Physical Comfort:** Providing blankets, water, or snacks can help partners feel nurtured and cared for.
- **Emotional Check-Ins:** Engaging in a conversation about the experience, discussing what was enjoyable, and addressing any discomfort can help process emotions and reinforce trust.

Seeking Professional Help

In some cases, individuals may benefit from seeking professional help to navigate their emotional landscape. This can include:

- **Therapy:** Engaging with a therapist who specializes in sexual health or kink can provide valuable insights and coping strategies.

- **Support Groups:** Connecting with others who share similar interests can alleviate feelings of isolation and provide a sense of community.

Conclusion

Emotional safety and support systems are fundamental to a fulfilling and consensual fisting experience. By fostering open communication, understanding emotional triggers, creating a supportive environment, prioritizing aftercare, and seeking professional help when needed, partners can navigate the complexities of fisting with confidence and care. Ultimately, emotional safety enhances intimacy and trust, allowing individuals to explore their desires in a nurturing and empowering manner.

Safely Navigating Intense Emotional States

Navigating intense emotional states during fisting play is an essential aspect of ensuring both physical and emotional safety. Engaging in such an intimate act can evoke a wide range of feelings, from pleasure and excitement to anxiety, fear, or vulnerability. Understanding how to manage these emotions effectively is crucial for a fulfilling and safe experience.

The Emotional Landscape of Fisting

When individuals engage in fisting, they may encounter various emotional states, including:

- **Euphoria:** The release of endorphins can create feelings of intense pleasure and joy, often leading to a heightened sense of connection with one's partner.
- **Vulnerability:** The act of fisting requires a significant level of trust and openness, which can make individuals feel exposed and emotionally vulnerable.
- **Anxiety:** Concerns about safety, performance, or potential pain can lead to heightened anxiety, which may inhibit relaxation and enjoyment.
- **Fear:** Fisting can trigger fears related to bodily harm or loss of control, especially for those who have past trauma or negative experiences related to intimacy.
- **Shame:** Societal taboos surrounding fisting can lead to feelings of shame or guilt, making it essential to address these emotions openly.

Theoretical Framework: Emotional Regulation

Emotional regulation theory posits that individuals can manage their emotional responses through various strategies. According to Gross (1998), emotional regulation can be categorized into two primary types: *antecedent-focused* and *response-focused* strategies.

$$\text{Emotional Regulation} = \text{Antecedent-Focused Strategies} + \text{Response-Focused Strategies} \tag{24}$$

Strategies for Navigating Intense Emotions

To navigate intense emotional states safely during fisting, consider the following strategies:

1. Establishing a Safe Word

A safe word is a predetermined signal that allows partners to pause or stop the activity if one person feels overwhelmed. This can be particularly helpful in managing anxiety or fear. Choose a word that is easy to remember and unlikely to be confused with other terms used during play.

2. Practicing Mindfulness Techniques

Mindfulness practices can help individuals stay present and grounded during fisting. Techniques such as deep breathing, body scanning, or focusing on sensations can help manage anxiety and promote relaxation.

$$\text{Mindfulness} = \frac{\text{Awareness of Present Moment}}{\text{Judgment of Experience}} \tag{25}$$

3. Engaging in Open Communication

Maintaining open lines of communication with your partner is vital. Discuss feelings before, during, and after the experience. This dialogue can help partners feel more secure and understood, thereby reducing anxiety and shame.

4. Utilizing Aftercare Practices

Aftercare involves providing emotional support and physical care after an intense experience. This can include cuddling, discussing feelings about the experience, or simply being present with each other. Aftercare can help individuals process their emotions and reaffirm their connection.

5. Recognizing and Validating Emotions

It's important to acknowledge and validate any emotions that arise during fisting. This includes recognizing feelings of fear, shame, or vulnerability without judgment. Understanding that these feelings are normal can help normalize the experience and reduce stigma.

6. Seeking Professional Support

For individuals who struggle with intense emotional states or have a history of trauma, seeking professional support from a therapist or counselor trained in sexual health or trauma-informed care can be beneficial. They can provide tools and strategies for managing emotions effectively.

Examples of Emotional Navigation

Example 1: Overcoming Anxiety Consider a scenario where a participant feels anxious about the physical act of fisting. They may express this anxiety to their partner and utilize a safe word to pause. Together, they can engage in a mindfulness exercise to help ground themselves, such as deep breathing, before resuming the activity.

Example 2: Managing Vulnerability In another instance, one partner may feel emotionally vulnerable after a particularly intense session. They can engage in aftercare by discussing their feelings and affirming their trust in each other. This dialogue can help both partners feel more secure and connected.

Conclusion

Navigating intense emotional states during fisting is a crucial aspect of the experience. By employing strategies such as establishing safe words, practicing mindfulness, engaging in open communication, and utilizing aftercare, individuals can create a safe and emotionally supportive environment. Understanding and managing emotions not only enhances the experience but also fosters deeper intimacy and trust between partners. Ultimately, the journey of exploring fisting should be one of empowerment, connection, and mutual respect.

Managing Emotional Triggers and Trauma Responses

Exploring fisting can evoke a range of emotional responses, particularly for individuals with histories of trauma or those who have experienced significant emotional triggers in their sexual lives. Understanding how to manage these emotional responses is crucial for ensuring a safe and fulfilling experience. This section aims to provide insights into recognizing, addressing, and navigating emotional triggers and trauma responses during fisting.

Understanding Emotional Triggers

An emotional trigger is a stimulus—such as a word, situation, or physical sensation—that evokes a strong emotional reaction, often related to past trauma. In the context of fisting, triggers may arise from physical sensations, the dynamics of power exchange, or even specific phrases or actions that resonate with past experiences. Recognizing these triggers is the first step in managing them effectively.

$$\text{Trigger} \rightarrow \text{Emotional Response} \rightarrow \text{Behavioral Reaction} \qquad (26)$$

For example, if a participant associates certain physical sensations with past trauma, they may experience anxiety or panic during a fisting session, leading to withdrawal or an inability to communicate their discomfort.

Identifying Personal Triggers

To manage emotional triggers, individuals should engage in self-reflection to identify their unique triggers. This process may involve:

- Keeping a journal to track emotional responses during intimate experiences.

- Reflecting on past experiences that may contribute to current emotional responses.

- Discussing feelings with a trusted partner or therapist to gain clarity.

By understanding their triggers, individuals can better prepare themselves for fisting experiences and communicate their needs to partners.

Communicating with Partners

Open communication with partners is essential in managing emotional triggers. This includes:

- Discussing potential triggers before engaging in fisting.
- Establishing safe words or signals that can be used to pause or stop the activity if a trigger arises.
- Encouraging partners to express their own triggers and emotional needs.

For instance, a partner may express that they feel anxious when certain words are used during play, allowing both partners to navigate the experience more safely and enjoyably.

Developing Coping Strategies

Having coping strategies in place can help individuals manage emotional triggers effectively. Some strategies include:

- **Grounding Techniques:** Techniques such as deep breathing, focusing on physical sensations, or using mindfulness practices can help individuals stay present and reduce anxiety. For example, during a fisting session, a participant might focus on the sensation of their feet on the ground or the texture of the sheets.
- **Positive Affirmations:** Repeating affirmations such as "I am safe" or "I am in control" can help reinforce a sense of security during intimate experiences.
- **Pre-Session Rituals:** Establishing a calming routine before engaging in fisting can help ease anxiety. This might include taking a warm bath, practicing yoga, or engaging in a shared meditation with a partner.

Recognizing Trauma Responses

Trauma responses can manifest in various ways, including emotional numbness, hyper-vigilance, dissociation, or sudden outbursts of anger or sadness. Recognizing these responses is crucial for both the individual and their partner to navigate emotional landscapes safely.

For example, if a participant suddenly becomes withdrawn during a fisting session, it may be a sign of dissociation. Partners should be prepared to pause and check in, allowing space for the individual to express their feelings and regain a sense of safety.

Aftercare and Emotional Support

Aftercare is a critical component of any BDSM or kink-related activity, including fisting. It involves providing emotional and physical care to one another post-session to facilitate a safe transition back to everyday life. Aftercare strategies may include:

- Engaging in gentle touch, cuddling, or skin-to-skin contact to promote feelings of safety and connection.

- Offering verbal reassurance, affirming that both partners are safe and cared for.

- Discussing the experience openly, including any emotional responses that arose during the session.

This post-session dialogue can help both partners process their experiences, reinforce trust, and address any emotional triggers that may have surfaced.

Seeking Professional Support

For individuals who struggle with managing emotional triggers or trauma responses, seeking professional help may be beneficial. Therapists specializing in trauma-informed care can provide tools and strategies tailored to individual needs. This may include:

- Trauma-focused therapy, such as Eye Movement Desensitization and Reprocessing (EMDR) or Cognitive Behavioral Therapy (CBT).

- Support groups for individuals exploring kink or BDSM, providing a safe space to share experiences and coping strategies.

- Workshops focused on emotional resilience and communication within intimate relationships.

Conclusion

Managing emotional triggers and trauma responses in the context of fisting is an essential aspect of ensuring a safe and fulfilling experience. By understanding personal triggers, communicating openly with partners, and employing effective coping strategies, individuals can navigate their emotional landscapes with confidence. Aftercare and professional support further enhance emotional safety and resilience, fostering deeper connections and intimacy in the exploration of fisting.

Building Trust and Resilience in Relationships

Building trust and resilience in relationships, particularly in the context of fisting, is a multifaceted endeavor that requires attention to emotional, psychological, and physical dimensions. Trust serves as the foundation of any intimate relationship, especially when exploring activities that challenge societal norms and personal boundaries. This section delves into the theoretical frameworks, potential challenges, and practical strategies for fostering trust and resilience among partners engaged in fisting.

Theoretical Frameworks of Trust

Trust is often conceptualized through various psychological theories. One prominent model is the *Trust Equation*, which posits that trust is a function of credibility, reliability, intimacy, and self-orientation:

$$\text{Trust} = \frac{\text{Credibility} + \text{Reliability} + \text{Intimacy}}{\text{Self-Orientation}} \tag{27}$$

Where: - **Credibility** refers to the partner's expertise and knowledge about fisting techniques and safety. - **Reliability** involves the consistency of actions and the ability to follow through on commitments. - **Intimacy** is the emotional closeness and openness between partners. - **Self-Orientation** denotes the extent to which one partner prioritizes their own needs over those of the other.

High levels of trust are achieved when partners exhibit credibility, reliability, and intimacy while minimizing self-orientation.

Challenges to Building Trust

Despite the importance of trust, several challenges can impede its development:

- **Fear of Vulnerability:** Engaging in fisting requires a significant degree of vulnerability. Partners may fear judgment or rejection, which can hinder open communication and honest expression of desires and boundaries.

- **Past Trauma:** Previous negative experiences, whether related to fisting or other forms of intimacy, can create barriers to trust. Individuals may carry emotional scars that affect their willingness to engage fully in new experiences.

- **Miscommunication:** Inadequate communication can lead to misunderstandings about desires, limits, and expectations. This misalignment can breed distrust and anxiety, undermining the safety of the experience.

- **Societal Stigma:** The taboo nature of fisting may lead to feelings of shame or secrecy, making it difficult for partners to discuss their experiences openly and honestly.

Strategies for Building Trust and Resilience

To cultivate trust and resilience in relationships, partners can implement the following strategies:

- **Open Communication:** Create a safe space for dialogue about desires, boundaries, and concerns. Use active listening techniques to ensure that each partner feels heard and validated. For example, partners can practice *reflective listening*, where one partner paraphrases what the other has said to confirm understanding.

- **Establishing Safe Words:** Safe words are essential in any intimate play, especially in fisting. They provide a clear signal to pause or stop, reinforcing the idea that consent can be revoked at any time. Discussing and agreeing upon safe words before engaging in fisting helps build a framework of trust.

- **Gradual Exploration:** Start with less intense forms of intimacy and gradually work towards fisting. This approach allows partners to build confidence in each other's abilities to communicate and respond to needs, fostering trust over time.

- **Aftercare Practices:** Aftercare is crucial following any intense intimate experience, including fisting. Engaging in aftercare practices—such as cuddling, discussing the experience, and providing emotional support—can strengthen the bond between partners and reinforce trust.

- **Educating Together:** Participating in workshops, reading literature, or attending classes on fisting techniques and safety can enhance both partners' knowledge and comfort levels. This shared educational journey can deepen intimacy and trust.

- **Addressing Emotional Responses:** Encourage partners to express their feelings before and after fisting. Discussing emotions such as excitement, anxiety, or even fear can help normalize these feelings and promote resilience within the relationship.

Examples of Building Trust in Practice

Consider a couple, Alex and Jamie, who are exploring fisting for the first time. They begin by having an open conversation about their desires, boundaries, and any fears they may have. They agree on a safe word—"red"—that will indicate when either partner needs to pause or stop.

Before engaging in fisting, they decide to practice relaxation techniques together, such as deep breathing exercises. This not only helps them feel more comfortable but also strengthens their emotional connection.

After their experience, they engage in aftercare by cuddling and discussing what they enjoyed and what could be improved. This debriefing allows them to process their feelings and reinforces their trust in each other.

Conclusion

Building trust and resilience in relationships, particularly when exploring activities like fisting, is an ongoing process that requires commitment, communication, and empathy. By understanding the theoretical underpinnings of trust, recognizing potential challenges, and implementing practical strategies, partners can foster a deeper connection that enhances their intimate experiences. Ultimately, a trusting relationship creates a safe space for exploration, growth, and mutual empowerment in the realm of sexuality.

Self-Care and Aftercare Practices

Aftercare is an essential component of any intimate experience, particularly in practices that push physical and emotional boundaries, such as fisting. It refers to the care and attention given to oneself and one's partner(s) following a session, ensuring emotional, physical, and psychological well-being. This section will explore the importance of aftercare, the various practices involved, and the underlying theories that support these practices.

The Importance of Aftercare

Aftercare serves multiple purposes:

- **Emotional Recovery:** Engaging in intense physical activities can elicit strong emotions. Aftercare provides a safe space to process these emotions, facilitating emotional recovery and reinforcing the bond between partners.
- **Physical Comfort:** Following a fisting session, one may experience physical discomfort or soreness. Aftercare can include physical comforts, such as hydration, nourishment, and soothing touch.
- **Reinforcement of Trust:** Aftercare practices reinforce trust and connection between partners, creating a safe environment where both individuals feel valued and cared for.
- **Psychological Integration:** Aftercare allows individuals to integrate their experiences, reflecting on what they enjoyed, what they might want to change, and how they can grow from the experience.

Self-Care Practices

Self-care is vital for individuals engaging in fisting, as it promotes overall well-being and prepares one for future experiences. Here are several self-care practices to consider:

Hydration and Nutrition

$$\text{Hydration Level} = \text{Water Intake (L)} \times \text{Activity Duration (h)} \quad (28)$$

After an intense session, it is crucial to rehydrate. Water helps flush out toxins and aids in recovery. Additionally, consuming a balanced meal can replenish energy levels and nutrients lost during the activity.

Physical Rest and Recovery Listening to your body is essential. Resting after a fisting session allows the body to recover and heal. This could involve lying down, taking a warm bath, or engaging in gentle stretching exercises to relieve tension.

PHYSICAL AND EMOTIONAL SAFETY

Emotional Reflection Taking time to reflect on the experience can be beneficial. Journaling about feelings, desires, and boundaries can help process emotions and prepare for future encounters. This practice fosters self-awareness and promotes personal growth.

Aftercare Practices

Aftercare should be tailored to the needs of both partners. Here are some examples of effective aftercare practices:

Physical Comfort - **Cuddling and Physical Touch:** Engaging in gentle, affectionate touch can provide comfort and reassurance. This can include cuddling, holding hands, or light massage. - **Warm Compresses:** Applying a warm compress to sore areas can help alleviate discomfort and promote relaxation.

Communication - **Post-Scene Check-Ins:** Partners should engage in open discussions about their experience. Questions to consider include:

- What did you enjoy the most?
- Were there any moments of discomfort?
- How can we improve our experience next time?

- **Validation and Reassurance:** Offering words of affirmation and support can reinforce emotional safety. Simple phrases like "I'm proud of you" or "Thank you for sharing this with me" can enhance feelings of connection.

Creating a Safe Space - **Environment:** Aftercare should occur in a comfortable, safe environment. This could involve dimming the lights, playing soft music, or using calming scents (e.g., lavender) to create a soothing atmosphere. - **Comfort Items:** Having comfort items on hand, such as blankets, pillows, or favorite snacks, can enhance the aftercare experience.

Theoretical Foundations of Aftercare

The significance of aftercare can be understood through various psychological and relational theories:

Attachment Theory Attachment theory posits that the bonds formed between individuals influence emotional responses and relationship dynamics. Aftercare strengthens these bonds by fostering security and trust, which are crucial for healthy relationships.

Polyvagal Theory Polyvagal theory emphasizes the role of the vagus nerve in emotional regulation and social connection. Engaging in aftercare practices can stimulate the parasympathetic nervous system, promoting relaxation and emotional safety.

Trauma-Informed Care Understanding trauma's impact on individuals is essential in intimate practices. Aftercare aligns with trauma-informed care principles by prioritizing safety, empowerment, and choice, allowing individuals to feel in control of their experiences.

Conclusion

In summary, self-care and aftercare practices are integral components of fisting experiences. These practices not only promote physical recovery but also foster emotional intimacy and trust between partners. By prioritizing self-care and engaging in meaningful aftercare, individuals can enhance their intimate experiences, leading to deeper connections and personal growth. Remember, the journey of exploration is ongoing, and nurturing oneself and one's partner(s) is key to a fulfilling and safe experience in the realm of fisting.

Finding Professional Help for Emotional Support

In the journey of exploring fisting, emotional support can be a crucial aspect of ensuring a safe and fulfilling experience. Engaging in such intimate practices often brings up complex feelings, and seeking professional help can provide valuable tools for navigating these emotions. This section discusses the importance of professional support, the types of professionals who can assist, and how to find the right fit for your needs.

The Importance of Professional Support

Exploring fisting and other forms of sexual expression can be both exhilarating and daunting. Individuals may encounter a variety of emotional responses, including excitement, anxiety, shame, or fear. These feelings can be amplified by societal stigma surrounding fisting and other non-conventional sexual practices. A professional therapist or counselor can help individuals process these emotions, providing a safe space to explore their feelings without judgment.

Types of Professionals Who Can Assist

When seeking professional help, it is essential to consider the type of support that aligns with your needs. Here are some types of professionals that can be beneficial:

- **Sex Therapists:** These professionals specialize in sexual health and intimacy issues. They can provide guidance on communication, consent, and emotional well-being related to sexual practices, including fisting.

- **Licensed Counselors or Psychologists:** Mental health professionals can assist individuals in addressing underlying emotional issues, trauma, or anxiety that may arise during their exploration of fisting.

- **Certified Sex Educators:** These individuals can offer educational resources and workshops focused on safe practices, consent, and communication, helping individuals feel more informed and confident.

- **Support Groups:** Peer-led support groups can provide a sense of community and shared experience, allowing individuals to connect with others who have similar interests and challenges.

How to Find the Right Professional

Finding the right professional can be a personal journey. Here are some steps to guide you in your search:

1. **Research Credentials:** Look for professionals with experience in sexual health, intimacy issues, and kink-aware practices. Verify their credentials and ensure they have a background in working with diverse sexual orientations and practices.

2. **Consider Specializations:** Some therapists may specialize in BDSM, kink, or alternative sexual practices. Seeking out those with this expertise can enhance the quality of support you receive.

3. **Ask About Their Approach:** During initial consultations, inquire about their therapeutic approach to issues related to sexual exploration. A

therapist who values consent, communication, and emotional safety will be better equipped to support your journey.

4. **Evaluate Comfort Level:** It is vital to feel comfortable and safe with your chosen professional. Trust your instincts; if a therapist does not align with your values or make you feel at ease, it is okay to seek someone else.

5. **Utilize Online Resources:** Websites such as the American Association of Sexuality Educators, Counselors, and Therapists (AASECT) can help you locate qualified professionals in your area. Additionally, online therapy platforms may offer access to sex-positive therapists.

Addressing Common Concerns

Individuals may have concerns about seeking professional help, such as fear of judgment or stigma. It is important to recognize that therapists are bound by confidentiality and ethical guidelines, which means they cannot disclose your personal information without consent. Moreover, a reputable therapist will approach your concerns with sensitivity and respect.

Another common concern is the cost of therapy. Many professionals offer sliding scale fees or accept insurance, making support more accessible. It is worthwhile to inquire about these options when searching for a therapist.

Examples of Situations Where Professional Help is Beneficial

1. **Navigating Emotional Triggers:** An individual may experience anxiety or distress when exploring fisting due to past trauma. A therapist can help them process these feelings and develop coping strategies.

2. **Building Communication Skills:** Partners may struggle with discussing their desires and boundaries. A sex therapist can facilitate conversations around consent and preferences, enhancing mutual understanding.

3. **Addressing Shame and Stigma:** Individuals may feel shame about their desires due to societal norms. Professional support can help reframe these feelings and foster self-acceptance.

4. **Aftercare and Emotional Processing:** Following a fisting session, individuals may experience a range of emotions. A therapist can assist in processing these feelings and provide guidance on aftercare practices.

Conclusion

Finding professional help for emotional support is an essential step in the journey of exploring fisting. By seeking guidance from qualified professionals, individuals can navigate their emotions, build healthy relationships, and enhance their overall experience. Remember, the path to self-discovery and sexual exploration is a personal one, and professional support can serve as a valuable resource along the way.

Beyond the Physical: Exploring the Emotional and Psychological Aspects of Fisting

Beyond the Physical: Exploring the Emotional and Psychological Aspects of Fisting

Beyond the Physical: Exploring the Emotional and Psychological Aspects of Fisting

Fisting, often regarded as a purely physical act, encompasses a rich tapestry of emotional and psychological dimensions that deserve exploration. Engaging in such an intimate practice can evoke a range of feelings, from exhilaration to vulnerability, and understanding these aspects can enhance the experience for all parties involved.

The Emotional Landscape of Fisting

Fisting can serve as a profound medium for emotional expression. The act itself often necessitates a high level of trust and vulnerability between partners. As intimacy deepens, individuals may find themselves confronting feelings they had previously suppressed. This emotional landscape can be understood through several psychological theories:

1. **Attachment Theory**: This theory posits that the bonds formed in early childhood influence adult relationships. In the context of fisting, individuals may seek to recreate feelings of safety and connection. A securely attached individual may feel more comfortable exploring fisting, viewing it as a way to deepen intimacy with a partner.

2. **The Polyvagal Theory**: This theory emphasizes the role of the vagus nerve in emotional regulation and social connection. Engaging in fisting can activate the parasympathetic nervous system, leading to feelings of calm and safety. This physiological response can enhance emotional bonding during the act.

3. **The Dual Control Model of Sexual Response**: This model suggests that sexual arousal is influenced by both excitatory and inhibitory factors. Fisting can stimulate both elements; the physical sensations can evoke excitement, while the emotional depth can provide a sense of safety and inhibition, creating a balanced experience.

Navigating Vulnerability and Trust

The act of fisting requires a unique level of vulnerability. Participants must communicate openly about their desires, limits, and fears. Establishing a safe space for dialogue is crucial. Here are some strategies to navigate this vulnerability:

- **Pre-Scene Discussions**: Before engaging in fisting, partners should have in-depth conversations about their emotional states, boundaries, and expectations. Discussing fears and desires can help mitigate anxiety and build trust.
- **Using Safe Words**: Safe words are essential in any BDSM or kink-related activity. They provide a mechanism for participants to communicate their comfort levels. Establishing clear safe words can empower individuals, allowing them to express discomfort without fear of judgment.
- **Aftercare Practices**: Aftercare is the process of attending to the emotional and physical needs of partners after an intense experience. This may include cuddling, discussing the experience, or simply being present. Engaging in aftercare can help solidify trust and reinforce emotional bonds.

Overcoming Fear and Shame

Many individuals carry societal stigma and personal shame surrounding practices like fisting. Addressing these feelings is crucial for a fulfilling experience. Here are some approaches:

- **Education and Awareness**: Understanding the anatomy and safety considerations of fisting can alleviate fears. Knowledge empowers individuals to engage in the practice confidently.
- **Therapeutic Support**: Seeking therapy can be beneficial for those grappling with shame or fear. A qualified therapist can help individuals unpack these feelings and develop healthier attitudes toward their desires.

BEYOND THE PHYSICAL: EXPLORING THE EMOTIONAL AND PSYCHOLOGICAL ASPECTS OF FISTING

- **Community Engagement**: Connecting with like-minded individuals can foster a sense of belonging and acceptance. Online forums, workshops, and local kink communities provide spaces to share experiences and learn from others.

The Connection Between Pain and Pleasure

Fisting can blur the lines between pain and pleasure. The psychological interplay between these sensations is complex and varies from person to person. Some individuals may find that the intensity of fisting enhances their pleasure, while others may experience discomfort. Understanding this connection can lead to more rewarding experiences:

- **Sensory Overload**: Engaging in fisting can create a state of sensory overload, where the body becomes acutely aware of sensations. This heightened awareness can lead to profound pleasure but may also trigger discomfort. Partners should communicate openly about their sensations during the act.
- **Emotional Release**: For some, fisting can serve as a form of emotional catharsis. The act of surrendering oneself to a partner can lead to the release of pent-up emotions, resulting in a sense of relief and pleasure.

Mutual Empowerment in Fisting Play

Fisting can be a powerful act of mutual empowerment. Participants often report feeling more in control of their bodies and desires. This empowerment can manifest in several ways:

- **Agency and Consent**: Engaging in fisting requires a high level of agency. Participants must actively negotiate their boundaries and desires, reinforcing their autonomy.
- **Body Positivity**: Fisting can challenge societal norms around body image and sexuality. By embracing their bodies and desires, individuals may develop a more positive self-image.
- **Exploration of Identity**: Fisting can serve as a means of exploring one's sexual identity. Participants may discover new facets of their desires and preferences, leading to personal growth.

Fisting as a Form of Active Meditation

For some, fisting can transcend the physical realm and become an act of active meditation. The focus required during the act can lead to a state of mindfulness, where individuals become acutely aware of their bodies and sensations. This meditative state can have several benefits:

- **Stress Reduction**: Engaging in fisting can provide an escape from daily stressors, allowing individuals to immerse themselves in the moment.
- **Enhanced Connection**: The mindfulness cultivated during fisting can enhance emotional and physical connections between partners, fostering intimacy and trust.
- **Self-Discovery**: The act of being present during fisting can lead to greater self-awareness and understanding of one's desires and boundaries.

Conclusion

Exploring the emotional and psychological aspects of fisting enriches the experience and fosters deeper connections between partners. By understanding the interplay of trust, vulnerability, and empowerment, individuals can navigate their fisting journeys with compassion and awareness. As we continue to explore the multifaceted nature of sexuality, embracing these emotional dimensions will pave the way for more fulfilling and authentic experiences.

The Intimacy and Vulnerability of Fisting

Intimacy as a Path to Self-Discovery

Intimacy, often viewed through the lens of romantic or sexual relationships, serves as a profound pathway to self-discovery. This section explores how the act of fisting, as an intimate practice, can facilitate a deeper understanding of oneself, one's desires, and one's emotional landscape.

Theoretical Framework

The exploration of intimacy can be grounded in various psychological and sociological theories. One such framework is the **Attachment Theory**, developed by John Bowlby and Mary Ainsworth, which posits that early relationships with caregivers shape our patterns of intimacy and connection in adulthood. Secure attachment fosters healthy relationships characterized by trust and open communication, while insecure attachment can lead to challenges in intimacy, such as fear of vulnerability or difficulty in expressing needs.

Additionally, the concept of **Self-Actualization**, as proposed by Abraham Maslow, suggests that intimacy is a vital component of achieving one's full potential. In Maslow's hierarchy of needs, love and belonging are foundational to self-esteem and ultimately to self-actualization. Engaging in intimate practices,

THE INTIMACY AND VULNERABILITY OF FISTING

such as fisting, can help individuals confront their desires and fears, leading to greater self-awareness and personal growth.

The Role of Vulnerability

Intimacy requires vulnerability, which can be challenging for many individuals. Brené Brown, a researcher on vulnerability and shame, emphasizes that embracing vulnerability is essential for forming deep connections. In the context of fisting, participants often navigate their fears and insecurities as they explore this intimate act. The willingness to be vulnerable can lead to profound insights about one's body, desires, and emotional responses.

$$V = \frac{D}{E} \qquad (29)$$

Where V represents vulnerability, D is the depth of emotional connection, and E is the external pressures or fears that may inhibit intimacy. As individuals engage in fisting, they may find that the act itself can diminish the fears represented by E, allowing for a greater exploration of D.

Experiential Learning and Self-Discovery

The practice of fisting can serve as a form of **experiential learning**, where individuals learn about themselves through direct experience. This process aligns with Kolb's Experiential Learning Cycle, which includes four stages: concrete experience, reflective observation, abstract conceptualization, and active experimentation.

1. **Concrete Experience**: Engaging in fisting provides a direct, embodied experience that can challenge preconceived notions about pleasure and intimacy. 2. **Reflective Observation**: After the experience, individuals may reflect on their feelings, sensations, and emotional responses, leading to insights about their desires and boundaries. 3. **Abstract Conceptualization**: Participants may theorize about their experiences, integrating new understandings of intimacy and self-awareness into their broader sexual identity. 4. **Active Experimentation**: Armed with new insights, individuals may choose to explore further, experimenting with different techniques, partners, or contexts in which to engage in fisting.

Addressing Challenges and Fears

While the journey of self-discovery through intimacy can be rewarding, it is not without challenges. Participants may confront fears related to body image, performance anxiety, or past trauma. Understanding these challenges is crucial for fostering a safe and supportive environment.

For example, an individual may feel apprehensive about their body during fisting. Engaging in open communication with partners about these feelings can help mitigate anxiety and enhance the intimate experience. Techniques such as **mindfulness** and **body positivity** can also play a role in addressing these challenges. Practicing mindfulness allows individuals to remain present during intimate moments, reducing anxiety and enhancing pleasure.

Case Studies and Real-Life Examples

Consider the case of Alex, who, after years of feeling disconnected from their body, decided to explore fisting with a trusted partner. Initially hesitant, Alex communicated their fears and boundaries, establishing a strong foundation of trust. Through the experience, Alex discovered a newfound appreciation for their body and sexual desires, leading to improved self-esteem and a deeper connection with their partner.

Another example is Jamie, who had previously experienced trauma related to intimacy. By gradually introducing fisting into their sexual repertoire, Jamie worked with a therapist to address their fears and insecurities. This process allowed Jamie to reclaim their body and agency, transforming a once-taboo act into a powerful tool for healing and self-discovery.

Conclusion

In conclusion, intimacy, particularly through practices like fisting, can serve as a profound pathway to self-discovery. By fostering vulnerability, encouraging experiential learning, and addressing challenges, individuals can unlock new dimensions of their sexual identity and emotional landscape. As individuals engage in intimate acts, they not only explore their desires but also embark on a journey toward greater self-awareness and personal growth. The act of fisting, when approached with intention, care, and communication, can illuminate the complexities of intimacy and the richness of human connection.

THE INTIMACY AND VULNERABILITY OF FISTING

Emotional Vulnerability and Trust

Emotional vulnerability is a critical component of intimacy and connection in any intimate relationship, particularly in the context of fisting. It involves the willingness to expose oneself emotionally, risking the potential for rejection or discomfort while simultaneously fostering a deeper bond with a partner. This section will explore the dynamics of emotional vulnerability, the importance of trust in fisting relationships, and how these elements contribute to a fulfilling and safe experience.

Understanding Emotional Vulnerability

Emotional vulnerability can be defined as the capacity to open oneself up to another person, sharing thoughts, feelings, and desires that may be difficult to express. Brené Brown, a prominent researcher on vulnerability, describes it as "uncertainty, risk, and emotional exposure" [?]. In the context of fisting, emotional vulnerability may manifest in several ways:

- **Sharing Fears and Desires:** Participants may need to communicate their fears about physical safety or emotional responses during fisting play. This sharing can enhance intimacy and create a supportive environment.

- **Expressing Limits and Boundaries:** Being open about personal limits and boundaries is essential for establishing a safe space. Vulnerability in this context means articulating what feels comfortable and what does not.

- **Navigating Emotional Responses:** Fisting can elicit intense emotional responses, including pleasure, fear, or even past trauma. Being able to express these feelings to a partner is crucial for mutual understanding and support.

The Role of Trust in Fisting

Trust is the foundation upon which emotional vulnerability is built. In fisting, where physical and emotional boundaries are tested, trust becomes paramount. Trust can be conceptualized through the following dimensions:

$$T = \frac{C + R + R_E}{3} \tag{30}$$

Where:

- T = Trust

- C = Consistency in behavior
- R = Reliability in communication
- R_E = Respect for emotional and physical boundaries

Each of these components plays a vital role in establishing and maintaining trust in a fisting relationship.

Building Trust through Communication

Effective communication is essential for building trust. Partners should engage in open dialogues about their experiences, desires, and concerns. Here are some strategies to enhance communication:

- **Active Listening:** Listening without interruption or judgment fosters a safe environment where both partners feel heard and valued.
- **Regular Check-ins:** Establishing regular times to discuss feelings and experiences can help partners stay attuned to each other's emotional states.
- **Nonverbal Cues:** Understanding body language and nonverbal signals can provide insight into a partner's emotional state, enhancing empathy and connection.

Navigating Emotional Vulnerability in Fisting Play

Fisting involves a unique interplay between physical sensations and emotional experiences. The following considerations can help partners navigate emotional vulnerability during fisting:

- **Pre-Scene Discussions:** Before engaging in fisting, partners should discuss their emotional states, desires, and any past experiences that might influence their current feelings.
- **Establishing Safe Words:** Safe words are essential for maintaining trust. They provide a clear signal for stopping or slowing down, allowing partners to prioritize emotional and physical safety.
- **Post-Scene Debriefing:** Aftercare is crucial for processing the experience. Partners should take time to discuss what felt good, what was challenging, and how they can support each other moving forward.

Examples of Emotional Vulnerability in Fisting

Consider the following scenarios that illustrate emotional vulnerability and trust in fisting:

- **Scenario 1: A New Experience**
  A couple decides to explore fisting for the first time. They engage in a pre-scene conversation where they discuss their fears, such as potential pain or feelings of inadequacy. By expressing these vulnerabilities, they create a supportive environment where both partners feel safe to explore their desires.

- **Scenario 2: Navigating Trauma**
  One partner has a history of trauma that resurfaces during fisting. They communicate their feelings of discomfort and the need for a break, demonstrating vulnerability. The other partner respects this need, fostering trust and emotional safety.

- **Scenario 3: Exploring Limits**
  During a session, one partner realizes they are feeling overwhelmed. They use their safe word, and the scene stops. Afterward, they discuss what led to that feeling, allowing for emotional processing and reinforcing trust in their relationship.

Conclusion

Emotional vulnerability and trust are integral to the experience of fisting. By fostering an environment of openness and respect, partners can navigate the complexities of their desires and fears. This journey into vulnerability not only enhances the fisting experience but also deepens the emotional connection between partners, ultimately leading to a more fulfilling and safe exploration of intimacy.

Overcoming Fear and Shame

The exploration of fisting, like many sexual practices, can evoke feelings of fear and shame. These emotions often stem from societal taboos, personal insecurities, and past experiences. Understanding and addressing these feelings is essential for a fulfilling and safe fisting experience.

The Roots of Fear and Shame

Fear and shame can manifest in various ways when considering fisting. Fear may arise from concerns about physical safety, the potential for injury, or the unknown aspects of the experience. Shame, on the other hand, often originates from internalized societal norms that label certain sexual practices as deviant or unacceptable.

$$\text{Fear} = f(\text{Perceived Risk, Lack of Knowledge}) \tag{31}$$

Where: - Perceived Risk refers to the individual's assessment of potential harm. - Lack of Knowledge reflects the absence of information about safe practices.

Shame can be more complex, often tied to personal history, body image issues, or previous negative experiences related to sexuality. The following equation illustrates the relationship between shame and its components:

$$\text{Shame} = f(\text{Social Conditioning, Personal Experience, Body Image}) \tag{32}$$

Where: - Social Conditioning includes cultural messages about sexuality. - Personal Experience relates to past encounters that may have been shaming or traumatic. - Body Image reflects how one perceives their own body in relation to societal standards.

Strategies for Overcoming Fear and Shame

To effectively navigate and overcome fear and shame, individuals can employ several strategies:

1. **Education and Knowledge** Gaining knowledge about fisting techniques, safety precautions, and anatomy can significantly reduce fear. Understanding the mechanics of fisting and how to engage in it safely can empower individuals, transforming fear into confidence.

$$\text{Confidence} = f(\text{Education, Preparation}) \tag{33}$$

Where: - Education encompasses learning about safe practices and anatomy. - Preparation involves setting boundaries, having discussions with partners, and ensuring a safe environment.

THE INTIMACY AND VULNERABILITY OF FISTING

2. Open Communication Discussing fears and concerns with partners fosters an environment of trust and understanding. Open communication can help partners navigate their feelings and establish clear boundaries, enhancing emotional safety.

$$\text{Trust} = f(\text{Communication}, \text{Vulnerability}) \tag{34}$$

Where: - Communication refers to the exchange of thoughts and feelings. - Vulnerability involves sharing personal fears and insecurities.

3. Mindfulness and Self-Compassion Practicing mindfulness can help individuals become aware of their fears without judgment. Techniques such as meditation, breathwork, and body awareness exercises can ground individuals, allowing them to process their emotions more effectively.

$$\text{Emotional Regulation} = f(\text{Mindfulness}, \text{Self-Compassion}) \tag{35}$$

Where: - Mindfulness is the practice of being present and aware. - Self-Compassion involves treating oneself with kindness and understanding.

4. Seeking Support Engaging with supportive communities, whether online or in person, can provide validation and encouragement. Sharing experiences with others who have navigated similar feelings can help normalize the emotions associated with fisting.

$$\text{Support} = f(\text{Community}, \text{Shared Experience}) \tag{36}$$

Where: - Community refers to groups that share similar interests or experiences. - Shared Experience reflects the commonality of navigating similar challenges.

5. Professional Guidance For individuals struggling with intense feelings of fear or shame, seeking the help of a therapist or sex educator can be beneficial. Professionals can provide tailored strategies to address these emotions and promote a healthier relationship with one's sexuality.

$$\text{Healing} = f(\text{Professional Support}, \text{Personal Effort}) \tag{37}$$

Where: - Professional Support involves guidance from trained individuals. - Personal Effort reflects the individual's commitment to personal growth.

Real-Life Examples

Consider the story of Jamie, who felt immense shame about her desire to explore fisting. Raised in a conservative environment, she internalized the belief that her desires were wrong. After educating herself about fisting, attending workshops, and engaging in open conversations with her partner, she began to dismantle her feelings of shame. With each positive experience, her confidence grew, allowing her to embrace her desires fully.

Similarly, Alex faced fears surrounding physical safety. By researching techniques and practicing with a trusted partner, Alex learned to listen to his body and communicate effectively, transforming fear into empowerment.

Conclusion

Overcoming fear and shame is a vital part of the fisting journey. By educating oneself, fostering open communication, practicing mindfulness, seeking support, and possibly engaging with professionals, individuals can navigate their emotions and embrace their desires. This journey not only enhances the experience of fisting but also contributes to a healthier relationship with one's own sexuality.

The Connection Between Pain and Pleasure

The interplay between pain and pleasure is a complex and multifaceted aspect of human sexuality, particularly in the context of fisting. Understanding this connection requires delving into both physiological and psychological dimensions, as well as the cultural narratives that shape our perceptions of these sensations.

Physiological Perspectives

From a physiological standpoint, pain and pleasure are processed in the brain through overlapping pathways. The body's response to pain involves the activation of nociceptors, which are specialized sensory neurons that respond to potentially damaging stimuli. When these nociceptors are activated, they send signals through the spinal cord to the brain, where they are interpreted as pain.

Conversely, pleasure is often associated with the release of neurotransmitters such as dopamine and endorphins. These chemicals not only enhance feelings of pleasure but can also modulate the perception of pain. This phenomenon is explained by the **Gate Control Theory of Pain**, proposed by Melzack and Wall in 1965. According to this theory, the nervous system can prioritize certain signals over others. When pleasurable sensations are experienced, they can effectively "close the gate" on pain signals, reducing the perception of discomfort.

$$P_{\text{perceived}} = S_{\text{input}} - G_{\text{pain}} + G_{\text{pleasure}} \tag{38}$$

Where:

- $P_{\text{perceived}}$ is the overall perception of sensation (pain or pleasure).
- S_{input} is the sensory input from the environment.
- G_{pain} is the gating effect of pain signals.
- G_{pleasure} is the gating effect of pleasurable sensations.

This equation highlights how the interplay between pain and pleasure can shape our overall sensory experience.

Psychological Perspectives

Psychologically, the connection between pain and pleasure can be understood through the lens of **sensory integration** and **contextual framing**. In many sexual practices, including fisting, the anticipation of pain can heighten arousal and pleasure. This phenomenon is often referred to as **masochism**, where individuals derive pleasure from the experience of pain.

The psychological mechanisms at play include: - **Conditioning**: Past experiences can condition individuals to associate certain types of pain with pleasure. For instance, if someone has experienced intense pleasure following a painful sensation in a consensual context, they may come to anticipate pleasure in similar future encounters. - **Cognitive appraisal**: The way individuals interpret and frame their experiences can significantly influence their perception of pain and pleasure. For example, someone may view the pain of fisting as a necessary part of achieving a deeper state of intimacy and connection, thereby transforming the experience into one of pleasure.

Cultural Narratives

Cultural narratives surrounding pain and pleasure also play a crucial role in shaping individual experiences. In many societies, pain is often stigmatized, while pleasure is celebrated. However, within the context of BDSM and kink communities, there exists a nuanced understanding that pain can be a pathway to pleasure. This perspective encourages individuals to explore their boundaries and embrace the full spectrum of their sensual experiences.

Examples and Case Studies

Consider the following examples that illustrate the connection between pain and pleasure in fisting:

1. **The Role of Endorphins**: Many individuals report experiencing a "high" after engaging in fisting, attributed to the release of endorphins during the experience. This biochemical response can create a sense of euphoria that transforms the initial discomfort into profound pleasure.

2. **The Experience of Subspace**: In BDSM contexts, participants may enter a state referred to as "subspace," characterized by a deep sense of relaxation and pleasure that often follows intense physical sensations, including pain. This altered state of consciousness can enhance the overall experience, allowing individuals to connect more deeply with their bodies and partners.

3. **Individual Variability**: It is important to recognize that the connection between pain and pleasure is highly individual. What one person may find pleasurable, another may find intolerable. This variability underscores the importance of communication and consent in all intimate encounters.

Conclusion

The connection between pain and pleasure is a rich area of exploration within the realm of fisting. By understanding the physiological, psychological, and cultural dimensions of this relationship, individuals can approach their experiences with greater awareness and intention. Embracing the complexity of these sensations can lead to deeper intimacy, personal growth, and a more fulfilling sexual journey. As we continue to navigate our desires and boundaries, let us celebrate the beautiful interplay of pain and pleasure as an integral part of our sexual expression.

Emotional Release and Catharsis

Emotional release and catharsis are integral components of the fisting experience, facilitating deeper connections and heightened states of intimacy between partners. This section delves into the theoretical underpinnings of emotional release, its practical implications in fisting, and the transformative power it holds for individuals and relationships.

Understanding Catharsis

The term *catharsis* originates from the Greek word *katharsis*, meaning "cleansing" or "purification." In psychological terms, catharsis refers to the process of releasing

THE INTIMACY AND VULNERABILITY OF FISTING

and thereby providing relief from strong or repressed emotions. Sigmund Freud introduced the concept in his work on psychoanalysis, suggesting that unexpressed emotions could lead to psychological distress. By expressing these emotions, individuals could achieve a sense of relief and emotional healing.

In the context of fisting, catharsis can manifest in various forms, including physical sensations, emotional expression, and psychological release. The act of fisting can serve as a conduit for exploring and expressing emotions that may otherwise remain unacknowledged or suppressed.

The Role of Emotional Release in Fisting

Fisting can evoke a range of emotions, from pleasure and excitement to fear and vulnerability. This emotional spectrum is essential to the experience, as it allows participants to engage deeply with their feelings and the sensations of their bodies. The physical act of fisting can trigger emotional responses due to the intense nature of the experience, which may include:

- **Vulnerability:** The act of allowing someone to penetrate you to such a degree can evoke feelings of vulnerability. This vulnerability can lead to emotional release as individuals confront and process their fears and insecurities.

- **Pleasure:** The pleasure derived from fisting can lead to a heightened emotional state, facilitating the release of built-up tension and stress. This pleasure can create a safe space for emotional expression.

- **Pain:** For some, the experience of pain during fisting can lead to a cathartic release. The connection between pain and pleasure is well-documented in BDSM practices, where the experience of pain can lead to a sense of liberation and emotional clarity.

The Psychological Mechanisms of Emotional Release

The psychological mechanisms behind emotional release during fisting can be understood through several theories:

1. **Affective Neuroscience:** This field examines how emotions are processed in the brain. The limbic system, particularly the amygdala, plays a crucial role in emotional responses. Engaging in intense physical activities, such as fisting, can stimulate the limbic system, leading to emotional release.

2. **Mind-Body Connection:** The mind-body connection is a vital aspect of emotional release. Engaging in physical sensations can help individuals reconnect

with their bodies, allowing them to experience and express emotions that may have been repressed. This connection can be particularly powerful in fisting, where the physical sensations can lead to emotional breakthroughs.

3. **Somatic Experiencing:** This therapeutic approach emphasizes the body's role in processing trauma and emotions. Fisting can serve as a form of somatic experiencing, allowing individuals to release pent-up emotions through physical sensations and experiences.

Examples of Emotional Release in Fisting

Several examples illustrate how emotional release can occur during fisting:

- **Crying or Laughing:** Participants may find themselves crying or laughing during or after a fisting session. These reactions can signify emotional release, allowing individuals to process feelings of joy, sadness, or relief.
- **Verbal Expression:** The act of fisting can prompt verbal expressions of emotions, such as affirmations, declarations of love, or even cries of frustration. This verbal communication can enhance intimacy and connection between partners.
- **Physical Reactions:** Physical reactions, such as shaking, trembling, or deep breathing, can indicate emotional release. These responses often occur when individuals confront intense emotions, allowing for a cathartic experience.

Facilitating Emotional Release in Fisting

To facilitate emotional release during fisting, consider the following strategies:

1. **Create a Safe Space:** Establish an environment where both partners feel safe to express their emotions freely. This can include setting the mood with soft lighting, comfortable seating, and ensuring privacy.

2. **Practice Open Communication:** Encourage open dialogue before, during, and after the fisting experience. Discuss emotional boundaries, triggers, and desires to foster a supportive atmosphere.

3. **Incorporate Aftercare:** Aftercare is a crucial component of any intense sexual experience. Engaging in aftercare practices, such as cuddling, talking, or providing physical comfort, can help partners process their emotions and reinforce their connection.

4. **Explore Breathwork:** Incorporating breathwork techniques during fisting can enhance emotional release. Deep, intentional breathing can help individuals stay grounded and connected to their bodies, facilitating the release of pent-up emotions.

5. **Encourage Reflection:** After the fisting experience, take time to reflect on the emotions that arose. Discussing these feelings can deepen intimacy and understanding between partners.

Conclusion

Emotional release and catharsis are powerful aspects of the fisting experience, allowing individuals to confront and process their emotions in a safe and supportive environment. By understanding the psychological mechanisms at play and implementing strategies to facilitate emotional expression, partners can enhance their fisting journey, fostering deeper intimacy and connection. As individuals explore the depths of their emotions through fisting, they may discover a profound sense of liberation and self-acceptance, ultimately enriching their sexual experiences and relationships.

Mutual Empowerment in Fisting Play

Mutual empowerment in fisting play is a profound aspect that transcends the physical act itself, weaving together elements of trust, vulnerability, and shared experience. This section explores how fisting can serve as a medium for both partners to experience empowerment, enhancing their connection and intimacy.

Theoretical Framework

The concept of mutual empowerment can be understood through various psychological and sociological lenses. One relevant theory is **Relational-Cultural Theory (RCT)**, which emphasizes the importance of relationships in fostering personal growth and well-being. According to RCT, empowerment emerges from the quality of relational dynamics, where both partners engage in a reciprocal exchange of support and respect. In the context of fisting, this dynamic is crucial as it allows individuals to explore their boundaries and desires in a safe environment.

Trust and Vulnerability

Empowerment in fisting is deeply rooted in trust. Engaging in such an intimate act requires both partners to feel safe and respected. Trust is built through open communication, where partners discuss their limits, desires, and fears. Vulnerability plays a significant role here; by exposing their desires and insecurities, individuals can foster a deeper connection.

For example, one partner may express a desire to explore deeper levels of penetration, while the other may have concerns about their physical limits. Through honest dialogue, they can negotiate boundaries that respect both partners' needs, ultimately leading to a more fulfilling experience.

Shared Experience and Connection

Fisting can create a shared experience that reinforces the bond between partners. The act itself requires a high level of coordination and awareness, which can enhance the sense of connection. When partners navigate the physical and emotional landscapes together, they cultivate a sense of mutual investment in each other's pleasure.

Consider a scenario where one partner is hesitant about the intensity of the experience. By communicating openly about their sensations and emotions, they can collaboratively adjust their approach, ensuring that both partners feel empowered in the moment. This shared journey not only enhances pleasure but also fosters a deeper emotional connection.

Empowerment Through Exploration

Engaging in fisting can also empower individuals to explore their bodies and desires in ways they may not have previously considered. This exploration can lead to greater body awareness and acceptance. The act of fisting challenges societal norms around sexuality and encourages individuals to reclaim their pleasure.

For instance, a person who has previously felt shame around their sexual desires may find empowerment in the act of fisting. By embracing this taboo, they can dismantle internalized stigma and cultivate a more positive relationship with their sexuality. This process of self-discovery can be profoundly liberating, allowing individuals to express their desires without fear of judgment.

Addressing Power Dynamics

While fisting can be an empowering experience, it is essential to recognize and navigate the inherent power dynamics involved. Fisting often occurs within the context of BDSM, where power exchange can be a significant factor. Partners must be aware of how power dynamics influence their interactions and ensure that empowerment is mutual.

In a dominant/submissive scenario, the dominant partner may have more control over the experience. However, it is crucial that the submissive partner feels empowered to communicate their needs and limits. This can be achieved through the use of safe words and ongoing check-ins, which allow for a continuous dialogue about comfort levels and desires.

Practical Examples of Empowerment in Fisting

1. **Negotiation of Limits**: Before engaging in fisting, partners can sit down and discuss what they are comfortable with. This negotiation process empowers both individuals to voice their desires and boundaries, setting the stage for a consensual and enjoyable experience.

2. **Feedback During Play**: During the act of fisting, partners can practice active listening. One partner may express pleasure or discomfort, and the other can respond accordingly. This real-time feedback loop fosters a sense of agency for both partners.

3. **Post-Play Reflection**: Aftercare is a crucial component of fisting play. Partners can engage in a debriefing session to discuss what they enjoyed and what could be improved. This reflection allows both individuals to feel heard and valued, reinforcing their empowerment.

Challenges to Mutual Empowerment

Despite the potential for empowerment, several challenges can arise during fisting play. Miscommunication, lack of trust, and differing expectations can hinder the mutual empowerment process. It is essential for partners to remain vigilant and address these challenges proactively.

For example, if one partner feels pressured to engage in fisting despite their discomfort, it can lead to feelings of disempowerment and resentment. To mitigate this, partners should continually check in with each other and ensure that consent is enthusiastic and ongoing.

Conclusion

Mutual empowerment in fisting play is a complex interplay of trust, vulnerability, and shared experiences. By fostering open communication, addressing power dynamics, and navigating challenges together, partners can enhance their connection and intimacy. As individuals explore their desires within a supportive framework, they not only empower themselves but also contribute to a more profound relational dynamic that celebrates both pleasure and connection.

Fisting as a Form of Active Meditation

Fisting, often regarded through the lens of physical intimacy, can also be approached as a profound form of active meditation. This perspective emphasizes the connection between physical sensations, emotional awareness, and mindfulness, allowing participants to experience heightened states of consciousness and presence. In this section, we will explore the theoretical underpinnings of fisting as an active meditative practice, address potential challenges, and provide practical examples for individuals seeking to incorporate this approach into their intimate experiences.

Theoretical Foundations

The concept of active meditation is rooted in the idea that mindfulness can be cultivated through physical activities that engage the body and mind simultaneously. According to Jon Kabat-Zinn, mindfulness is defined as "the awareness that arises from paying attention, on purpose, in the present moment, and non-judgmentally." In the context of fisting, this awareness can be enhanced through the following mechanisms:

- **Sensory Awareness:** Fisting invites participants to focus on the myriad sensations experienced during the act. This includes the warmth of skin, the texture of the body, and the subtle shifts in pressure and movement. By concentrating on these sensations, individuals can cultivate a deeper awareness of their own bodies and their partners.

- **Breath Control:** The practice of breath control is a common element in both meditation and fisting. Participants can use their breath to center themselves, synchronize their movements, and create a rhythm that enhances the overall experience. Focusing on inhalation and exhalation can help to ground individuals in the moment, reducing anxiety and promoting relaxation.

- **Mind-Body Connection:** Fisting requires a keen awareness of both physical and emotional states. This connection can facilitate a deeper understanding of one's own limits and desires, fostering a sense of empowerment and self-acceptance. Engaging in fisting as a meditative practice encourages individuals to explore their bodies in a non-judgmental manner, leading to increased body positivity and self-love.

THE INTIMACY AND VULNERABILITY OF FISTING

Challenges and Considerations

While fisting can serve as an active meditation, there are challenges that practitioners may encounter. These include:

- **Distraction:** In a world filled with distractions, it can be challenging to maintain focus during intimate acts. Participants may find their thoughts wandering to external concerns or internal judgments. To counteract this, establishing a safe and comfortable environment is crucial. Dimming the lights, playing soft music, or using aromatherapy can help create a conducive space for meditation.

- **Emotional Barriers:** Emotional vulnerability is a significant aspect of both fisting and meditation. Participants may experience fear, shame, or anxiety that can hinder their ability to be present. Engaging in open communication with partners about these feelings can help build trust and create a supportive atmosphere. Practicing self-compassion and acknowledging these emotions as part of the journey is essential.

- **Physical Limitations:** The physical nature of fisting requires awareness of one's own body and limits. Practitioners should be mindful of their comfort levels and any potential pain or discomfort. This awareness can be cultivated through regular practice, allowing individuals to gradually explore their boundaries while remaining attuned to their bodies.

Practical Examples

To integrate fisting as a form of active meditation into intimate experiences, consider the following practices:

- **Setting Intentions:** Before engaging in fisting, take a moment to set intentions for the experience. This could involve expressing desires for deeper connection, exploration of sensations, or simply a commitment to being present. Sharing these intentions with partners can enhance the shared experience and foster a sense of unity.

- **Mindful Breathing:** Begin the session with a few minutes of mindful breathing. Focus on inhaling deeply through the nose and exhaling slowly through the mouth. Encourage partners to synchronize their breath, creating a shared rhythm that can enhance the overall experience. This practice can help ground individuals and prepare them for the journey ahead.

- **Sensory Exploration:** As the fisting experience unfolds, encourage participants to focus on the sensations they are experiencing. This could involve verbalizing feelings, such as warmth, pressure, or pleasure. Engaging in this sensory exploration can deepen the meditative state and enhance emotional connection.

- **Post-Session Reflection:** After the fisting session, take time to reflect on the experience. This could involve discussing feelings, sensations, and any emotional responses that arose. Engaging in this debriefing allows participants to integrate their experiences and cultivate a deeper understanding of their bodies and desires.

Conclusion

In conclusion, fisting can serve as a powerful form of active meditation, fostering a deep connection between the body, mind, and emotions. By cultivating sensory awareness, practicing breath control, and embracing the mind-body connection, individuals can transform their intimate experiences into profound journeys of self-discovery and empowerment. While challenges may arise, the potential for personal growth and emotional healing through this practice is immense. As individuals navigate their fisting journeys, they are encouraged to embrace the process with curiosity, compassion, and a commitment to mindfulness.

Exploring the Sacred and Spiritual Aspects of Fisting

Fisting, often viewed through the lens of physical pleasure and erotic exploration, can also be approached as a deeply spiritual and sacred practice. This perspective invites individuals to engage with their bodies and their partners in a way that transcends mere physicality, allowing for profound emotional and spiritual connections. In this section, we will explore various theories and practices that highlight the sacred and spiritual dimensions of fisting, addressing potential challenges and providing examples to illustrate these concepts.

Theoretical Foundations

The exploration of the sacred aspects of fisting can be framed within several theoretical perspectives:

1. **Tantric Philosophy**: Tantric practices emphasize the union of body, mind, and spirit. In this context, fisting can be seen as a form of sacred intimacy that allows partners to connect on multiple levels. The act of fisting can be viewed

as a way to merge energies, facilitating a deeper understanding of oneself and one's partner. The focus on breath, intention, and presence in Tantric practices can enhance the spiritual experience of fisting, transforming it into a meditative act.

2. **Somatic Experiencing**: This therapeutic approach emphasizes the connection between body sensations and emotional experiences. Engaging in fisting with a focus on somatic awareness allows individuals to explore their physical sensations while also processing emotional responses. This can lead to a deeper understanding of personal boundaries, trauma, and healing, making the act of fisting a transformative experience.

3. **Sacred Sexuality**: This concept encompasses various spiritual traditions that view sexuality as a sacred expression of life force energy. Within this framework, fisting is not merely a physical act but a celebration of the divine within the body. Practitioners may engage in rituals or meditative practices before, during, or after fisting to honor the sacredness of the experience.

Challenges and Considerations

While exploring the sacred aspects of fisting can be enriching, it is essential to acknowledge potential challenges:

- **Cultural Stigmas**: Many cultures view fisting as taboo or deviant, which can create internal conflict for individuals seeking to integrate spirituality with their sexual practices. Overcoming societal stigma requires a commitment to personal authenticity and the courage to challenge conventional beliefs.

- **Emotional Vulnerability**: Engaging in fisting as a sacred act may bring up deep-seated emotions, including fear, shame, or trauma. It is crucial for partners to establish a safe space for exploration, using tools such as consent, communication, and aftercare to navigate these emotional landscapes.

- **Misunderstanding of Spirituality**: Some individuals may conflate spirituality with specific religious practices, leading to misconceptions about what constitutes a sacred act. It is vital to define spirituality in a way that resonates personally, allowing for a more inclusive understanding of sacredness in sexual practices.

Practical Examples

To illustrate the sacred and spiritual aspects of fisting, consider the following practices:

1. **Setting Intentions**: Before engaging in fisting, partners can take a moment to set intentions for their experience. This might involve expressing

desires, fears, or what they hope to gain from the encounter. By articulating these intentions, individuals can create a shared focus that enhances the spiritual connection.

2. **Mindful Breathing**: Incorporating mindful breathing techniques can deepen the spiritual experience of fisting. Partners can synchronize their breath, using inhalations and exhalations to create a rhythmic flow that enhances intimacy. This practice encourages presence and connection, transforming the act into a shared meditation.

3. **Ritualistic Elements**: Some individuals may choose to incorporate ritualistic elements into their fisting practice. This could include lighting candles, playing specific music, or using essential oils to create a sacred atmosphere. These elements can help frame the experience as a spiritual journey, inviting a sense of reverence.

4. **Post-Experience Reflection**: After engaging in fisting, partners can take time to reflect on their experience. This could involve discussing feelings, sensations, and insights gained during the act. Engaging in this reflective practice can help solidify the spiritual aspects of the experience and foster deeper emotional connections.

Conclusion

Exploring the sacred and spiritual aspects of fisting allows individuals to engage with their bodies and their partners in a transformative way. By integrating theories from Tantric philosophy, somatic experiencing, and sacred sexuality, practitioners can elevate fisting from a purely physical act to a deeply meaningful exploration of intimacy and connection. While challenges may arise, the rewards of such exploration can lead to profound personal growth and enhanced relationships. Embracing the sacred dimensions of fisting invites individuals to honor their bodies, their partners, and the spiritual journey that unfolds through this intimate practice.

Developing Emotional Resilience and Growth

Emotional resilience is the ability to adapt to stressful situations and recover from adversity. In the context of fisting, where vulnerability and intimacy are deeply intertwined, developing emotional resilience can enhance both personal growth and relational dynamics. This section explores the pathways to cultivating resilience, addressing potential challenges, and providing actionable strategies for growth.

Understanding Emotional Resilience

Emotional resilience is often defined as the capacity to maintain psychological well-being in the face of stress or trauma. According to [?], resilience involves a dynamic process of positive adaptation in response to adversity. This concept can be applied to fisting practices, where individuals may encounter emotional challenges related to vulnerability, trust, and intimacy.

Theoretical Frameworks

One relevant theoretical framework is the **Resilience Theory**, which posits that resilience can be developed through various protective factors, such as social support, emotional regulation, and self-efficacy [?]. In the context of fisting, these factors can be cultivated through:

- **Social Support:** Building a supportive community of partners and friends who understand and respect the nuances of fisting can provide emotional safety and validation.

- **Emotional Regulation:** Learning techniques to manage emotions, such as mindfulness and cognitive restructuring, can help individuals navigate intense feelings that may arise during fisting.

- **Self-Efficacy:** Developing confidence in one's ability to communicate needs and boundaries fosters a sense of control and empowerment.

Common Challenges

While exploring fisting, individuals may face several emotional challenges, including:

- **Fear of Vulnerability:** The act of fisting requires a high level of trust, which can trigger fears of rejection or emotional exposure.

- **Shame and Stigma:** Societal attitudes towards fisting can evoke feelings of shame, impacting self-acceptance and emotional well-being.

- **Post-Scene Emotional Processing:** Aftercare is essential for emotional resilience; however, individuals may struggle to process their feelings post-scene, leading to unresolved emotions.

Strategies for Developing Resilience

To foster emotional resilience in the context of fisting, consider the following strategies:

1. **Engage in Open Communication:** Establishing clear communication with partners about feelings, boundaries, and experiences can mitigate fears and enhance trust. Utilize active listening techniques to validate each other's experiences.

2. **Practice Mindfulness:** Mindfulness techniques, such as meditation and body awareness exercises, can help individuals stay present and manage anxiety during fisting. Practicing mindfulness can enhance the mind-body connection, allowing for a deeper exploration of sensations and emotions.

3. **Create a Safe Space for Reflection:** After a fisting session, engage in debriefing conversations with partners to reflect on the experience. Discuss what felt pleasurable, what was challenging, and how to improve future encounters.

4. **Develop a Support Network:** Seek out peer support groups or online communities focused on fisting and sexual exploration. Sharing experiences and advice can normalize feelings and foster a sense of belonging.

5. **Seek Professional Guidance:** Consider therapy or counseling, especially if past traumas impact current experiences. A therapist can provide tools for emotional regulation and resilience-building.

Examples of Resilience in Fisting

Consider a scenario where a couple explores fisting for the first time. They engage in thorough discussions about boundaries and desires beforehand, establishing a safe word. During the experience, one partner feels overwhelmed. Instead of pushing through, they communicate their discomfort, demonstrating emotional resilience. After the session, they engage in aftercare, reflecting on their feelings and reinforcing their connection.

Another example is a person who has faced stigma regarding their sexual preferences. By joining a supportive community, they learn to embrace their desires and share their experiences, transforming feelings of shame into empowerment and self-acceptance.

Conclusion

Developing emotional resilience in the context of fisting is a multifaceted process involving open communication, emotional regulation, and community support. By addressing challenges and implementing strategies for growth, individuals can enhance their experiences and foster deeper connections with themselves and their partners. Embracing vulnerability through fisting can ultimately lead to profound personal growth and a richer understanding of intimacy.

Building Intimacy and Connection with Partners

Building intimacy and connection with partners through fisting can be a profound and transformative experience. This section explores the theoretical underpinnings of intimacy, the potential challenges that may arise, and practical strategies to foster a deeper bond during fisting play.

Theoretical Framework of Intimacy

Intimacy is often defined as a close familiarity or friendship; it is a feeling of closeness and connection that transcends mere physical interaction. According to the *Intimacy Theory* proposed by Derlega and Grzelak (1979), intimacy can be conceptualized through three dimensions: emotional, physical, and intellectual.

1. **Emotional Intimacy**: This involves sharing feelings, thoughts, and vulnerabilities with one another. Emotional intimacy can enhance the sense of safety during fisting, allowing partners to explore their desires without fear of judgment.

2. **Physical Intimacy**: Physical closeness, such as through touch, can deepen the bond between partners. In the context of fisting, the physical act itself can serve as a vehicle for expressing affection and trust.

3. **Intellectual Intimacy**: Engaging in open discussions about desires, boundaries, and fantasies contributes to a deeper understanding of each partner's needs and preferences. This dialogue is essential for ensuring that both partners feel heard and valued.

Challenges in Building Intimacy

While fisting can enhance intimacy, several challenges may arise:

- **Fear of Vulnerability**: The act of fisting requires a significant level of trust and vulnerability. Partners may fear being judged or rejected, which can hinder emotional connection.

- **Miscommunication**: Lack of clear communication regarding desires and boundaries can lead to misunderstandings. This can create discomfort and erode trust between partners.
- **Physical Discomfort**: If one partner experiences pain or discomfort during fisting, it can disrupt the flow of intimacy and lead to feelings of inadequacy or frustration.
- **Emotional Triggers**: For some, the physical act of fisting may evoke past traumas or emotional responses that can complicate the experience. Recognizing and addressing these triggers is crucial for maintaining intimacy.

Strategies for Fostering Intimacy

To cultivate intimacy and connection during fisting, consider the following strategies:

1. **Establish Open Communication**: Prior to engaging in fisting, partners should have an open dialogue about their desires, boundaries, and any concerns. Utilizing active listening techniques can help partners feel understood and supported. For example, using phrases like "I hear you" or "That makes sense" can validate feelings.

2. **Create a Safe Environment**: Setting the scene for fisting can enhance comfort and intimacy. Dim lighting, soft music, and a clean, inviting space can help partners feel relaxed.

3. **Engage in Pre-Play Rituals**: Engaging in rituals such as massage, kissing, or cuddling can build emotional and physical intimacy before transitioning to fisting. These activities can help partners feel more connected and attuned to one another.

4. **Utilize Safe Words and Signals**: Establishing safe words or signals can promote a sense of security. Knowing that either partner can pause or stop the activity allows for a more relaxed exploration.

5. **Practice Aftercare**: Aftercare is essential for reinforcing intimacy post-fisting. This can include cuddling, discussing the experience, or simply being present with one another. Aftercare helps partners process their emotions and reinforces the bond created during play.

6. **Explore Emotional Vulnerability**: Encourage partners to share their feelings about the experience, including any fears or insecurities that arose. This exchange can deepen emotional intimacy and enhance connection.

7. **Incorporate Sensual Touch**: During fisting, partners can maintain intimacy by incorporating sensual touch in other areas of the body. This can help balance the physical intensity of fisting with tenderness and affection.

8. **Be Patient and Attentive**: Patience is key in building intimacy. Taking time to explore and respond to each other's cues fosters a deeper connection. Partners should be attentive to each other's reactions and adjust their approach accordingly.

Case Study: The Journey of Sarah and Alex

Consider the example of Sarah and Alex, a couple who sought to deepen their intimacy through fisting. Initially, both partners felt apprehensive about the experience, fearing potential discomfort and emotional vulnerability. They began by engaging in open discussions about their desires and boundaries, which laid the groundwork for trust.

Before their first experience, they created a cozy environment with soft lighting and calming music. They also established safe words, ensuring that both felt secure in their exploration. During the act, they focused on maintaining communication, checking in with each other frequently.

Afterward, they engaged in aftercare, sharing their feelings about the experience. This discussion allowed them to process their emotions and reinforced their connection. Over time, Sarah and Alex found that fisting became a powerful tool for enhancing their intimacy, allowing them to explore deeper emotional and physical connections.

Conclusion

Building intimacy and connection through fisting is a multifaceted process that requires open communication, trust, and vulnerability. By understanding the theoretical framework of intimacy, recognizing potential challenges, and implementing effective strategies, partners can create a fulfilling and intimate experience. Fisting can serve not only as a physical exploration but also as a pathway to deeper emotional bonds and mutual understanding, ultimately enriching the relationship.

Fisting and Power Dynamics

Understanding Power Dynamics in BDSM and Kink

Power dynamics in BDSM and kink encompass a complex interplay of authority, control, and submission that can manifest in various ways during sexual play. Understanding these dynamics is crucial for participants to engage in safe, consensual, and fulfilling experiences. This section explores the theoretical frameworks, practical implications, and examples of power dynamics within BDSM and kink, highlighting the importance of consent, negotiation, and emotional intelligence.

Theoretical Frameworks

The study of power dynamics in BDSM often draws from several theoretical perspectives, including:

- **Foucault's Theory of Power:** Michel Foucault's work on power relations emphasizes that power is not merely held by one individual over another but is a complex network of relationships that can shift and change. In BDSM, power exchange is often negotiated and agreed upon, allowing both parties to experience empowerment within defined boundaries.

- **Transactional Analysis:** This psychological theory posits that interactions can be understood in terms of three ego states: Parent, Adult, and Child. In BDSM, participants may switch between these states, with the Dominant often embodying the Parent and the Submissive embodying the Child. Understanding these roles can enhance communication and emotional connection.

- **Social Exchange Theory:** This theory suggests that human relationships are formed through the exchange of resources, which can include emotional support, physical pleasure, and the negotiation of power. In BDSM, the exchange is often explicit, with both parties agreeing on the terms of their interaction, thus reinforcing trust and mutual satisfaction.

Types of Power Dynamics

Power dynamics in BDSM can be categorized into several types, each with distinct characteristics:

- **Dominance and Submission (D/s):** This dynamic involves one partner (the Dominant) taking control while the other (the Submissive) willingly relinquishes power. This relationship can be temporary (during a scene) or ongoing (in a Total Power Exchange relationship).

- **Master and Slave (M/s):** This is a more intense form of D/s, where the Master has total control over the Slave's actions, decisions, and sometimes even thoughts. This dynamic requires a high level of trust and clear communication about limits and boundaries.

- **Switching:** Some individuals may identify as "switches," meaning they can take on both Dominant and Submissive roles depending on the context and partner. This flexibility allows for a richer exploration of power dynamics.

Consent and Negotiation

Central to any power dynamic in BDSM is the concept of consent. Consent must be informed, enthusiastic, and ongoing. Participants should engage in thorough negotiation before any scene, discussing boundaries, safe words, and expectations.

$$\text{Consent} = \text{Informed} + \text{Enthusiastic} + \text{Ongoing} \qquad (39)$$

This equation underscores that consent is not a one-time agreement but a continuous dialogue throughout the experience. Safe words, such as "red" for stop and "yellow" for slow down, provide a mechanism for the Submissive to communicate their comfort level during play.

Challenges and Misconceptions

Despite the consensual nature of BDSM, misconceptions persist regarding power dynamics:

- **Abuse vs. BDSM:** A common misconception is that BDSM inherently involves abuse. In reality, BDSM is predicated on consent and mutual agreement, differentiating it from abusive relationships where consent is absent or coerced.
- **Gender Roles:** Power dynamics are often mistakenly viewed through a heteronormative lens, suggesting that men must always be Dominant and women Submissive. In practice, power dynamics are fluid and can exist across all genders and sexual orientations.

Examples of Power Dynamics in Practice

To illustrate the application of power dynamics in BDSM, consider the following scenarios:

- **Scene Negotiation:** A couple discusses their desire to explore a D/s dynamic. The Dominant expresses a wish to bind and blindfold the Submissive, while the Submissive communicates a boundary regarding the use of pain. They agree on a safe word and establish a safe environment for their exploration.

- **Role Reversal:** In a switching scenario, two partners may alternate roles during a session. One partner may begin as the Dominant, guiding the other through a series of commands, before switching to a Submissive role, allowing the other partner to take control. This fluidity enriches their experience and enhances understanding of each other's desires.

Conclusion

Understanding power dynamics in BDSM and kink is essential for fostering safe, consensual, and pleasurable experiences. By engaging in open communication, thorough negotiation, and continuous consent, participants can explore the depths of intimacy and trust that power exchange offers. As individuals navigate these dynamics, they contribute to a culture that values respect, autonomy, and the celebration of diverse sexual expressions.

In summary, power dynamics in BDSM are not merely about control but are rich, multifaceted interactions that require emotional intelligence, clear communication, and mutual respect. By appreciating the complexities of these dynamics, participants can engage in more fulfilling and transformative experiences.

Consent and Negotiation in Power Exchange Relationships

In the realm of power exchange relationships, particularly those that involve fisting, the principles of consent and negotiation become paramount. Understanding how to navigate these dynamics not only enhances the safety and enjoyment of all parties involved but also fosters trust and intimacy. This section will delve into the theoretical underpinnings of consent, the nuances of negotiation in power exchange scenarios, and practical examples to illustrate these concepts.

Theoretical Framework of Consent

Consent is a foundational element in any sexual relationship, especially in BDSM and kink contexts. According to the *Enthusiastic Consent* model, consent should be given freely, enthusiastically, and can be revoked at any time. This model contrasts with the traditional view of consent as a mere absence of "no," emphasizing that an affirmative, informed agreement is essential for all activities.

The *Negotiation Model* of consent further elaborates this concept by advocating for clear communication about desires, boundaries, and limits before engaging in any sexual activity. This model is particularly relevant in power exchange relationships, where dynamics of dominance and submission can complicate the negotiation process.

Negotiation in Power Exchange Relationships

Negotiation in power exchange relationships involves a careful and respectful dialogue about the roles each partner will play, the activities they wish to engage in, and the boundaries that must be respected. Here are key components of effective negotiation:

- **Open Communication:** Partners should create a safe space for discussing their desires, fears, and limits. This includes sharing past experiences, preferences, and any relevant emotional or physical considerations.

- **Establishing Roles:** Clearly defining the roles of dominant and submissive partners can help set the stage for the negotiation. Each partner should express their expectations regarding their roles and what they hope to achieve through the power exchange.

- **Setting Boundaries:** It is crucial to establish explicit boundaries regarding what is acceptable and what is not. This includes discussing hard limits (activities that are off-limits) and soft limits (activities that may require negotiation or gradual exploration).

- **Safe Words:** The use of safe words is a critical component of negotiation. A safe word is a predetermined word or phrase that can be used to pause or stop the activity immediately. Common examples include "red" for stop and "yellow" for slow down or check-in.

- **Aftercare Planning:** Aftercare refers to the support and care provided to partners following a scene. Discussing aftercare needs during the negotiation process ensures that both partners feel safe and cared for after engaging in intense activities.

Common Problems in Consent and Negotiation

Despite the importance of consent and negotiation, challenges can arise in power exchange relationships. Some common problems include:

- **Miscommunication:** Ambiguities in communication can lead to misunderstandings about desires and boundaries. It is crucial for partners to ask clarifying questions and confirm understanding.

- **Assumptions:** Partners may make assumptions about each other's comfort levels or desires based on their own experiences. This can lead to situations where one partner feels pressured to engage in activities they are not comfortable with.

- **Power Imbalance:** In power exchange dynamics, the dominant partner may inadvertently exert pressure on the submissive partner to agree to activities. It is essential for the dominant partner to remain aware of their influence and ensure that consent is genuinely given.

- **Fear of Rejection:** Submissive partners may fear that expressing their limits or desires will lead to rejection or disappointment from the dominant partner. Creating a non-judgmental space for discussion can help mitigate this fear.

Practical Examples

To illustrate effective negotiation in power exchange relationships, consider the following scenarios:

> **Example**
>
> **Scenario 1: Establishing Boundaries**
> Alice and Bob are exploring fisting as part of their power exchange dynamic. During their negotiation, Alice expresses her desire to try fisting but also shares her fear of pain. Bob listens attentively and reassures her that they can take things slowly. They agree on a safe word and establish a boundary that they will only proceed if Alice feels comfortable at every step.
> **Outcome:** By openly discussing her fears and establishing clear boundaries, Alice feels empowered and safe, enhancing their trust and intimacy.

> **Example**
>
> **Scenario 2: Aftercare Planning**
> Cathy and David engage in a fisting scene that involves intense sensations. Before the scene, they discuss aftercare, with Cathy expressing her need for physical closeness and reassurance afterward. David agrees to hold her and provide verbal affirmations post-scene.
> **Outcome:** The aftercare plan helps Cathy feel emotionally supported, allowing her to process the experience positively.

Conclusion

The dynamics of consent and negotiation in power exchange relationships, particularly in the context of fisting, require intentionality, clarity, and mutual respect. By adhering to the principles of enthusiastic consent and engaging in thorough negotiation, partners can create a safe and pleasurable environment that fosters intimacy and trust. Recognizing and addressing potential problems can further enhance the experience, ensuring that both partners feel valued and respected in their exploration of desires.

In summary, effective consent and negotiation are not merely procedural steps; they are integral to the emotional and psychological safety of all involved in power exchange relationships. By prioritizing these elements, partners can embark on their fisting journeys with confidence and mutual understanding.

Dominance, Submission, and Fisting

The intersection of dominance, submission, and fisting creates a unique dynamic that can enhance the experience of both partners involved. Understanding this interplay not only enriches the practice but also deepens the emotional and psychological connections between participants.

Understanding Power Dynamics in BDSM and Kink

Power dynamics are fundamental to BDSM and kink, where participants engage in consensual exchanges of power. Fisting, as a form of kink, often incorporates elements of dominance and submission (D/s). In this context, the dominant partner may take control of the fisting process, guiding the submissive partner through the experience. The psychological aspect of D/s can heighten arousal and deepen intimacy, making the act of fisting more than just a physical endeavor.

Consent and Negotiation in Power Exchange Relationships

Consent is paramount in any BDSM practice, including fisting. Before engaging in fisting, it is essential for partners to negotiate boundaries, limits, and safe words. This negotiation should include discussions about the roles each partner wishes to embody, the level of trust involved, and any specific desires or fears. For example, a dominant partner might express a desire to explore deeper insertion, while the submissive partner may need to establish limits on pain and discomfort.

The negotiation process can be framed through the following equation, which emphasizes the balance of power and consent:

$$\text{Power Exchange} = \text{Consent} + \text{Communication} + \text{Trust} \qquad (40)$$

This equation illustrates that a healthy power exchange relies on mutual understanding and respect for each partner's needs.

Dominance, Submission, and Fisting Techniques

Incorporating D/s dynamics into fisting can manifest in various techniques and approaches. For instance, the dominant partner may dictate the pace and depth of the fisting, allowing the submissive partner to surrender control. This can enhance feelings of vulnerability and trust, which are essential components of a fulfilling D/s relationship.

A common technique involves the dominant partner using verbal commands to guide the submissive partner's actions, such as:

- **Slow down:** This command can help the submissive partner regulate their sensations and maintain comfort.

- **Push deeper:** This encourages the submissive partner to explore their limits, fostering a sense of surrender.

- **Let go:** This phrase can be used to help the submissive partner release tension and fully embrace the experience.

The use of these commands not only enhances the physical experience but also reinforces the psychological aspects of D/s play.

Tapping into Roleplay and Fantasy

Roleplay is a powerful tool within D/s dynamics, allowing partners to explore different personas and scenarios. For example, a dominant partner may take on the role of a "master" or "mistress," while the submissive partner might embody a "pet" or "slave." This roleplay can add layers of excitement and anticipation to the fisting experience.

Fantasy scenarios can also enhance the emotional connection. Consider a scene where the dominant partner uses fisting as a means of "training" the submissive partner to submit fully. This can create a sense of purpose and direction within the scene, heightening both partners' arousal.

Exploring Dominance and Submission Through Fisting

Fisting can serve as a physical manifestation of dominance and submission. The act itself requires a high level of trust, as the submissive partner must feel safe enough to allow their partner to take control of their body. This trust can lead to profound emotional experiences, as the submissive partner may feel a sense of liberation in surrendering to their dominant partner.

Additionally, the physical sensations associated with fisting can amplify feelings of submission. The fullness created by a hand inside the body can evoke a sense of being "owned" or "filled," enhancing the psychological aspects of submission.

Aftercare and Emotional Support in Power Play

Aftercare is an essential component of any BDSM encounter, particularly in scenes involving intense physical and emotional experiences like fisting. Aftercare involves the dominant partner providing emotional and physical support to the submissive partner post-scene. This can include:

- **Physical care:** Ensuring the submissive partner is comfortable, hydrated, and relaxed.

- **Emotional support:** Engaging in gentle conversation to help the submissive partner process their experience and feelings.

- **Reassurance:** Affirming the submissive partner's worth and the consensual nature of the experience.

The importance of aftercare cannot be overstated; it helps to mitigate any emotional fallout and reinforces the bond between partners.

Finding Balance and Equitable Power Exchange

While D/s dynamics can enhance the fisting experience, it is crucial to maintain a balance between dominance and submission. Both partners should feel empowered to express their needs and desires. An equitable power exchange allows for flexibility, where the roles can shift depending on the partners' preferences and comfort levels.

In conclusion, the interplay between dominance, submission, and fisting offers a rich landscape for exploration. By understanding the dynamics at play, partners can create a fulfilling and safe experience that deepens their connection and enhances their sexual repertoire. As with all aspects of BDSM, communication, consent, and trust are the cornerstones of a successful fisting experience within a D/s framework.

Tapping into Roleplay and Fantasy

Roleplay and fantasy are integral components of human sexuality, providing avenues for exploration, expression, and connection. In the context of fisting, these elements can enhance the experience, deepen intimacy, and allow individuals to explore desires that may be difficult to express in everyday life. This section delves into the dynamics of roleplay and fantasy, their psychological underpinnings, and practical considerations for incorporating them into fisting experiences.

Understanding Roleplay and Fantasy

Roleplay involves adopting specific roles or personas during sexual activities, allowing individuals to step outside their everyday identities. Fantasy, on the other hand, is a mental construct—an imaginative scenario that may or may not involve real-life dynamics. Both practices serve as powerful tools for sexual expression, enabling participants to explore desires, boundaries, and power dynamics in a safe and consensual environment.

Psychological Frameworks   From a psychological perspective, roleplay and fantasy can be understood through various theories, including:

- **Psychodynamic Theory:** This approach emphasizes the unconscious mind, where repressed desires and conflicts may manifest through fantasy. Engaging in roleplay can help individuals confront these unconscious urges in a controlled manner.
- **Cognitive-Behavioral Theory:** This theory posits that thoughts influence feelings and behaviors. By creating and engaging in fantasies, individuals can reshape their perceptions of pleasure, intimacy, and vulnerability.

- **Social Learning Theory:** This theory suggests that behaviors are learned through observation and imitation. In the realm of sexuality, individuals may adopt roleplay scenarios they have encountered in media, literature, or personal experiences, shaping their desires and preferences.

Common Themes in Fisting Roleplay

When incorporating roleplay into fisting, several themes often emerge, reflecting broader sexual dynamics:

- **Power Exchange:** Roleplay scenarios often involve dominant and submissive dynamics, where one partner takes on a more assertive role while the other surrenders control. Fisting can amplify this power exchange, heightening sensations of vulnerability and trust.
- **Medical Play:** Some individuals may find the idea of medical roleplay appealing, incorporating elements of examination and care into their fisting experiences. This can involve the use of sterile environments, medical instruments, or even roleplaying as a doctor and patient.
- **Fantasy Characters:** Engaging in roleplay as fictional characters—whether from literature, film, or mythology—can provide a playful and imaginative context for fisting. This might involve embodying characters with specific traits or attributes, enhancing the overall experience through storytelling.

Incorporating Roleplay and Fantasy into Fisting

To effectively incorporate roleplay and fantasy into fisting experiences, consider the following practical strategies:

1. Communication and Consent   Before engaging in roleplay, open and honest communication is essential. Discuss desires, boundaries, and potential scenarios with your partner(s) to ensure everyone is on the same page. Establishing safe words and signals can help navigate the intensity of the experience while maintaining trust and safety.

2. Setting the Scene   Creating an environment that aligns with the chosen fantasy can enhance the experience. This may involve using props, costumes, or specific lighting to evoke the desired atmosphere. For example, if engaging in medical play, consider incorporating medical instruments and sterile settings to heighten authenticity.

3. Embracing the Role   Once the scene is set, fully embrace the chosen role. This may involve adopting specific behaviors, language, or mannerisms that align with the character or dynamic. Allow yourself to immerse in the fantasy, letting go of inhibitions and embracing the exploration of desires.

4. Debriefing After the Scene   After engaging in roleplay, take time to debrief with your partner(s). Discuss what worked well, what could be improved, and how each person felt during the experience. This reflection can enhance emotional intimacy and provide insights for future explorations.

Potential Challenges and Considerations

While roleplay and fantasy can enhance fisting experiences, several challenges may arise:

- **Miscommunication:** Without clear communication, misunderstandings can occur, leading to discomfort or emotional distress. Regular check-ins and discussions about boundaries are crucial.

- **Emotional Triggers:** Engaging in certain fantasies may inadvertently trigger past trauma or emotional discomfort. Participants should remain aware of their emotional states and be prepared to pause or stop if needed.

- **Societal Stigma:** Roleplay and fantasy can be stigmatized, leading to feelings of shame or embarrassment. Embracing these practices requires self-acceptance and a supportive environment where individuals feel safe to express their desires.

Conclusion

Tapping into roleplay and fantasy can significantly enrich the experience of fisting, providing opportunities for exploration, intimacy, and connection. By understanding the psychological frameworks, common themes, and practical considerations, individuals can navigate the complexities of desire and enhance their sexual experiences. Ultimately, the key to successful roleplay lies in communication, consent, and a willingness to embrace vulnerability and exploration in a safe and trusting environment.

Exploring Dominance and Submission Through Fisting

The practice of fisting can serve as a profound exploration of dominance and submission (D/s) dynamics, providing a unique context in which power exchange is negotiated, experienced, and expressed. This section aims to elucidate how fisting intertwines with the principles of D/s relationships, examining the psychological, emotional, and physical dimensions of this intimate act.

Understanding D/s Dynamics

Dominance and submission are foundational concepts in BDSM (Bondage, Discipline, Dominance, Submission, Sadism, and Masochism). They involve a consensual power exchange where one partner (the dominant) takes control, while the other (the submissive) relinquishes it. This dynamic is often characterized by trust, communication, and mutual respect. The psychological underpinnings of D/s relationships can be traced back to the work of theorists such as [1], who argue that the act of submission can lead to profound emotional release and a sense of belonging.

Fisting as a Tool for Power Exchange

Fisting can amplify the D/s experience by heightening sensations of vulnerability and control. The act of fisting itself—where one partner's hand is inserted into another's body—can be seen as an ultimate expression of dominance. The dominant partner is in control of the pace, depth, and intensity, while the submissive partner must surrender to the sensations and trust the dominant's guidance.

$$\text{Power Exchange} = \text{Trust} + \text{Communication} + \text{Consent} \quad (41)$$

This equation illustrates that the essence of power exchange relies on the foundational elements of trust, communication, and consent. Without these components, the D/s dynamic can become harmful rather than pleasurable.

Psychological Aspects of D/s in Fisting

The psychological effects of engaging in fisting within a D/s framework can be multifaceted. For the submissive, the act of surrendering control can lead to feelings of liberation and catharsis. Research shows that submission can evoke a sense of safety and acceptance, allowing individuals to explore their desires without fear of judgment [2]. Conversely, for the dominant partner, fisting can provide a sense of empowerment and responsibility. The dominant must navigate the submissive's limits, ensuring that the experience remains safe and consensual.

Communication and Negotiation

Effective communication is crucial in D/s relationships, particularly when exploring fisting. Prior to engaging in fisting, partners should discuss their boundaries, desires, and safe words. This negotiation process can be framed within the context of the following questions:

- What are your limits regarding fisting?
- How do you want to feel during this experience?
- What safe words or signals will we use?
- How will we check in with each other during the act?

By addressing these questions, both partners can establish a clear understanding of each other's needs and expectations, fostering a safe environment for exploration.

Physical Considerations in D/s Fisting

From a physical standpoint, fisting requires a heightened awareness of the body and its responses. The dominant partner must be attuned to the submissive's physical cues, recognizing signs of discomfort or distress. This attentiveness can enhance the D/s dynamic, as it reinforces the dominant's role in ensuring the submissive's safety.

$$\text{Physical Awareness} = \text{Observation} + \text{Feedback} + \text{Adaptation} \tag{42}$$

This equation highlights the importance of being observant, receptive to feedback, and adaptable to the submissive's needs during the fisting experience.

Exploring Roleplay and Fantasy

Fisting can also serve as a canvas for roleplay and fantasy within D/s dynamics. Partners may choose to enact specific scenarios, such as a dominant character asserting control over a submissive one. This roleplay can enhance the emotional and psychological aspects of the experience, allowing participants to delve deeper into their desires and fantasies.

For example, a scene might involve the dominant partner asserting their authority through verbal commands, guiding the submissive through the process of fisting. This interplay of power can heighten arousal and deepen the connection between partners.

Aftercare and Emotional Support

Aftercare is an essential component of any BDSM activity, particularly in fisting, where emotional and physical boundaries can be tested. Aftercare involves providing support and care to each other post-scene, allowing both partners to process their experiences. This can include cuddling, discussing feelings, or simply being present for one another.

The emotional connection fostered through aftercare can solidify the D/s dynamic, reinforcing trust and intimacy. Partners may engage in reflective conversations about what they enjoyed, what could be improved, and how they felt during the experience.

Challenges and Considerations

While fisting can be an empowering exploration of D/s dynamics, it is not without its challenges. Issues such as miscommunication, lack of trust, or failure to respect boundaries can lead to negative experiences. Partners must remain vigilant about consent and continuously check in with each other, ensuring that both individuals feel safe and respected throughout the process.

Additionally, it is crucial to recognize the potential for emotional triggers or trauma to surface during intense experiences. Acknowledging these vulnerabilities and having a plan for addressing them can enhance the overall experience.

Conclusion

In conclusion, exploring dominance and submission through fisting can be a deeply rewarding experience for partners willing to engage in this intimate act. By understanding the psychological, emotional, and physical dimensions of D/s dynamics, partners can create a safe and pleasurable environment for exploration. Through effective communication, negotiation, and aftercare, fisting can serve as a powerful tool for deepening trust and intimacy within a D/s relationship. As with all BDSM practices, the key lies in mutual respect, consent, and a shared desire for exploration.

Bibliography

[1] Smith, J. (2021). *The Psychology of Kink: Understanding BDSM Relationships*. Kink Press.

[2] Johnson, A. (2022). *Emotional Safety in BDSM: Building Trust and Connection*. Safe Space Publishing.

Aftercare and Emotional Support in Power Play

Aftercare is a crucial component of any BDSM or kink experience, particularly in the context of power play, such as fisting. It involves the care and attention given to partners after a scene, ensuring that both physical and emotional needs are addressed. This section will explore the importance of aftercare, the various forms it can take, and how it contributes to the overall health and satisfaction of participants in power dynamics.

The Importance of Aftercare

Aftercare serves several essential functions in the aftermath of an intense scene:

- **Physical Recovery:** After engaging in any form of BDSM, including fisting, the body may need time to recover. This can include hydration, nourishment, and any necessary medical attention for physical injuries. For example, a partner may need to apply soothing creams to areas that have experienced friction or trauma.

- **Emotional Regulation:** Engaging in power play can elicit strong emotional responses, ranging from exhilaration to vulnerability. Aftercare provides a safe space for partners to process these emotions. For instance, discussing feelings of euphoria or discomfort can help partners navigate their emotional landscapes post-scene.

- **Reinforcement of Trust:** Aftercare reinforces the trust established during the scene. It reassures partners that their well-being is a priority. This can be as simple as cuddling or as involved as a thorough debriefing of the scene.

- **Closure and Integration:** Aftercare allows participants to integrate their experiences, reflecting on what they enjoyed and what could be improved. This reflection can enhance future encounters and deepen the connection between partners.

Forms of Aftercare

Aftercare can take many forms, and it is essential to tailor it to the individual needs of each partner. Here are some common methods of aftercare:

- **Physical Comfort:** This can include cuddling, providing blankets, or offering a warm drink. The physical presence of a partner can be incredibly grounding after an intense experience.

- **Verbal Reassurance:** Engaging in gentle conversation can help partners feel secure. Phrases such as "You did amazing" or "I'm so proud of you" can reinforce positive feelings.

- **Debriefing:** Discussing the scene in detail can help partners understand their experiences. Questions to consider include:
  - What did you enjoy the most?
  - Was there anything that felt uncomfortable or unexpected?
  - How can we improve our communication for next time?

- **Emotional Support:** Some partners may require more emotional support than others. This can include active listening or providing a safe space for emotional expression. For example, one partner may need to cry or express feelings of vulnerability without fear of judgment.

- **Physical Care:** Attending to any physical needs, such as cleaning wounds or applying ointments, can be crucial. Ensuring that both partners feel physically cared for can enhance emotional connection.

Challenges in Aftercare

While aftercare is essential, it can also present challenges. Some common issues include:

- **Miscommunication:** Partners may have different expectations regarding aftercare. It is vital to communicate needs and preferences before engaging in a scene to ensure everyone is on the same page.

- **Emotional Disconnect:** After an intense scene, one partner may feel elated while the other feels emotionally drained. Recognizing these differences and addressing them sensitively is crucial to maintaining a healthy dynamic.

- **Inadequate Aftercare:** Sometimes, partners may overlook aftercare due to fatigue or emotional overwhelm. This can lead to feelings of neglect or abandonment, which can harm the relationship. Establishing a clear aftercare plan can mitigate this risk.

Examples of Effective Aftercare

To illustrate effective aftercare practices, consider the following scenarios:

- **Scenario 1:** After a fisting scene, one partner feels anxious and needs reassurance. The other partner wraps them in a blanket, offers a warm drink, and engages them in light conversation about their favorite moments from the scene. This approach helps ease anxiety and fosters a sense of security.

- **Scenario 2:** Following a particularly intense scene, a partner experiences emotional release and begins to cry. The other partner provides a safe space for emotional expression, holding them close and validating their feelings. This act of empathy reinforces trust and connection.

- **Scenario 3:** After a scene, partners sit together to discuss their experiences. They take turns sharing what they enjoyed and what they might want to explore differently in the future. This debriefing not only enhances communication but also builds anticipation for future encounters.

Conclusion

Aftercare is an integral part of power play that ensures both partners feel safe, valued, and connected after an intense experience. By prioritizing aftercare, participants can foster trust, promote emotional well-being, and enhance the overall satisfaction of their BDSM experiences. It is essential to recognize that aftercare is not a one-size-fits-all approach; understanding and addressing the unique needs of each partner is key to successful aftercare. As partners engage in ongoing communication and reflection, they can cultivate deeper intimacy and a more profound connection, ultimately enriching their journey together in the realm of power dynamics and fisting.

Finding Balance and Equitable Power Exchange

In the realm of fisting and other BDSM practices, the dynamics of power exchange play a crucial role in shaping the experiences of those involved. Finding balance and equitable power exchange is essential to ensure that all parties feel safe, respected, and empowered throughout their journey. This section explores the theoretical underpinnings of power dynamics, the challenges that can arise, and practical strategies for achieving a harmonious balance.

Theoretical Foundations of Power Dynamics

Power dynamics in BDSM contexts can be understood through the lens of various theories, including social exchange theory, which posits that human relationships are formed based on the perceived costs and benefits involved. In a BDSM context, participants negotiate the terms of their engagement, weighing the emotional, physical, and psychological costs against the anticipated rewards.

The power exchange can be categorized into three primary types:

- **Dominance and Submission (D/s):** This dynamic involves one partner (the Dominant) taking control over the other (the Submissive), often with explicit consent and predefined limits. The Submissive willingly relinquishes some degree of power, which can lead to heightened feelings of trust and intimacy.

- **Switching:** Some individuals may identify as 'switches,' meaning they enjoy taking on both Dominant and Submissive roles depending on the context and partners involved. This fluidity can enhance the experience by allowing participants to explore different facets of their sexuality and relationship dynamics.

- **Master/Slave Dynamics:** This is a more intense form of power exchange, where one partner (the Master) assumes complete control over the other (the Slave). This dynamic requires a high level of trust, communication, and negotiation to ensure that both partners feel safe and respected.

Challenges in Power Exchange

While power exchange can be exhilarating and fulfilling, it also presents unique challenges. Some common issues include:

- **Miscommunication:** Failure to communicate effectively about desires, boundaries, and limits can lead to misunderstandings and potential harm. It is vital to establish clear lines of communication from the outset.

- **Power Imbalance:** An unequal distribution of power can lead to feelings of resentment, discomfort, or even abuse. Both partners must actively engage in the negotiation process to ensure that power dynamics remain equitable.

- **Emotional Vulnerability:** The act of surrendering control can evoke intense emotions. It is essential for both Dominants and Submissives to recognize and address these feelings, ensuring that emotional safety is prioritized.

- **Societal Stigma:** Participants in power exchange dynamics may face societal judgment or stigma, which can impact their self-esteem and willingness to engage openly in these practices. Building a supportive community can help mitigate these effects.

Strategies for Achieving Balance

To foster equitable power exchange, consider the following strategies:

- **Open Communication:** Establish ongoing dialogue about desires, boundaries, and limits. Use tools like check-ins before, during, and after scenes to ensure that both parties feel comfortable and respected.

- **Negotiation:** Prior to engaging in any power exchange activities, negotiate the terms clearly. Discuss what each partner is comfortable with, including safe words, limits, and aftercare needs.

- **Mutual Respect:** Acknowledge and honor each partner's autonomy and agency. Power exchange should never come at the expense of one partner's well-being or dignity.

- **Education and Training:** Engage in workshops or training sessions to deepen your understanding of power dynamics and BDSM practices. Knowledge can empower both partners to navigate their experiences more effectively.

- **Aftercare:** Prioritize aftercare to address the emotional and physical needs of both partners following a scene. This practice reinforces trust and connection, helping to maintain balance in the relationship.

Examples of Equitable Power Exchange

Consider the following scenarios that illustrate the principles of equitable power exchange:

- **Scenario 1: A D/s Relationship** - In a Dominance and submission relationship, both partners agree on specific roles. The Dominant partner may take the lead during scenes, but they consistently check in with the Submissive, ensuring that they are comfortable and consenting to the activities. The Submissive has the right to withdraw consent at any time, and the Dominant respects this boundary.

- **Scenario 2: Switching Roles** - A couple enjoys switching roles during their play. They take turns being the Dominant and Submissive, allowing each partner to experience both sides of the dynamic. They communicate openly about their preferences and boundaries, ensuring that both feel fulfilled and empowered in their chosen roles.

- **Scenario 3: Master/Slave Dynamic** - In a Master/slave relationship, the Master may have significant control over the Slave's daily activities. However, they establish a detailed contract outlining the Slave's limits, desires, and safe words. The Master regularly checks in with the Slave to ensure their emotional well-being and to adjust the dynamic as needed.

In conclusion, finding balance and equitable power exchange in fisting and BDSM practices is essential for fostering a safe and fulfilling experience. By prioritizing communication, mutual respect, and education, partners can create a dynamic that honors the desires and boundaries of everyone involved. Ultimately, the goal is to cultivate a relationship where both partners feel empowered, respected, and connected, allowing for deeper intimacy and exploration.

Safely Navigating Edge Play and Extreme Scenarios

Edge play refers to activities that push the boundaries of what is considered safe, sane, and consensual in BDSM and kink practices. It can include a wide variety of practices, including fisting, that explore physical and psychological limits. While edge play can be thrilling and rewarding, it requires a heightened awareness of safety, communication, and emotional readiness. In this section, we will explore the key considerations for safely navigating edge play and extreme scenarios, focusing on the intricacies of fisting.

Understanding Edge Play

Edge play is often defined by its inherent risks, which can be physical, emotional, or psychological. Engaging in edge play requires a deep understanding of oneself and one's partner(s), as well as a commitment to maintaining safety and consent throughout the experience. It is crucial to recognize that the thrill of edge play can sometimes lead to a temporary suspension of fear, making it essential to have clear safety protocols in place.

Theoretical Framework

The practice of edge play can be analyzed through several theoretical lenses, including:

- **Risk-Aware Consensual Kink (RACK):** This framework emphasizes the importance of understanding and accepting the risks involved in kink practices. Participants should engage in informed consent, ensuring that all parties are aware of potential dangers and agree to proceed.

- **The Psychology of Risk-Taking:** Research suggests that individuals are often drawn to risk-taking behavior due to the release of neurotransmitters such as dopamine and adrenaline. This physiological response can enhance feelings of pleasure and excitement, but it also necessitates careful consideration of the potential for harm.

- **Power Dynamics:** Edge play often involves complex power dynamics, where one partner may take on a more dominant role while the other submits. Understanding these dynamics is crucial for maintaining consent and emotional safety during intense experiences.

Identifying Risks in Edge Play

When engaging in fisting as an edge play activity, several risks must be considered:

- **Physical Risks:** These include potential injuries such as tears, bruising, or internal damage. It is vital to understand the anatomy involved in fisting to minimize these risks. For example, proper hand positioning and the use of ample lubrication can significantly reduce the likelihood of injury.

- **Psychological Risks:** Edge play can trigger intense emotional responses, including fear, anxiety, or trauma. Participants should engage in thorough pre-scene discussions to ensure that all emotional triggers are identified and addressed.

- **Consent Violations:** Given the heightened emotions and adrenaline associated with edge play, it is essential to have clear communication protocols in place. This includes establishing safe words, signals, and aftercare practices to ensure all participants feel safe and cared for.

Practical Strategies for Safety

To navigate edge play safely, consider the following strategies:

1. **Pre-Scene Negotiation:** Before engaging in any edge play, have an open and honest discussion with your partner(s) about limits, desires, and concerns. This conversation should include a review of safe words and signals, as well as any specific risks associated with fisting.

2. **Establishing Safe Words:** Safe words are essential in edge play. Choose a word or phrase that is easy to remember and communicate, even in an intense state. Common examples include "red" for stop and "yellow" for slow down or check-in.

3. **Continuous Communication:** During the scene, maintain an ongoing dialogue with your partner(s). This can include verbal check-ins or non-verbal signals to ensure that everyone is comfortable and consensually engaged in the experience.

4. **Aftercare:** Aftercare is a crucial component of any BDSM scene, particularly in edge play. It involves providing emotional and physical support to one another post-scene. This can include cuddling, discussing the experience, or addressing any physical discomfort.

5. **Educate Yourself:** Knowledge is power. Engage in educational resources, workshops, and discussions about fisting and edge play to better understand techniques, risks, and safety measures. This could involve reading literature, attending seminars, or connecting with experienced practitioners.

Case Studies and Examples

To illustrate the principles of safely navigating edge play, consider the following hypothetical scenarios:

- **Scenario 1: The Novice Fister**
  A couple decides to explore fisting for the first time. They engage in a thorough pre-scene negotiation, discussing boundaries, desires, and safe words. During the scene, they maintain open communication, and the receiving partner uses the safe word to indicate discomfort. The dominant partner stops immediately, checks in, and they switch to a different activity for the remainder of the session. Aftercare includes cuddling and discussing what worked and what didn't.

- **Scenario 2: Experienced Practitioners**
  A more experienced couple engages in edge play with fisting as a central focus. They have established a high level of trust and communication. They decide to incorporate elements of bondage into their scene, which heightens the intensity. They have a clear plan for aftercare and agree to check in frequently. The receiving partner uses a non-verbal signal to indicate they need a break, which is respected immediately, showcasing their commitment to safety and consent.

- **Scenario 3: Group Play**
  In a group setting, participants discuss their limits and establish a clear framework for consent before beginning. They agree on a safe word that everyone understands. As the scene progresses, one participant feels overwhelmed and uses the safe word. The entire group stops, reassures the participant, and takes a break to regroup and discuss feelings. This emphasizes the importance of communication in group dynamics.

Conclusion

Navigating edge play and extreme scenarios, particularly in the context of fisting, requires a strong foundation of trust, communication, and safety awareness. By understanding the risks involved and implementing practical strategies for safety, participants can explore the thrilling aspects of edge play while minimizing potential harm. Remember, the essence of kink lies in the mutual enjoyment and empowerment of all participants, making safety and consent paramount in every encounter.

Exploring Psychological Dominance and Submission

The exploration of psychological dominance and submission within the context of fisting involves a nuanced understanding of power dynamics, consent, and emotional interplay. This section delves into the theoretical frameworks that underpin these dynamics, potential challenges faced by participants, and practical examples that illuminate the complexities of this interplay.

Theoretical Frameworks

Psychological dominance and submission can be understood through various theoretical lenses, including:

- **Social Exchange Theory:** This theory posits that relationships are formed based on the perceived costs and benefits. In the context of BDSM, individuals may engage in dominant or submissive roles to derive psychological satisfaction and fulfillment, which can be viewed as an exchange of power. The equation can be illustrated as:

$$S = B - C$$

  where S is satisfaction, B is benefits, and C is costs.

- **Attachment Theory:** This psychological framework suggests that early relationships with caregivers shape our future relational patterns. In BDSM dynamics, individuals might reenact or explore their attachment styles, finding comfort in the structure of dominance and submission. Secure attachment can foster trust, while insecure attachment may lead to challenges in navigating power dynamics.

- **The BDSM Continuum:** This model illustrates a spectrum of dominance and submission, ranging from consensual power exchange to coercive control. Understanding where one falls on this continuum can help participants navigate their experiences and intentions, ensuring that their interactions remain consensual and safe.

- **Foucault's Power Dynamics:** Michel Foucault's theories on power suggest that power is not merely held but is relational and contextual. In BDSM, power exchange is consensual and negotiated, allowing participants to explore their desires while maintaining agency. This perspective emphasizes the importance of communication and consent in establishing boundaries and understanding roles.

Challenges and Considerations

Engaging in psychological dominance and submission can present various challenges, including:

- **Miscommunication:** One of the most significant risks in power dynamics is the potential for miscommunication regarding limits, desires, and consent. Clear and open dialogue is crucial to ensure that all parties are aligned in their expectations and boundaries.

- **Emotional Vulnerability:** Submissives often place themselves in vulnerable positions, which can trigger past traumas or insecurities. Dominants must be attuned to their partner's emotional state and provide reassurance and support throughout the experience.

- **Role Confusion:** Participants may struggle with their identities within the dynamic, particularly if they switch roles frequently. Establishing a clear understanding of each person's role, desires, and boundaries can help mitigate confusion.

- **Aftercare Needs:** Aftercare is an essential aspect of BDSM that involves providing emotional and physical support following a scene. Both dominants and submissives may require aftercare to process their experiences and reinforce their connection.

Examples of Psychological Dynamics in Fisting

To illustrate the complexities of psychological dominance and submission in fisting, consider the following scenarios:

- **Scenario 1: The Trust Fall**
  In this scenario, a submissive partner expresses a desire to explore fisting as a means of deepening their trust in the dominant partner. The dominant partner takes on the role of a guide, slowly introducing the submissive to the sensations of fisting while emphasizing the importance of communication. They establish a safe word, allowing the submissive to maintain control over the experience. This dynamic fosters a sense of safety and trust, enhancing the emotional connection between partners.

- **Scenario 2: The Role Reversal**
  A couple who typically engages in a dominant-submissive dynamic decides

to explore role reversal. The dominant partner, accustomed to leading, finds themselves in a submissive role during a fisting session. This experience challenges their perceptions of power and control, allowing them to explore vulnerability and emotional release. The submissive partner, now in a dominant role, learns to navigate the responsibilities of leading, ensuring their partner's safety and comfort throughout the experience.

- Scenario 3: The Emotional Release
A submissive partner experiences a cathartic release during a fisting session, where the physical sensations intertwine with emotional processing. The dominant partner remains attuned to their partner's needs, providing verbal affirmations and physical support. This scenario exemplifies how fisting can serve as a conduit for emotional expression, allowing individuals to explore their feelings of vulnerability, trust, and empowerment.

Conclusion

Exploring psychological dominance and submission in the context of fisting is a multifaceted journey that requires open communication, trust, and a deep understanding of one's own desires and boundaries. By navigating these dynamics thoughtfully, participants can cultivate rich, fulfilling experiences that enhance their emotional and psychological connections. As with all aspects of BDSM, the key lies in mutual respect, consent, and a commitment to ongoing dialogue and education.

Building Trust and Communication in Power Dynamics

Building trust and effective communication in power dynamics is essential for a fulfilling and safe fisting experience. Power exchange can heighten intimacy and pleasure, but it also requires a solid foundation of trust and open dialogue between partners. In this section, we will explore the theoretical underpinnings of trust in power dynamics, common challenges that arise, and practical strategies for fostering trust and communication.

Theoretical Framework

Trust is a multifaceted construct that plays a critical role in any intimate relationship, particularly in those involving power dynamics. According to Mayer, Davis, and Schoorman's model of trust, three key components contribute to trustworthiness: ability, benevolence, and integrity [?].

$$\text{Trustworthiness} = f(\text{Ability, Benevolence, Integrity}) \qquad (43)$$

- **Ability** refers to the partner's skills and competencies, which in the context of fisting, includes knowledge of techniques and safety practices. - **Benevolence** involves the partner's genuine care for the other's well-being, crucial in ensuring emotional and physical safety during play. - **Integrity** relates to the partner's adherence to moral and ethical principles, including honoring boundaries and consent.

Understanding these components can help partners navigate their dynamics and establish a deeper level of trust.

Common Challenges

Despite the best intentions, challenges can arise in power dynamics that may undermine trust and communication. Some common issues include:

1. **Miscommunication:** Power dynamics often involve nuanced negotiations about desires and boundaries. Misunderstandings can lead to feelings of betrayal or discomfort. 2. **Fear of Vulnerability:** Engaging in power exchange can evoke fears of exposure or rejection, making it difficult for partners to express their needs and concerns. 3. **Power Imbalance:** If one partner feels they have significantly more power, they may struggle to communicate openly, fearing that their partner will not take their concerns seriously. 4. **Past Trauma:** Previous negative experiences related to power dynamics can create barriers to trust, making it essential to approach communication with sensitivity.

Strategies for Building Trust and Communication

To overcome these challenges, partners can adopt several strategies:

1. **Establish Clear Boundaries** Initiate discussions about personal boundaries before engaging in power dynamics. Use clear language and encourage both partners to express their limits. This process not only clarifies expectations but also fosters a sense of safety.

2. **Use Active Listening Techniques** Active listening is crucial for effective communication. Partners should practice reflecting back what they hear, asking clarifying questions, and validating each other's feelings. This technique helps ensure that both partners feel heard and understood.

3. Create a Safe Word and Signals Establishing a safe word and non-verbal signals provides an immediate way to communicate discomfort or the need to pause. This practice reinforces the idea that both partners have equal power to halt the scene, enhancing trust.

4. Engage in Regular Check-Ins Regularly scheduled check-ins, both during and after scenes, allow partners to discuss their experiences, feelings, and any adjustments needed for future encounters. This practice can help identify and address any issues before they escalate.

5. Foster Emotional Vulnerability Encourage an environment where both partners can express their vulnerabilities without judgment. Sharing fears, desires, and past experiences can deepen intimacy and trust.

6. Prioritize Aftercare Aftercare is an essential component of power dynamics, providing emotional support and reassurance post-play. Engaging in aftercare rituals can help partners reconnect and solidify trust, reinforcing the idea that both partners care for each other's well-being.

7. Educate Together Engaging in educational opportunities, such as workshops or reading materials on power dynamics and fisting safety, can enhance both partners' understanding and skills. This shared learning experience can strengthen the bond and trust between partners.

Examples of Effective Communication in Power Dynamics

Consider the following scenarios that illustrate effective communication in power dynamics:

- **Scenario 1:** During a pre-scene discussion, Partner A expresses a desire to explore deeper penetration but also shares a past experience of discomfort. Partner B listens actively and suggests a gradual approach, using a safe word to pause if needed. This dialogue builds trust and ensures both partners feel safe exploring their desires.

- **Scenario 2:** After a fisting session, Partner A feels overwhelmed and shares this with Partner B. Instead of dismissing these feelings, Partner B validates them and offers comfort through aftercare practices, such as cuddling and discussing the experience. This approach reinforces the trust that both partners are committed to each other's emotional safety.

Conclusion

Building trust and communication in power dynamics is an ongoing process that requires intentionality and care. By establishing clear boundaries, practicing active listening, and prioritizing aftercare, partners can create a safe and fulfilling environment for exploring fisting and power exchange. Remember, trust is not a one-time achievement but a continuous journey that evolves with each interaction. Embrace the process, and allow your connection to deepen as you navigate the complexities of power dynamics together.

Fisting for Healing and Emotional Recovery

The Therapeutic Potential of Fisting

Fisting, often considered a taboo or extreme sexual practice, possesses significant therapeutic potential that can contribute to emotional healing, self-discovery, and the reclamation of bodily autonomy. This section explores the therapeutic aspects of fisting, emphasizing its role in trauma recovery, emotional release, and the enhancement of intimate connections.

Understanding the Therapeutic Framework

The therapeutic potential of fisting can be understood through various psychological and somatic frameworks. Notably, the work of Dr. Bessel van der Kolk in *The Body Keeps the Score* highlights how trauma is stored in the body and how physical experiences can facilitate healing. Fisting, as a deeply embodied practice, can serve as a means of reconnecting with one's body, allowing individuals to process and release stored trauma.

Reclaiming Agency and Empowerment

Fisting can be a powerful act of reclaiming agency over one's body. For individuals who have experienced trauma, particularly sexual trauma, engaging in consensual fisting can represent a profound shift from victimhood to empowerment. The act of choosing to engage in fisting allows individuals to assert control over their bodies and sexual experiences. This reclamation is crucial for healing, as it fosters a sense of autonomy and self-efficacy.

Emotional Release and Catharsis

The act of fisting can facilitate emotional release and catharsis. Many individuals report experiencing intense emotions during or after fisting, ranging from pleasure to vulnerability, and even anger or sadness. This emotional spectrum can be understood through the lens of somatic psychology, which posits that physical sensations and emotional experiences are interconnected. Engaging in fisting can provide a safe space for individuals to explore and express these emotions, ultimately leading to a sense of relief and release.

Navigating Pain and Pleasure

Fisting often involves navigating the complex relationship between pain and pleasure. This interplay can be therapeutic, as it encourages individuals to confront their discomfort and explore their limits. The concept of *edge play*—pushing boundaries while maintaining safety—can be applied here. By understanding and communicating about pain thresholds, individuals can develop a deeper awareness of their bodies and emotional states. This exploration can lead to increased resilience and a more nuanced understanding of personal boundaries.

Fisting as a Form of Active Meditation

Engaging in fisting can also be likened to a form of active meditation. The focus required during the practice encourages mindfulness, allowing individuals to be present in their bodies and sensations. This mindfulness can promote relaxation and reduce anxiety, contributing to overall emotional well-being. The rhythmic nature of fisting can create a meditative state, where individuals can experience a sense of flow and connection with themselves and their partners.

Therapeutic Techniques and Approaches

To harness the therapeutic potential of fisting, practitioners may consider incorporating specific techniques and approaches:

- **Trauma-Informed Practices:** Recognizing the impact of trauma on the body and mind, practitioners should create a safe environment that prioritizes consent and communication. This includes discussing triggers and establishing safe words.

- **Mindfulness and Breathwork:** Encouraging mindfulness and breath awareness during fisting can enhance the experience, allowing individuals to stay connected to their bodies and emotions. Techniques such as deep breathing can help manage anxiety and promote relaxation.

- **Aftercare:** Providing aftercare following a fisting session is essential for emotional and physical well-being. This may involve cuddling, verbal affirmations, or engaging in soothing activities to help individuals process their experiences.

- **Integration Sessions:** Following fisting experiences, individuals may benefit from integration sessions, where they can discuss their feelings and insights with a therapist or trusted partner. This can facilitate emotional processing and reinforce the therapeutic aspects of the experience.

Case Studies and Examples

Consider the case of *Alex*, a survivor of sexual trauma who found empowerment through fisting. Initially hesitant, Alex explored fisting with a trusted partner in a safe environment. The experience allowed Alex to reclaim agency over their body, leading to significant emotional release and a newfound sense of empowerment. Following the session, Alex engaged in aftercare, which facilitated further emotional processing and integration.

Another example is *Jordan*, who utilized fisting as a therapeutic tool in conjunction with somatic therapy. Through guided sessions, Jordan was able to confront and release stored emotions, ultimately leading to a deeper understanding of their relationship with pleasure and pain. The integration of mindfulness techniques enhanced Jordan's experience, allowing for a profound sense of healing.

Conclusion

The therapeutic potential of fisting extends beyond mere physical pleasure; it encompasses emotional healing, empowerment, and self-discovery. By approaching fisting with intentionality, mindfulness, and a focus on consent, individuals can unlock its profound benefits. As society continues to evolve in its understanding of sexuality and healing, fisting may emerge as a valuable tool in therapeutic contexts, fostering deeper connections with oneself and others.

In summary, the therapeutic aspects of fisting underscore the importance of body awareness, emotional release, and the reclamation of agency. As we navigate the complexities of human sexuality, it is essential to recognize and embrace the healing potential that lies within our most intimate experiences.

Trauma-Informed Approaches to Fisting

Trauma-informed care is a framework that recognizes the widespread impact of trauma on individuals and emphasizes the importance of creating a safe and supportive environment. When exploring fisting, it is crucial to adopt a trauma-informed approach to ensure that all participants feel secure, respected, and empowered. This section will discuss the principles of trauma-informed care, the potential trauma-related issues that may arise during fisting, and practical strategies for implementing these approaches.

Understanding Trauma

Trauma can result from various experiences, including physical, emotional, or sexual abuse, neglect, and significant life stressors. The effects of trauma can manifest in numerous ways, influencing an individual's emotional, psychological, and physical well-being. According to the *American Psychological Association*, trauma can lead to symptoms such as anxiety, depression, hypervigilance, and dissociation. These symptoms can impact a person's ability to engage in intimate activities, including fisting.

Principles of Trauma-Informed Care

1. **Safety**: Establishing a sense of physical and emotional safety is paramount. Participants should feel secure in their environment, knowing they can express their needs and boundaries without fear of judgment or violation.

2. **Trustworthiness and Transparency**: Open communication about intentions, boundaries, and expectations fosters trust. Participants should be encouraged to voice their concerns and desires, and all interactions should be characterized by honesty and integrity.

3. **Peer Support**: Encouraging connections with others who have shared experiences can provide a sense of belonging and validation. Peer support can help individuals process their feelings and experiences related to trauma.

4. **Collaboration**: Empowering individuals to take an active role in their fisting journey promotes autonomy and agency. This collaborative approach ensures that all participants have a say in the activities and can negotiate the terms of engagement.

5. **Empowerment**: Focusing on strengths and resilience rather than deficits helps individuals reclaim their sense of control. Empowerment can be fostered through education about their bodies, consent, and safe practices.

6. **Cultural, Historical, and Gender Issues**: Recognizing and respecting the diverse backgrounds and identities of participants is essential. This includes understanding how cultural and historical contexts shape individuals' experiences of trauma and intimacy.

Potential Trauma-Related Issues in Fisting

When engaging in fisting, various trauma-related issues may arise, including:

- **Triggers**: Certain physical sensations, positions, or contexts may evoke memories of past trauma. It is essential for participants to identify their triggers and communicate them clearly.
- **Dissociation**: Individuals with a history of trauma may experience dissociation during intense physical experiences, leading to a sense of detachment from their bodies. This can create confusion or anxiety during fisting.
- **Fear of Vulnerability**: The intimate nature of fisting can heighten feelings of vulnerability, which may be challenging for individuals with trauma histories. Participants may struggle with feelings of shame or inadequacy.
- **Trust Issues**: Past betrayals or violations can lead to difficulties in trusting partners during intimate acts. This can create barriers to communication and engagement in fisting.

Implementing Trauma-Informed Approaches in Fisting

To ensure a trauma-informed experience during fisting, consider the following strategies:

1. **Pre-Session Communication**: Before engaging in fisting, have an open and honest conversation about each participant's experiences, boundaries, and potential triggers. Discuss safe words, signals, and what to do if someone feels uncomfortable at any point.
2. **Establish a Safe Environment**: Create a physical space that feels secure and comfortable. This includes ensuring privacy, minimizing distractions, and providing supportive tools (e.g., pillows, blankets) to enhance comfort.
3. **Focus on Consent**: Emphasize the importance of enthusiastic consent. Remind participants that they have the right to withdraw consent at any time and that their comfort and safety are the top priority.
4. **Encourage Mindfulness**: Incorporate mindfulness techniques to help participants stay present and aware of their bodies. This can include breathing exercises, body scans, or grounding techniques to reduce anxiety and enhance connection.

5. **Aftercare**: Aftercare is essential for emotional processing and healing. Provide time for participants to discuss their experiences, feelings, and any challenges that arose during the session. This can help reinforce trust and connection.

6. **Seek Professional Support**: Encourage individuals to seek therapy or counseling if they have unresolved trauma that may impact their fisting experiences. A trauma-informed therapist can provide valuable support and coping strategies.

Case Example

Consider a scenario where two partners, Alex and Jamie, are exploring fisting for the first time. Alex has a history of sexual trauma, which makes them particularly sensitive to feelings of vulnerability and trust.

Before their session, Alex and Jamie engage in a thorough discussion about Alex's past experiences, identifying specific triggers and establishing safe words. They decide to create a safe space by dimming the lights, playing soothing music, and having pillows available for comfort.

During the session, Jamie remains attentive to Alex's verbal and non-verbal cues, checking in frequently to ensure Alex feels safe and comfortable. When Alex begins to feel overwhelmed, they use their safe word, and Jamie immediately stops, providing reassurance and space for Alex to process their feelings.

After the session, they engage in aftercare, discussing what went well and what could be improved. Alex expresses gratitude for Jamie's understanding and support, reinforcing their trust and connection.

By adopting a trauma-informed approach, Alex and Jamie are able to navigate the complexities of fisting while prioritizing emotional safety and mutual respect.

Conclusion

Implementing trauma-informed approaches to fisting is essential for creating a safe and supportive environment for all participants. By recognizing the potential impact of trauma, prioritizing communication and consent, and fostering empowerment, individuals can explore fisting in a way that honors their experiences and promotes healing. This approach not only enhances the physical experience but also deepens emotional connection and intimacy, paving the way for a fulfilling and transformative journey in fisting.

Reclaiming Power and Agency Through Fisting

Fisting, often perceived as a taboo or extreme sexual act, can serve as a powerful medium for individuals to reclaim their sense of power and agency over their bodies and sexual experiences. This reclamation is particularly significant in a society that frequently imposes restrictive narratives on sexuality, pleasure, and bodily autonomy. In this section, we will explore the psychological and emotional dimensions of fisting as a means of empowerment, drawing on relevant theories and examples to illustrate its potential for healing and self-discovery.

Understanding Power and Agency

Power and agency are fundamental concepts in the context of sexual expression. Power refers to the ability to influence or control one's own life and circumstances, while agency is the capacity to act independently and make choices. In sexual contexts, reclaiming power and agency often involves overcoming societal norms, personal fears, and past traumas that can inhibit one's ability to fully engage in and enjoy sexual experiences.

The Therapeutic Potential of Fisting

Fisting can act as a therapeutic tool for individuals seeking to reclaim their bodies and sexual identities. For many, the act of fisting transcends mere physicality; it becomes a profound exploration of trust, vulnerability, and empowerment. This therapeutic potential can be understood through several psychological theories:

- **Feminist Theory:** Feminist perspectives emphasize the importance of bodily autonomy and the right to pleasure. Fisting can challenge traditional narratives that often marginalize women's sexual desires, allowing individuals to assert their needs and preferences.

- **Trauma-Informed Care:** Recognizing that many individuals carry trauma related to their bodies or sexuality, a trauma-informed approach emphasizes safety, empowerment, and choice. Fisting, when approached consensually and safely, can facilitate a reclaiming of bodily autonomy and a positive re-engagement with one's sexuality.

- **Embodiment Theory:** This theory posits that our physical experiences are integral to our sense of self. Engaging in fisting can enhance body awareness, allowing individuals to reconnect with their bodies in a pleasurable and affirming way.

Navigating Personal Histories and Trauma

For many individuals, past experiences can create barriers to sexual expression. These may include histories of sexual trauma, societal stigmas, or internalized shame. Fisting can provide a unique opportunity to confront and navigate these challenges.

$$\text{Empowerment} = (\text{Awareness} + \text{Consent} + \text{Communication}) \times \text{Trust} \quad (44)$$

In this equation, empowerment is achieved through a combination of awareness of one's desires, the establishment of consent, effective communication, and the presence of trust between partners. Engaging in fisting can serve as a means of reclaiming one's narrative, transforming past experiences of powerlessness into acts of agency and choice.

Examples of Reclamation Through Fisting

1. **Personal Narratives:** Many individuals report that fisting has allowed them to explore their bodies in ways that were previously inaccessible. For instance, a person who has experienced sexual trauma may find that fisting, when done in a safe and consensual environment, helps them reclaim a sense of control over their body and sexual pleasure.

2. **Community and Connection:** Fisting can foster a sense of community among practitioners. Engaging with others who share similar interests can create a supportive environment where individuals feel empowered to explore their desires without judgment. This communal aspect can enhance feelings of belonging and acceptance, further reinforcing one's agency.

3. **Workshops and Education:** Many sex-positive workshops now include fisting as part of their curriculum, emphasizing safety, consent, and communication. Participants often leave these workshops feeling more empowered and knowledgeable about their bodies and desires, illustrating how education can facilitate reclamation.

The Role of Aftercare in Reclamation

Aftercare is a crucial component of any intense sexual experience, including fisting. It involves the emotional and physical care provided to partners after engaging in potentially intense or vulnerable activities. Aftercare can reinforce feelings of safety and trust, allowing individuals to process their experiences and reaffirm their agency.

$$\text{Aftercare} = (\text{Physical Comfort} + \text{Emotional Support}) \times \text{Trust} \qquad (45)$$

In this equation, aftercare is essential for maintaining the emotional well-being of participants and reinforcing the trust established during the act of fisting. By ensuring that both partners feel cared for and respected, aftercare can transform the experience into one of empowerment rather than vulnerability.

Conclusion: Embracing Empowerment through Fisting

Reclaiming power and agency through fisting is a multifaceted process that can lead to profound personal growth and healing. By understanding the psychological underpinnings of power dynamics, navigating personal histories, and engaging in supportive community practices, individuals can transform their experiences into powerful acts of self-affirmation. As we continue to explore the complexities of sexual expression, it is essential to recognize fisting not merely as a physical act but as a journey toward empowerment, intimacy, and self-discovery.

Fisting as a Form of Sexual Healing

Fisting, often regarded as a taboo or extreme sexual practice, can serve as a powerful tool for sexual healing and empowerment. This section explores the therapeutic potential of fisting, emphasizing its role in reclaiming agency, processing trauma, and fostering deeper intimacy between partners.

The Therapeutic Potential of Fisting

Engaging in fisting can facilitate profound experiences of connection and vulnerability, allowing individuals to explore their bodies in ways that promote healing. The act itself can be viewed through the lens of somatic therapy, which emphasizes the connection between the body and emotional well-being. According to [?], somatic therapies focus on bodily sensations and experiences to help individuals process trauma. Fisting, as a tactile and immersive experience, may enable participants to confront and release pent-up emotions, leading to catharsis and emotional release.

The therapeutic benefits of fisting can be understood through the framework of the **Polyvagal Theory** [?], which posits that safety and connection are essential for emotional regulation. When practiced consensually and safely, fisting can create a safe space for individuals to explore their boundaries and desires, fostering a sense of security that is conducive to healing. This safety allows individuals to access deeper emotional states, facilitating a journey toward self-discovery and healing.

Reclaiming Power and Agency Through Fisting

For many individuals, particularly those who have experienced trauma or abuse, fisting can be an act of reclamation. Engaging in a practice that may have once been associated with feelings of powerlessness can transform the experience into one of empowerment. By establishing clear boundaries and engaging in open communication, participants can redefine their relationship with their bodies and sexuality.

The act of fisting can symbolize a reclaiming of agency, as individuals take control of their sexual experiences. This empowerment can be particularly significant for survivors of sexual trauma. As noted by [?], the process of reclaiming one's body and sexuality is a crucial aspect of healing from trauma. By choosing to engage in fisting on their own terms, individuals can assert their autonomy and redefine their narratives around pleasure and pain.

Processing and Resolving Emotional Wounds

Fisting can also serve as a means of processing and resolving emotional wounds. The intensity of the experience may catalyze emotional release, allowing individuals to confront feelings of shame, guilt, or anger. This process can be likened to **exposure therapy**, where individuals gradually confront their fears in a safe environment. In the context of fisting, this exposure can lead to desensitization of negative associations with intimacy and touch.

For example, an individual who has experienced trauma related to penetration may find that engaging in fisting allows them to reclaim their body in a way that feels empowering and safe. Through careful and consensual exploration, they can navigate their fears and gradually expand their comfort zone, ultimately leading to healing and integration of their experiences.

Fisting and Body-Based Therapies

Integrating fisting into body-based therapies can enhance the healing process. Techniques such as mindfulness and breathwork can be employed alongside fisting to deepen the emotional and physical experience. Mindfulness practices encourage individuals to remain present with their sensations, fostering a heightened awareness of their bodies and emotional states.

Incorporating breathwork into fisting can also facilitate emotional release. As individuals engage in deep, intentional breathing, they may find it easier to process intense emotions that arise during the experience. This combination of physical and emotional awareness can create a holistic healing experience that honors both the body and mind.

Peer Support and Group Therapy for Fisters

The communal aspect of fisting can further enhance its therapeutic potential. Engaging in peer support or group therapy settings allows individuals to share their experiences, fostering a sense of belonging and understanding. As noted by [?], group therapy can provide individuals with the opportunity to learn from others, gain new perspectives, and feel less isolated in their experiences.

Participating in workshops or support groups specifically focused on fisting can create a safe space for individuals to explore their desires and concerns. This shared exploration can lead to greater acceptance of one's sexuality and a reduction in feelings of shame or stigma.

Fisting in the Context of Sex Therapy

Sex therapists may incorporate fisting into their practice as a means of addressing issues related to intimacy, trust, and pleasure. By guiding clients through the process of safe and consensual fisting, therapists can help individuals explore their boundaries and desires in a supportive environment. This therapeutic approach can foster open communication between partners, enhancing their emotional connection and intimacy.

In conclusion, fisting can serve as a powerful form of sexual healing, allowing individuals to reclaim their bodies, process emotional wounds, and foster deeper connections with their partners. By integrating fisting into therapeutic practices, individuals can embark on a journey of self-discovery and empowerment, ultimately leading to a more fulfilling and liberated sexual experience.

Navigating Intergenerational Trauma in Fisting Play

Intergenerational trauma refers to the transmission of the effects of trauma from one generation to another. This phenomenon can profoundly impact individuals' sexual experiences, including practices such as fisting. Understanding how intergenerational trauma manifests in fisting play is crucial for fostering a safe and supportive environment for exploration.

Theoretical Framework

The concept of intergenerational trauma is rooted in several psychological theories, including attachment theory and the social learning theory. Attachment theory posits that early relationships with caregivers shape an individual's ability to form secure attachments later in life [?]. When caregivers experience trauma, their responses can create an environment of fear, anxiety, or neglect, affecting their children's emotional and relational development.

Social learning theory suggests that behaviors, including sexual practices and attitudes, are learned through observation and imitation [?]. If children observe their caregivers engaging in unhealthy sexual dynamics or experiencing trauma, they may internalize these patterns, which can influence their own sexual behaviors, desires, and boundaries.

Problems Associated with Intergenerational Trauma

1. **Fear and Anxiety**: Individuals with a history of intergenerational trauma may experience heightened anxiety or fear surrounding intimacy and vulnerability. This can create barriers to fully engaging in fisting play, where trust and openness are essential.

2. **Shame and Guilt**: Feelings of shame or guilt may arise from internalized beliefs about sexuality that have been passed down through generations. This can lead to conflicts between desires for exploration and ingrained beliefs about what is acceptable.

3. **Difficulty with Boundaries**: Trauma can disrupt an individual's ability to establish and maintain healthy boundaries. In fisting play, where consent and limits are paramount, this can lead to challenges in communication and the potential for crossing personal boundaries.

4. **Reenactment of Trauma**: Some individuals may unconsciously reenact traumatic experiences during sexual encounters, including fisting. This can manifest as a desire to regain control or process unresolved feelings related to the original trauma.

Examples of Intergenerational Trauma in Fisting Play

1. **Family Dynamics**: An individual raised in a household where sexual expression was stigmatized may approach fisting with trepidation, fearing judgment or rejection. For example, a person may feel conflicted about their desire to explore fisting due to their upbringing, where open discussions about sexuality were discouraged.

2. **Cultural Influences**: In cultures with strict norms surrounding sexuality, individuals may carry the weight of these beliefs into their intimate relationships. For instance, someone from a conservative background might struggle with feelings of shame when considering fisting, viewing it as a taboo act that contradicts their cultural teachings.

3. **Previous Trauma**: A person who has experienced sexual trauma may find themselves triggered during fisting play, especially if they have not adequately processed their experiences. This can lead to emotional withdrawal or panic during what should be an intimate experience.

Strategies for Navigating Intergenerational Trauma

1. **Open Communication**: Establishing a foundation of open dialogue with partners is essential. Discussing feelings, fears, and past experiences can help create a safe space for exploration. Utilizing tools such as active listening and non-judgmental responses can foster trust.

2. **Therapeutic Support**: Seeking therapy, particularly trauma-informed therapy, can provide individuals with tools to navigate their experiences and emotions. Therapists can help clients process intergenerational trauma and develop healthier coping mechanisms for intimacy.

3. **Setting Boundaries**: Clearly defining personal boundaries and limits before engaging in fisting play can help individuals feel more secure. Discussing safe words and signals ensures that all parties feel comfortable and respected throughout the experience.

4. **Mindfulness Practices**: Incorporating mindfulness techniques can assist individuals in grounding themselves during fisting play. Practicing awareness of bodily sensations and emotions can help mitigate anxiety and allow for a more enjoyable experience.

5. **Education and Empowerment**: Educating oneself about fisting techniques, safety, and emotional aspects can empower individuals to engage in fisting play with confidence. Understanding the mechanics and emotional implications can demystify the practice and reduce fear.

Conclusion

Navigating intergenerational trauma in fisting play requires awareness, compassion, and intentionality. By understanding the ways trauma can influence sexual expression and relationships, individuals can create healthier dynamics that honor their desires while addressing past wounds. Fostering open communication, seeking therapeutic support, and establishing clear boundaries are vital steps in transforming fisting from a potential source of anxiety into an empowering and liberating experience.

Processing and Resolving Emotional Wounds

Engaging in fisting can elicit a wide range of emotional responses, particularly for individuals with past traumas or unresolved emotional wounds. Understanding how to process and resolve these emotional wounds is essential for fostering a safe and fulfilling fisting experience. This section will explore the psychological theories relevant to emotional healing, the common issues that may arise, and practical strategies to address these challenges.

Theoretical Frameworks

Several psychological theories provide insight into the processing and resolution of emotional wounds. Key frameworks include:

- **Attachment Theory:** This theory posits that early relationships with caregivers shape our ability to form secure attachments in adulthood. In the context of fisting, individuals with insecure attachment styles may struggle with trust and vulnerability, making it essential to establish a safe environment.

- **Trauma-Informed Care:** This approach emphasizes understanding the impact of trauma on an individual's life. Recognizing triggers, creating safety, and promoting empowerment are critical components that can enhance the fisting experience for those with trauma histories.

- **Somatic Experiencing:** This therapeutic approach focuses on the body's sensations and experiences as a pathway to healing trauma. Somatic techniques can help individuals reconnect with their bodies and process emotional wounds that may arise during fisting.

Common Emotional Issues

When exploring fisting, individuals may encounter various emotional issues, including:

- **Fear and Anxiety:** Concerns about vulnerability, bodily harm, or the potential for emotional distress can create anxiety. This fear may stem from past experiences of trauma or negative associations with intimacy.

- **Shame and Guilt:** Engaging in fisting may provoke feelings of shame or guilt, particularly if individuals internalize societal taboos surrounding sexual practices. These feelings can hinder the ability to enjoy the experience fully.

- **Trust Issues:** Individuals with a history of betrayal or abandonment may struggle to trust their partners during fisting. This lack of trust can lead to heightened anxiety and difficulty in surrendering to the experience.

- **Emotional Triggers:** Certain sensations or scenarios during fisting may trigger memories of past trauma, leading to overwhelming emotional responses. Recognizing these triggers is vital for managing emotional reactions.

Strategies for Processing Emotional Wounds

To effectively process and resolve emotional wounds associated with fisting, consider the following strategies:

- **Establish a Safe Space:** Create an environment where both partners feel secure and comfortable. This includes open communication about limits, desires, and boundaries. Establishing safe words and signals can help navigate any discomfort that arises.

- **Engage in Pre-Scene Discussions:** Prior to engaging in fisting, partners should have open conversations about their emotional histories, triggers, and any concerns. This dialogue fosters understanding and builds trust.

- **Practice Mindfulness Techniques:** Mindfulness can help individuals stay present and grounded during fisting. Techniques such as deep breathing, body scans, and focusing on sensations can aid in processing emotions as they arise.

- **Utilize Aftercare Practices:** Aftercare is crucial in addressing emotional wounds. This may involve physical comfort, verbal affirmations, or simply spending time together to process the experience. Discussing feelings post-scene can help partners understand each other's emotional states.

- **Seek Professional Support:** For individuals with significant emotional wounds or trauma histories, working with a therapist who specializes in trauma-informed care can be beneficial. Therapy can provide tools for processing emotions and building resilience.

- **Journaling and Reflection:** Encouraging individuals to keep a journal of their experiences can help in processing emotions. Reflecting on feelings before and after fisting sessions can illuminate patterns and facilitate healing.

- **Gradual Exposure:** For those with intense fears or anxieties, gradual exposure to fisting can help desensitize emotional responses. Starting with less invasive forms of intimacy and slowly progressing can build confidence and trust.

- **Community Support:** Engaging with supportive communities, whether online or in-person, can provide a sense of belonging and understanding. Sharing experiences with others who have similar journeys can foster healing and connection.

Examples of Processing Emotional Wounds

Consider the following scenarios that illustrate the importance of processing emotional wounds in the context of fisting:

- **Scenario 1: Trust Building** - A couple, Alex and Jamie, decide to explore fisting after discussing their desires. Jamie has a history of abandonment issues and feels anxious about surrendering control. They establish a safe word and agree to take breaks if Jamie feels overwhelmed. By openly communicating throughout the experience, Jamie is able to gradually build trust and feel more secure.

- **Scenario 2: Managing Triggers** - During a fisting session, Sam experiences a sudden wave of anxiety triggered by a specific sensation. Recognizing this as a trigger, they communicate with their partner and take a break. After discussing the feelings that arose, they realize the sensation reminded Sam of a past trauma. This awareness allows them to process the emotion and adjust their approach in future sessions.

- **Scenario 3: Aftercare and Reflection** - After a fisting session, Taylor and Morgan engage in aftercare, discussing what felt good and what was challenging. Taylor expresses feelings of shame that surfaced during the experience. Morgan reassures Taylor and emphasizes the importance of their shared exploration. This post-scene debriefing fosters emotional intimacy and helps Taylor process their feelings.

Conclusion

Processing and resolving emotional wounds is a vital aspect of exploring fisting safely and consensually. By understanding the emotional complexities involved, establishing a supportive environment, and utilizing effective strategies, individuals can navigate their emotional landscapes and enhance their fisting experiences. Ultimately, this journey can lead to greater intimacy, trust, and self-discovery, enriching both personal and shared sexual explorations.

Fisting and Body-Based Therapies

Fisting, as an intimate and deeply physical practice, can intersect with various forms of body-based therapies, offering unique opportunities for healing, self-exploration, and empowerment. This section delves into the therapeutic potential of fisting, exploring how it can be integrated into body-based therapeutic practices to foster emotional recovery, enhance body awareness, and promote holistic well-being.

Understanding Body-Based Therapies

Body-based therapies encompass a wide range of practices that prioritize the connection between the mind and body. These therapies, including somatic experiencing, bodywork, and trauma-informed approaches, emphasize the role of physical sensations, movement, and touch in healing emotional and psychological wounds. The foundational premise of body-based therapies is that the body holds memories and experiences that can affect mental and emotional health.

The Therapeutic Potential of Fisting

Fisting can serve as a powerful tool for therapeutic exploration. The act of fisting, when approached with consent, care, and intention, can create a profound sense of connection between partners. This connection can facilitate emotional release and catharsis, allowing individuals to confront and process feelings that may have been suppressed or unacknowledged.

1. **Emotional Release and Catharsis** The physical act of fisting can trigger intense emotional responses, leading to catharsis. For some, the experience may evoke feelings of joy, empowerment, or liberation, while for others, it may bring forth repressed emotions such as sadness or anger. This emotional release can be therapeutic, providing a safe space to explore and express feelings that have been difficult to articulate.

2. **Reclaiming Power and Agency** For individuals who have experienced trauma, fisting can symbolize a reclamation of power and agency over one's body. Engaging in fisting can help individuals redefine their relationship with their bodies, transforming a potentially traumatic experience into one of empowerment and choice. This process can be particularly healing for those who have felt disempowered in their sexual experiences.

Integrating Fisting into Body-Based Therapies

To effectively integrate fisting into body-based therapies, practitioners must prioritize safety, consent, and emotional support. Here are several approaches to consider:

1. **Somatic Experiencing** Somatic experiencing is a therapeutic approach that focuses on the body's sensations to process trauma. Incorporating fisting into somatic therapy can help clients reconnect with their bodies and explore physical sensations in a safe and supportive environment. Therapists may guide clients through breathwork and grounding techniques to facilitate a deeper awareness of their bodily experiences during fisting.

2. **Bodywork and Massage Therapy** Integrating fisting into bodywork or massage therapy can enhance the therapeutic experience. Practitioners can focus on the pelvic floor and surrounding muscles, using fisting as a means to release tension and promote relaxation. This can be particularly beneficial for individuals experiencing pelvic pain or discomfort, as fisting can help increase blood flow and improve muscle elasticity.

3. **Trauma-Informed Approaches** When working with individuals who have experienced trauma, it is essential to adopt a trauma-informed approach. This includes establishing a safe and trusting environment, allowing clients to set their own boundaries, and prioritizing consent at every stage of the process. Fisting can

be introduced as a therapeutic option, with clients encouraged to communicate their needs and desires openly.

Challenges and Considerations

While fisting can offer therapeutic benefits, it is essential to acknowledge potential challenges and considerations:

1. Emotional Triggers Fisting may evoke strong emotional reactions, which can be both positive and negative. Practitioners should be prepared to navigate these emotional responses and provide support to clients as they process their feelings. It is crucial to create a safe space for clients to express their emotions and to offer aftercare following fisting sessions.

2. Physical Risks As with any intimate practice, there are physical risks associated with fisting. Practitioners must emphasize the importance of safety protocols, including proper hygiene, lubrication, and communication about limits. Educating clients on the physical aspects of fisting can help mitigate risks and enhance the overall experience.

3. Consent and Boundaries Consent is paramount in any therapeutic context, especially when incorporating fisting. Practitioners should encourage open dialogue about consent, boundaries, and comfort levels, ensuring that clients feel empowered to express their needs and desires throughout the process.

Examples of Fisting in Body-Based Therapy

To illustrate the therapeutic potential of fisting, consider the following examples:

1. Empowerment Workshops Some body-based therapy workshops incorporate fisting as a means of exploring empowerment and body positivity. Participants engage in discussions about consent, boundaries, and body image before practicing fisting techniques in a safe and supportive environment. This approach encourages participants to reclaim their bodies and cultivate a sense of agency.

2. Individual Therapy Sessions In individual therapy sessions, a therapist may introduce fisting as a tool for exploring body awareness and emotional release. The therapist guides the client through breathwork and mindfulness exercises, allowing them to connect with their physical sensations during fisting. This process can facilitate emotional healing and promote a deeper understanding of the mind-body connection.

Conclusion

Fisting, when approached with care, consent, and intention, can be a valuable addition to body-based therapies. By fostering emotional release, reclaiming power, and enhancing body awareness, fisting can support individuals on their healing journeys. Practitioners must prioritize safety, communication, and emotional support to ensure that clients can explore this intimate practice in a therapeutic context. As we continue to expand our understanding of the mind-body connection, integrating fisting into body-based therapies offers new avenues for healing and self-discovery.

Fisting in the Context of Sex Therapy

Fisting, often regarded as a taboo practice, can serve as a powerful tool within the realm of sex therapy. This section explores how fisting can be integrated into therapeutic practices, the potential benefits, and the considerations therapists must keep in mind when addressing this subject with clients.

The Therapeutic Potential of Fisting

Fisting can facilitate profound emotional and physical experiences, enabling individuals to explore their bodies and boundaries in a safe and consensual environment. The therapeutic potential of fisting lies in its ability to:

- Enhance body awareness and acceptance.
- Promote open communication about desires and boundaries.
- Foster intimacy and trust between partners.
- Provide a means for emotional release and catharsis.

Therapists may utilize fisting as a method to help clients confront fears, shame, or trauma related to their bodies and sexuality. By creating a safe space for exploration, clients can work through their emotions and build resilience.

Addressing Concerns and Misconceptions

When introducing fisting into sex therapy, it's crucial to address common concerns and misconceptions. Many individuals may associate fisting with pain or injury. Educating clients about the importance of preparation, consent, and communication can alleviate these fears. For instance, therapists can explain:

- The significance of gradual exploration and warming up.
- The necessity of using ample lubrication and proper hygiene.
- How to establish safe words and signals to ensure comfort and safety.

By demystifying the practice, clients may feel more empowered to explore fisting as a healthy expression of their sexuality.

Integrating Fisting into Therapeutic Practices

Therapists can integrate fisting into their practices through various approaches, such as:

- **Psychoeducation:** Providing clients with information on anatomy, pleasure, and safety can help them make informed decisions about their sexual practices.
- **Role-Playing:** Engaging clients in role-playing scenarios can help them practice communication and boundary-setting in a controlled environment.
- **Mindfulness Techniques:** Encouraging clients to practice mindfulness during fisting can enhance their connection to their bodies and promote emotional awareness.

Case Studies and Examples

To illustrate the therapeutic benefits of fisting, consider the following hypothetical case studies:

Case Study 1: Overcoming Trauma A client who experienced sexual trauma may find it challenging to engage in intimate relationships. Through sex therapy, the therapist introduces fisting as a means of reclaiming agency over their body. With careful guidance, the client gradually explores fisting, focusing on their comfort levels and boundaries. This process fosters a sense of empowerment, allowing the client to reconnect with their body and sexuality.

Case Study 2: Enhancing Intimacy A couple struggling with intimacy issues may benefit from incorporating fisting into their sexual repertoire. The therapist facilitates discussions about desires and boundaries, encouraging the couple to communicate openly. As they explore fisting together, they experience increased trust and vulnerability, leading to a deeper emotional connection.

Ethical Considerations in Therapy

When addressing fisting in the context of sex therapy, therapists must adhere to ethical guidelines, including:

- **Informed Consent:** Clients should be fully informed about the potential risks and benefits of fisting before engaging in any exploration.
- **Cultural Sensitivity:** Recognizing that attitudes toward fisting may vary across different cultures and communities is essential. Therapists should approach the topic with sensitivity and openness.
- **Professional Boundaries:** Therapists must maintain appropriate boundaries and avoid any dual relationships that could compromise the therapeutic process.

Conclusion

Fisting, when approached with care and understanding, can be a valuable component of sex therapy. By fostering open communication, addressing fears, and promoting body positivity, therapists can help clients navigate their sexual desires in a safe and empowering manner. As societal attitudes toward sexuality continue to evolve, integrating practices like fisting into therapeutic contexts can contribute to a more holistic understanding of sexual health and well-being.

$$\text{Therapeutic Outcome} = \text{Body Awareness} + \text{Communication} + \text{Emotional Release} \tag{46}$$

Peer Support and Group Therapy for Fisters

Peer support and group therapy can play a crucial role in the journey of individuals exploring fisting as a form of sexual expression. This section delves into the significance of community support, the therapeutic benefits of group dynamics, and practical considerations for those seeking to engage in peer-led or facilitated therapeutic environments.

The Importance of Community Support

The exploration of fisting can often evoke a range of emotions, including excitement, vulnerability, and sometimes even shame. Engaging with a community of like-minded individuals can help mitigate feelings of isolation and provide a safe space for sharing experiences. Community support serves several essential functions:

- **Validation:** Sharing experiences with peers can validate feelings and desires that may be stigmatized or misunderstood by broader society. This affirmation can reduce internalized shame and encourage self-acceptance.

- **Shared Knowledge:** Group settings allow for the exchange of knowledge and experiences. Members can share techniques, safety practices, and emotional coping strategies, enriching the collective understanding of fisting.

- **Emotional Support:** Engaging in discussions about experiences can foster emotional resilience. Members can provide comfort and reassurance, helping each other navigate the complexities of their journeys.

Therapeutic Benefits of Group Dynamics

Group therapy can offer unique therapeutic benefits distinct from one-on-one therapy. The dynamics of a group can facilitate deeper connections and understanding among participants. Some key therapeutic aspects include:

- **Normalization of Experiences:** Hearing others share similar experiences can normalize feelings of anxiety, fear, or excitement related to fisting. This normalization can diminish feelings of being "different" or "abnormal."

- **Role Modeling:** Participants can observe and learn from the coping mechanisms and strategies employed by others. This role modeling can inspire individuals to adopt healthier approaches to their own challenges.

- **Collective Empowerment:** Group settings can foster a sense of collective empowerment, where participants support each other's growth and exploration. This empowerment can be particularly significant in a context where societal stigma exists.

Facilitating Peer Support Groups

Creating a supportive peer group requires intentionality and care. Here are some considerations for establishing a successful peer support group for fisters:

- **Establishing Ground Rules:** Setting clear guidelines for confidentiality, respect, and consent is essential. This creates a safe environment where participants feel comfortable sharing personal experiences.

- **Inclusive Practices:** Ensure that the group is inclusive and respectful of diverse identities and experiences. This may involve actively seeking out participants from various backgrounds and orientations.

- **Facilitator Training:** If the group is facilitated, the leader should have training in group dynamics and an understanding of the emotional complexities surrounding fisting. This training can help navigate sensitive topics and foster a supportive atmosphere.

Examples of Peer Support Initiatives

Several organizations and communities have successfully implemented peer support initiatives for individuals exploring fisting and other sexual practices. These examples can serve as inspiration for creating similar groups:

- **Online Forums:** Many online platforms host forums where individuals can discuss their experiences with fisting. These forums often include moderated discussions, allowing members to ask questions and share insights in a safe space.

- **Local Meetups:** Some communities organize regular meetups for individuals interested in fisting. These gatherings provide opportunities for socialization, education, and skill-sharing in a relaxed environment.

- **Workshops and Retreats:** Specialized workshops focusing on fisting techniques, safety, and emotional aspects can provide structured learning opportunities. Retreats may offer immersive experiences where participants can engage deeply with their interests in a supportive setting.

Addressing Challenges in Peer Support

While peer support can be immensely beneficial, it is essential to recognize and address potential challenges:

- **Conflict Resolution:** Conflicts may arise within groups due to differing opinions or experiences. Establishing protocols for conflict resolution can help maintain a positive environment.

- **Navigating Emotional Triggers:** Discussions around fisting may trigger past traumas for some participants. It is vital for facilitators to be aware of these dynamics and to provide support or resources for individuals who may need additional help.

- **Maintaining Boundaries:** Participants should be encouraged to communicate their boundaries clearly. This includes discussing what topics are comfortable to explore and what should be avoided.

Conclusion

Peer support and group therapy for fisters can provide invaluable resources for individuals exploring the nuances of fisting. By fostering a sense of community, sharing knowledge, and offering emotional support, these groups can help individuals navigate their journeys with greater confidence and safety. As the stigma surrounding fisting continues to be challenged, the importance of supportive spaces cannot be overstated. Engaging in peer support not only enhances personal exploration but also contributes to broader efforts to destigmatize and normalize diverse sexual practices.

Sacred Sexuality and Fisting for Spiritual Healing

The intersection of sacred sexuality and fisting presents a unique opportunity for individuals to explore their spirituality through the lens of physical intimacy. Sacred sexuality refers to the practice of engaging in sexual experiences that are deeply connected to one's spiritual beliefs and personal growth. This section will delve into how fisting can be integrated into sacred sexuality, facilitating spiritual healing and transformation.

Theoretical Foundations

Sacred sexuality is rooted in various spiritual traditions, including Tantra, Shamanism, and certain branches of Neo-Paganism. These traditions emphasize the connection between sexual energy and spiritual awakening. Sexual energy, often referred to as *Kundalini* in Tantric practices, is believed to be a powerful force that can lead to higher states of consciousness when harnessed correctly. Fisting, as a form of intimate exploration, can serve as a conduit for this energy, allowing practitioners to transcend the physical and connect with their spiritual selves.

Transformative Experiences

Engaging in fisting as a sacred sexual practice can lead to profound experiences of emotional release and spiritual awakening. The act itself, when performed with intention and mindfulness, can create a space for participants to explore vulnerability, trust, and surrender. This process can be likened to a form of active meditation, where the focus on breath and bodily sensations allows individuals to enter altered states of consciousness.

For example, a couple may choose to incorporate fisting into their sacred sexuality practice by setting a clear intention for their session. They might begin with a ritualistic preparation, such as lighting candles, playing soft music, or engaging in breathing exercises. This intentionality transforms the act of fisting from a purely physical experience into a spiritual journey, fostering a deeper connection between partners.

Healing Through Intimacy

Fisting can also serve as a powerful tool for emotional and spiritual healing. Many individuals carry trauma related to their bodies, sexuality, or past relationships. The intimate nature of fisting allows for a safe space to confront and release these traumas. The process of surrendering to another person during fisting can create a sense of safety and acceptance, allowing for the healing of deep-seated emotional wounds.

Consider a scenario where an individual who has experienced sexual trauma engages in fisting as a form of reclaiming their body. Through this practice, they can learn to experience pleasure in a controlled and consensual environment, gradually rebuilding their relationship with their body and sexuality. The act of fisting, when approached with care and sensitivity, can facilitate a journey toward self-acceptance and empowerment.

Challenges and Considerations

While the integration of fisting into sacred sexuality can be transformative, it is essential to approach this practice with caution and awareness. The potential for emotional triggers and past trauma to resurface must be acknowledged. Participants should engage in thorough communication before exploring fisting, discussing boundaries, fears, and desires openly.

Additionally, the spiritual aspect of fisting requires a commitment to mindfulness and presence. Practitioners should be aware of their own emotional states and those of their partners, ensuring that the experience remains consensual and supportive. Utilizing aftercare practices post-session can help individuals process their experiences and reinforce emotional safety.

Examples of Sacred Fisting Practices

Several practices can be adopted to integrate fisting into sacred sexuality effectively:

- **Ritualistic Preparation:** Create a sacred space by incorporating elements such as crystals, incense, or sacred texts that resonate with your spiritual beliefs. This environment can enhance the spiritual experience of fisting.

- **Mindful Breathing:** Engage in synchronized breathing exercises before and during the fisting experience. This practice can help both partners maintain a connection to their bodies and the present moment, fostering a deeper sense of intimacy.

- **Setting Intentions:** Before beginning, partners can take a moment to express their intentions for the session. This could involve personal goals for healing, connection, or exploration, creating a shared focus that deepens the experience.

- **Post-Session Reflection:** After the session, partners can engage in a debriefing ritual, sharing their feelings and sensations experienced during fisting. This practice reinforces emotional connection and allows for any necessary healing discussions.

Conclusion

Integrating fisting into sacred sexuality practices can be a deeply enriching experience, offering pathways for emotional healing and spiritual growth. By approaching this practice with intention, mindfulness, and open communication, individuals can explore the profound connection between their bodies and their spiritual selves. As with any intimate practice, the key lies in creating a safe and supportive environment that honors the complexities of human sexuality and the sacredness of shared experiences.

Exploring Fisting in Different Relationships and Communities

Exploring Fisting in Different Relationships and Communities

Exploring Fisting in Different Relationships and Communities

Fisting, often considered a taboo or niche sexual practice, can be explored across various types of relationships and communities. Understanding the dynamics of fisting within different contexts can enhance the experience, promote safety, and foster deeper intimacy. This section aims to illuminate the multifaceted nature of fisting, examining how it manifests in heterosexual relationships, LGBTQ+ partnerships, and BDSM or kink communities.

The Dynamics of Fisting Across Relationships

Fisting is not merely a physical act; it is deeply intertwined with emotional, psychological, and social dimensions. Each relationship type brings its unique set of dynamics, which can influence how fisting is approached, understood, and practiced.

Heterosexual Relationships In heterosexual relationships, fisting may be approached with a blend of curiosity and apprehension. Traditional gender roles and societal expectations can create barriers to open communication about desires and boundaries. Research indicates that many heterosexual couples may struggle with discussing sexual preferences due to fear of judgment or misunderstanding. For example, a study by [Smith(2020)] highlights that women often feel pressure to conform to normative sexual behaviors, which can stifle their exploration of practices like fisting.

To navigate these challenges, couples should prioritize open dialogue. Establishing a safe space for discussing fantasies can help couples overcome societal stigma. Utilizing tools such as consent checklists and safe words can facilitate communication and ensure that both partners feel comfortable exploring fisting.

LGBTQ+ Relationships In LGBTQ+ communities, fisting often holds a different cultural significance. It can serve as a powerful expression of identity and liberation from heteronormative constraints. The historical context of fisting within gay male communities, for instance, has roots in sexual liberation movements, where it emerged as a form of intimacy and connection.

[Jones(2019)] notes that fisting can also be a way to challenge societal norms surrounding masculinity and sexuality. In LGBTQ+ relationships, discussions around fisting may incorporate themes of empowerment and self-acceptance. However, challenges still exist, particularly concerning stigma and discrimination from outside the community. Open discussions about desires and boundaries remain critical in fostering a safe environment for exploration.

BDSM and Kink Communities Within BDSM and kink communities, fisting often takes on a more structured approach, emphasizing consent, negotiation, and safety. The principles of Risk-Aware Consensual Kink (RACK) and Safe, Sane, and Consensual (SSC) guide practitioners in navigating the complexities of power dynamics and physical limits. Fisting can be integrated into BDSM scenes as a form of power exchange, where the act itself becomes a manifestation of trust and vulnerability.

[Taylor(2021)] emphasizes that in these communities, fisting is frequently accompanied by aftercare practices, which are essential for emotional and physical recovery post-scene. This integration of care highlights the importance of emotional safety, particularly in activities that can evoke intense feelings or trauma responses.

Challenges and Considerations

While fisting can be a fulfilling and intimate experience, it is essential to acknowledge the challenges that may arise within different relationships and communities.

Communication Barriers One of the most significant barriers to exploring fisting is communication. Partners may fear vulnerability, leading to unexpressed desires or misconceptions about the practice. For example, a partner may assume that their desire to fist is unacceptable or that it will be met with rejection. This fear can prevent open dialogue and limit exploration.

Stigma and Misconceptions Stigma surrounding fisting can also create challenges. Misconceptions about the act—such as it being inherently dangerous or associated with violence—can deter individuals from exploring it. Educational resources and community support can help dispel these myths, fostering a more informed and accepting environment.

Physical and Emotional Safety Physical safety is paramount when exploring fisting, regardless of the relationship context. Partners should engage in thorough discussions about boundaries, limits, and safe practices. Emotional safety is equally important, as fisting can evoke intense feelings. Acknowledging and addressing these emotions can enhance the experience and strengthen the bond between partners.

Conclusion

Exploring fisting within various relationships and communities offers opportunities for growth, intimacy, and self-discovery. By fostering open communication, addressing stigma, and prioritizing safety, individuals can navigate the complexities of fisting in a way that honors their desires and builds deeper connections. As societal norms continue to evolve, the potential for fisting to serve as a bridge for intimacy and empowerment remains significant, inviting individuals to embrace their sexuality in all its forms.

Bibliography

[Smith(2020)] Smith, J. (2020). *Breaking the Silence: Communication in Heterosexual Relationships*. Journal of Sexual Health, 12(3), 45-60.

[Jones(2019)] Jones, A. (2019). *Fisting and Identity: Exploring LGBTQ+ Sexual Practices*. Sexuality Research and Social Policy, 16(4), 299-310.

[Taylor(2021)] Taylor, R. (2021). *The Art of Aftercare in BDSM: Emotional Recovery and Safety*. Kink Studies Journal, 5(2), 67-82.

Fisting in Heterosexual Relationships

Overcoming Heteronormative Taboos and Myths

In contemporary discussions surrounding sexuality, particularly in the realm of kink and BDSM, the act of fisting often encounters a myriad of heteronormative taboos and myths. These societal constructs can inhibit exploration and enjoyment of this intimate practice among heterosexual couples. Understanding and dismantling these barriers is crucial for fostering a more inclusive and liberated sexual experience.

Defining Heteronormativity

Heteronormativity refers to the cultural bias that privileges heterosexual relationships and norms, often marginalizing other sexual orientations and practices. This framework posits heterosexuality as the default mode of sexual expression, leading to the stigmatization of non-conforming behaviors, such as fisting.

Common Myths about Fisting in Heterosexual Contexts

One prevalent myth is the belief that fisting is inherently violent or aggressive. This misconception can stem from media portrayals that emphasize the extremes of kink without providing context about consent, communication, and mutual pleasure. In reality, fisting, like any sexual activity, can be a deeply intimate and consensual act when approached with care and understanding.

Another myth is the idea that fisting is only for those who identify with the LGBTQ+ community. This notion perpetuates the false belief that heterosexual couples should adhere strictly to traditional sexual practices. In truth, fisting can be a fulfilling exploration of intimacy for all couples, regardless of sexual orientation.

Addressing Stigma through Education

Education plays a pivotal role in overcoming these taboos. By providing accurate information about fisting, couples can dispel myths and foster a more open dialogue about desires and boundaries. Resources such as workshops, literature, and community discussions can help normalize the practice and encourage individuals to explore their fantasies without shame.

For example, couples can engage in conversations that explore their interests in fisting, addressing any fears or misconceptions they may have. This dialogue can include discussing previous experiences, setting boundaries, and establishing safe words to ensure comfort and safety throughout the experience.

The Role of Consent and Communication

Central to overcoming taboos is the emphasis on consent and communication. Establishing a foundation of trust allows couples to explore fisting in a way that feels safe and pleasurable. This process involves:

- **Active Listening:** Partners should practice active listening to understand each other's perspectives and feelings about fisting. This ensures that both individuals feel heard and respected.

- **Setting Boundaries:** Discussing personal limits and comfort levels is essential. Each partner should feel empowered to express their boundaries without fear of judgment.

- **Establishing Safe Words:** Safe words provide a mechanism for partners to communicate when they need to pause or stop an activity. This practice reinforces the importance of consent and mutual respect.

Challenging Cultural Narratives

Cultural narratives surrounding sexuality often emphasize penetrative intercourse as the primary means of sexual fulfillment. Fisting challenges this narrative by offering alternative pathways to pleasure. By embracing fisting, heterosexual couples can redefine their sexual experiences and explore new dimensions of intimacy.

Conclusion

Overcoming heteronormative taboos and myths surrounding fisting is essential for fostering a more inclusive and fulfilling sexual landscape. Through education, open communication, and a commitment to consent, couples can navigate these barriers and explore fisting as a legitimate expression of intimacy and pleasure. By challenging societal norms, we not only empower ourselves but also contribute to a broader cultural acceptance of diverse sexual practices.

In summary, the journey towards embracing fisting within heterosexual relationships requires a conscious effort to dismantle ingrained taboos and myths. As we cultivate understanding and acceptance, we pave the way for deeper connections and enriched sexual experiences, ultimately enhancing our intimate lives.

Communication and Consent in Heterosexual Fisting

In the realm of sexual exploration, particularly in the context of fisting, effective communication and clear consent are paramount. This section will delve into the nuances of communication and consent specifically within heterosexual relationships, addressing common challenges, theoretical frameworks, and practical examples to facilitate a safe and pleasurable experience.

The Importance of Communication

Communication serves as the foundation of any healthy sexual relationship. In fisting, where boundaries are often tested and vulnerability is heightened, clear and open dialogue is essential. Effective communication involves not only expressing desires and limits but also actively listening to one's partner. According to [1], understanding one's own body and desires is crucial for conveying these to a partner, thus fostering a supportive and informed environment.

Theoretical Frameworks Theories of communication in intimate relationships, such as the **Interpersonal Process Model of Intimacy**, emphasize that intimacy is built through self-disclosure and partner responsiveness [Reis(2004)]. In the context of fisting, partners must engage in self-disclosure regarding their comfort levels, fears, and desires. This transparency not only enhances intimacy but also establishes a framework for consent.

Establishing Consent

Consent in fisting is not a one-time agreement; it is an ongoing conversation that evolves throughout the experience. [Perel(2017)] posits that consent should be enthusiastic, informed, and revocable at any time. In heterosexual fisting, this means that both partners must be aware of the physical and emotional implications of the act and agree to engage in it willingly.

Types of Consent 1. **Explicit Consent:** This involves clear verbal agreements before engaging in fisting. For example, one partner may say, "I want to try fisting tonight, but let's discuss our boundaries first."

2. **Informed Consent:** Partners should discuss the risks involved and ensure that both parties understand what fisting entails, including potential physical discomfort and emotional vulnerability.

3. **Ongoing Consent:** Throughout the act, partners should check in with each other. Phrases like "How does that feel?" or "Do you want to continue?" can help maintain an open line of communication.

Common Challenges and Solutions

Despite the importance of communication and consent, several challenges may arise in heterosexual relationships when exploring fisting:

1. **Fear of Vulnerability** Many individuals may fear being vulnerable during such an intimate act. This can lead to reluctance in expressing boundaries or desires. To mitigate this, partners should create a safe space where vulnerability is welcomed. Engaging in warm-up activities, such as gentle touch or other forms of intimacy, can help ease anxiety.

2. **Misunderstandings About Consent** There is often confusion regarding what constitutes consent, particularly in the context of BDSM and kink practices. It is crucial to clarify that consent must be given freely and without coercion. Partners

should engage in discussions about safe words, which can be used to pause or stop the activity if discomfort arises. A commonly used safe word is "red," indicating a complete stop, while "yellow" can signify a need to slow down or check in.

3. **Power Dynamics**   In heterosexual relationships, traditional gender roles may influence communication patterns, potentially leading to imbalances in consent discussions. It is essential to recognize these dynamics and strive for equality in conversations about fisting. Both partners should feel empowered to voice their needs and concerns without fear of judgment.

Practical Examples

To illustrate effective communication and consent in heterosexual fisting, consider the following scenarios:

Scenario 1: Pre-Scene Discussion   Before engaging in fisting, partners might sit down to discuss their experiences, fears, and desires. One partner may express, "I've read about fisting and I'm curious, but I'm also nervous about pain. Can we talk about how to make it pleasurable for both of us?" This dialogue not only establishes consent but also opens the door for collaboration on techniques and boundaries.

Scenario 2: Checking In During the Act   As the act progresses, one partner may say, "I'm feeling a bit overwhelmed; can we take a break?" This check-in is crucial for ensuring ongoing consent and comfort. The other partner should respond with understanding and reassurance, fostering an environment where both feel safe to express their feelings.

Conclusion

In conclusion, communication and consent are fundamental to exploring fisting safely and enjoyably within heterosexual relationships. By fostering an environment of open dialogue, establishing clear consent, and addressing common challenges, partners can engage in a fulfilling and consensual fisting experience. The journey of exploration is enhanced when both partners feel heard, respected, and empowered to express their desires and boundaries.

Bibliography

[Nagoski(2015)] Nagoski, E. (2015). *Come as You Are: The Surprising New Science that Will Transform Your Sex Life.* Simon & Schuster.

[Perel(2017)] Perel, E. (2017). *The State of Affairs: Rethinking Infidelity.* HarperCollins.

[Reis(2004)] Reis, H. T. (2004). *The Interpersonal Process Model of Intimacy.* In J. M. H. (Ed.), *Handbook of Personal Relationships* (pp. 367-389). Wiley.

Pleasure and Sensation in Heterosexual Fisting

Fisting, often regarded as one of the most intimate forms of sexual exploration, invites participants to navigate a complex landscape of pleasure and sensation. In heterosexual relationships, the dynamics of pleasure during fisting can be particularly nuanced, intertwining physical sensations with emotional connectivity. Understanding these elements is vital for creating a fulfilling and safe experience.

Physiological Responses to Fisting

Fisting involves the insertion of the hand into the vagina or anus, which can elicit a variety of physiological responses. The vagina, for instance, is rich in nerve endings, particularly in the G-spot area, which can be stimulated during fisting. Research indicates that the G-spot, when stimulated, can lead to heightened sexual arousal and even orgasm for some individuals [?].

The pelvic floor muscles also play a crucial role in the experience of pleasure during fisting. Engaging these muscles can enhance sensation, and awareness of their contraction and relaxation can lead to increased pleasure. Techniques such as Kegel exercises can strengthen these muscles, thereby enhancing sexual satisfaction [?].

Emotional and Psychological Dimensions

The emotional landscape of fisting is equally important. Engaging in this form of intimacy requires a foundation of trust and communication between partners. The act itself can evoke feelings of vulnerability, which may lead to emotional release and catharsis. For many, fisting transcends mere physicality, becoming a profound exploration of intimacy and connection.

In heterosexual relationships, societal norms often dictate how pleasure is expressed and experienced. This can create barriers to fully embracing fisting, as individuals may grapple with feelings of shame or embarrassment. Overcoming these societal taboos is essential for partners to explore their desires openly. As Esther Perel emphasizes, the erotic is often rooted in the interplay of intimacy and distance; thus, the vulnerability of fisting can foster deeper connections [?].

Navigating Sensation: Pleasure vs. Pain

Understanding the fine line between pleasure and pain is paramount in the practice of fisting. The sensation of fullness can be pleasurable, but it is crucial to differentiate between pleasurable stretching and potential pain or injury. Participants should engage in ongoing communication about their comfort levels and boundaries.

The use of safe words can be an effective tool for managing sensations during fisting. Establishing a clear signal allows the receiving partner to communicate their limits without hesitation. This practice not only enhances safety but also reinforces the trust necessary for exploring deeper levels of intimacy.

Techniques for Enhancing Pleasure

To maximize pleasure during heterosexual fisting, several techniques can be employed:

- **Warm-Up:** Begin with gentle external stimulation to relax the body and increase arousal. This may include kissing, caressing, or using fingers to explore erogenous zones.

- **Lubrication:** Generous application of lubricant is essential for comfort and pleasure. Water-based or silicone-based lubricants can reduce friction and enhance sensations.

- **Gradual Insertion:** Start with one or two fingers, allowing the receiving partner to acclimate to the sensation before progressing to the full hand. This gradual approach can help prevent discomfort and build anticipation.

- **Varying Movements:** Experiment with different hand shapes and movements. Curving the fingers or using a fist can create diverse sensations within the vaginal canal or rectum.

- **Communication:** Maintain an open dialogue throughout the experience. Check in regularly to ensure that both partners are comfortable and enjoying the process.

Common Challenges and Solutions

Despite the potential for pleasure, some challenges may arise during heterosexual fisting:

- **Physical Discomfort:** If the receiving partner experiences pain, it is essential to stop immediately. Adjusting technique, angle, or lubrication can often alleviate discomfort.

- **Emotional Barriers:** Address any feelings of shame or fear that may surface. Open discussions about desires and boundaries can help partners navigate these emotions.

- **Lack of Trust:** Building trust takes time. Engaging in smaller acts of intimacy can help partners feel more secure before progressing to fisting.

Conclusion

Pleasure and sensation in heterosexual fisting are deeply intertwined with trust, communication, and emotional connection. By understanding the physiological, emotional, and psychological aspects of fisting, partners can create a safe and pleasurable experience that enhances their intimacy. As with any sexual exploration, the journey of fisting is best approached with care, openness, and mutual respect.

Gender Dynamics and Power Play in Heterosexual Fisting

In the exploration of fisting within heterosexual relationships, it is crucial to understand the intricate interplay of gender dynamics and power play. Fisting, often perceived as a taboo or extreme sexual practice, can serve as a lens through which to examine broader societal constructs of gender, power, and sexuality. This section delves into the ways these dynamics manifest in heterosexual fisting scenarios, supported by relevant theories and examples.

Theoretical Frameworks

To comprehend the gender dynamics at play in heterosexual fisting, we can draw upon several theoretical frameworks, including feminist theory, queer theory, and psychoanalytic perspectives.

Feminist Theory Feminist theory posits that societal norms and power structures shape sexual experiences and expressions. In the context of heterosexual fisting, the act can challenge traditional gender roles, allowing for a re-negotiation of power between partners. For instance, the submissive partner may experience empowerment through surrendering control, while the dominant partner navigates the responsibility that comes with this power.

Queer Theory Queer theory expands the understanding of sexuality beyond binary definitions, emphasizing fluidity and the spectrum of sexual experiences. In heterosexual fisting, this perspective encourages the exploration of non-normative sexual practices that may defy traditional heterosexual scripts, allowing individuals to engage in power dynamics that may be unexpected within a heteronormative framework.

Psychoanalytic Perspectives From a psychoanalytic viewpoint, the act of fisting can evoke deep emotional responses tied to intimacy, vulnerability, and trust. The dynamics of dominance and submission in fisting may also reflect unconscious desires and fears, where the act becomes a means of exploring repressed aspects of one's sexuality.

Challenges and Misconceptions

While fisting can be a site of empowerment and exploration, it is also fraught with challenges and misconceptions, particularly regarding gender dynamics.

Misconceptions about Gender Roles One prevalent misconception is that fisting inherently reinforces traditional gender roles, with men as dominant and women as submissive. However, this binary view overlooks the diverse ways individuals can express power and vulnerability in their sexual relationships. For example, a woman may take on a dominant role in fisting, guiding her partner's experience and actively participating in the dynamics of power exchange.

Communication Barriers Effective communication is vital in navigating the complexities of gender dynamics in fisting. Partners may encounter challenges in expressing their desires and boundaries due to societal conditioning around gendered communication styles. For instance, women may feel pressured to prioritize their partner's pleasure over their own, while men may struggle to articulate their vulnerabilities. It is essential to foster an environment where both partners feel empowered to communicate openly, ensuring that the act of fisting is consensual and fulfilling for all involved.

Examples of Gender Dynamics in Fisting

To illustrate the complexities of gender dynamics and power play in heterosexual fisting, consider the following examples:

Example 1: Re-negotiating Power In a heterosexual couple, the woman expresses a desire to explore fisting as a way to deepen intimacy. Initially, her partner is hesitant, feeling pressure to conform to traditional gender norms that dictate men should be dominant. However, through open communication, they establish a safe space to discuss their fantasies and boundaries. The woman takes the lead during the experience, guiding her partner and actively participating in the power exchange. This dynamic allows both partners to explore their desires while challenging preconceived notions of gender roles.

Example 2: Vulnerability and Trust In another scenario, a man who has traditionally held a dominant role in his sexual relationships expresses a desire to experience submission through fisting. His partner, understanding the emotional weight of this request, ensures that they establish clear boundaries and safe words. As they engage in fisting, the man discovers a newfound vulnerability, allowing him to connect with his partner on a deeper level. This experience not only enhances their intimacy but also challenges the societal expectation that men must always be dominant.

The Role of Aftercare

Aftercare is an essential component of any BDSM or kink practice, including fisting. It involves the emotional and physical care provided to partners after an intense sexual experience. In the context of heterosexual fisting, aftercare can help to reinforce the trust and connection established during the act.

Emotional Aftercare Emotional aftercare may include verbal reassurance, cuddling, or discussing the experience to process feelings and reinforce the bond between partners. It is particularly important in heterosexual fisting, where the dynamics of power can evoke intense emotional responses. Partners should feel safe to express their feelings and any vulnerabilities that arose during the experience.

Physical Aftercare Physical aftercare involves tending to any physical discomfort or needs that may arise from fisting. This may include hydration, hygiene practices, and addressing any soreness or injuries. Ensuring that both partners feel cared for physically reinforces the mutual respect and connection essential in navigating power dynamics.

Conclusion

In conclusion, the exploration of gender dynamics and power play in heterosexual fisting reveals a rich tapestry of experiences that challenge traditional notions of sexuality. By understanding the theoretical frameworks, addressing misconceptions, and embracing open communication, partners can navigate the complexities of power dynamics in a way that fosters intimacy, trust, and mutual empowerment. Fisting, when approached with care and respect, can serve as a profound exploration of the intersection of gender, power, and sexuality, ultimately enriching the sexual experiences of those involved.

Addressing Stigma and Discrimination in Heterosexual Fisting

Fisting, as a sexual practice, often faces a significant amount of stigma and discrimination, particularly within heterosexual relationships. This stigma can stem from a variety of sources, including cultural norms, misconceptions about sexuality, and societal beliefs about what constitutes acceptable sexual behavior. Understanding and addressing these stigmas is crucial for fostering a more open and accepting discourse around fisting, allowing individuals to explore their desires without fear of judgment or discrimination.

Cultural Norms and Misconceptions

Cultural narratives surrounding heterosexuality often paint a picture of conventional sexual practices that prioritize penetration through vaginal intercourse. Fisting, which challenges these norms by introducing an alternative form of intimacy and pleasure, can be seen as deviant or taboo. This perception is often reinforced by media portrayals that sensationalize or misrepresent fisting, leading to further misconceptions. For instance, many people mistakenly believe that fisting is inherently dangerous or abusive, overlooking the importance of consent, communication, and safety practices that can make fisting a pleasurable and fulfilling experience.

Impact of Stigma on Individuals and Relationships

The stigma surrounding fisting can lead to feelings of shame and isolation for those who are interested in exploring this practice. Individuals may internalize societal judgments, leading to a reluctance to communicate their desires to partners. This lack of communication can prevent couples from fully exploring their sexual compatibility and can hinder the development of trust and intimacy in their relationships. Research suggests that open communication about sexual desires is essential for relationship satisfaction [?]. Therefore, addressing stigma is not only about changing societal perceptions but also about empowering individuals to express their needs without fear.

Examples of Stigmatization

Consider a heterosexual couple where one partner expresses interest in fisting. The receiving partner may feel apprehensive due to societal stigma, fearing that their interest will be seen as abnormal or that it will change how their partner perceives them. This stigma can manifest in various ways, including derogatory comments or jokes about the practice, reinforcing feelings of shame. Furthermore, individuals may face judgment from peers or family members if their sexual practices are revealed, leading to a culture of silence around alternative sexual expressions.

Strategies for Addressing Stigma

To combat stigma and discrimination surrounding heterosexual fisting, several strategies can be employed:

1. **Education and Awareness:** Increasing knowledge about fisting through workshops, literature, and open discussions can demystify the practice.

Educational initiatives should focus on the importance of consent, safety, and communication, as well as the positive aspects of fisting as an expression of intimacy.

2. **Community Building:** Creating supportive communities where individuals can share experiences and learn from one another can help normalize fisting. These communities can provide a safe space for individuals to discuss their desires and concerns without fear of judgment.

3. **Challenging Stereotypes:** Actively working to dismantle stereotypes associated with fisting can help reduce stigma. This can be done by promoting positive representations of fisting in media and literature, showcasing it as a valid and pleasurable sexual practice.

4. **Encouraging Open Communication:** Partners should be encouraged to discuss their sexual interests openly. Establishing a culture of communication can help mitigate feelings of shame and foster a deeper connection between partners.

5. **Advocacy:** Engaging in advocacy efforts to promote sexual rights and destigmatize alternative sexual practices can lead to broader societal change. This includes challenging discriminatory laws and practices that marginalize individuals based on their sexual preferences.

Conclusion

Addressing the stigma and discrimination surrounding heterosexual fisting is essential for creating an inclusive environment where individuals can explore their sexuality freely. By fostering education, community, and open communication, we can challenge societal norms and empower individuals to embrace their desires without fear. The journey towards acceptance is ongoing, but each step taken contributes to a more compassionate understanding of diverse sexual expressions.

Navigating Heterosexual Fisting in Monogamous Relationships

In the context of monogamous relationships, fisting can be a deeply intimate act that fosters connection, trust, and exploration between partners. This section will delve into the unique dynamics of heterosexual fisting within monogamous partnerships, addressing the challenges and joys that can arise when incorporating this practice into a committed relationship.

Understanding the Dynamics

Heterosexual relationships often come with societal expectations regarding sexual roles and behaviors. Fisting, as a practice that challenges conventional sexual norms, can provoke a range of emotions and responses. Understanding these dynamics is crucial for partners wishing to explore fisting safely and consensually.

Communication is Key Effective communication is the cornerstone of any healthy relationship, particularly when introducing new sexual practices. Partners should engage in open discussions about their desires, boundaries, and concerns related to fisting. This can include:

- Discussing personal motivations for wanting to explore fisting.
- Establishing clear boundaries and limits before engaging in the act.
- Sharing any fears or apprehensions about the experience.
- Creating a safe word or signal to ensure that either partner can pause or stop the activity at any time.

Addressing Societal Taboos

Fisting can be viewed as taboo, particularly in heterosexual contexts where traditional sexual practices are often emphasized. This stigma can lead to feelings of shame or embarrassment for individuals who wish to explore fisting. It is essential for partners to:

- Acknowledge societal pressures and personal beliefs that may influence their perceptions of fisting.
- Engage in conversations that normalize the practice and emphasize its consensual nature.
- Explore educational resources together to demystify fisting and reduce feelings of shame.

Creating a Safe Environment

Safety and comfort are paramount when exploring fisting. Partners should take the time to create a conducive environment that fosters relaxation and trust. Considerations include:

- Choosing a private space where both partners feel secure and free from interruptions.

- Setting the mood with soft lighting, music, or aromatherapy to enhance relaxation.

- Having all necessary supplies, such as lubricant, gloves, and towels, readily available to minimize distractions and maintain hygiene.

Physical Preparation and Techniques

Before engaging in fisting, both partners should prioritize physical preparation. This includes:

Warming Up Warming up is essential for comfort and safety. Partners should engage in foreplay that allows for gradual arousal and relaxation of the body. Techniques may include:

- Manual stimulation of erogenous zones to increase blood flow and sensitivity.

- Incorporating gentle stretching of the vaginal or anal opening with fingers or toys.

- Using plenty of lubricant to facilitate ease of movement and reduce friction.

Techniques for Successful Fisting When both partners feel ready, they can begin the fisting process. Key techniques to keep in mind include:

- Starting with one or two fingers to gauge comfort levels before gradually introducing the entire hand.

- Maintaining open communication throughout the process, checking in with each other frequently.

- Experimenting with different angles and movements to find what feels pleasurable for both partners.

Emotional Considerations

Fisting can evoke a range of emotions, from pleasure to vulnerability. Partners should be prepared to navigate these feelings together. This may involve:

- Engaging in aftercare practices post-fisting to reinforce emotional connection and support.

- Discussing the experience afterward, sharing what felt good and any discomfort that may have arisen.
- Recognizing that emotions may surface during the act, and being willing to address them openly.

Potential Challenges

While exploring fisting can be rewarding, it may also present challenges. Common issues include:

Physical Discomfort If either partner experiences pain or discomfort during fisting, it is crucial to stop immediately. Pain can be an indicator of potential injury or that the body is not adequately prepared for the act. Partners should:

- Respect each other's limits and prioritize safety over exploration.
- Revisit the warming-up process if discomfort arises, ensuring that both partners feel relaxed and ready.

Navigating Emotional Triggers Fisting can sometimes trigger past traumas or emotional responses. To address this, partners should:

- Be aware of each other's emotional histories and potential triggers.
- Approach the experience with sensitivity and care, allowing for breaks or pauses as needed.

Conclusion

Navigating heterosexual fisting in monogamous relationships can be a fulfilling journey of exploration, intimacy, and trust. By fostering open communication, addressing societal taboos, and prioritizing safety and emotional well-being, partners can create a rewarding experience that deepens their connection. As with any sexual practice, the key lies in mutual respect, consent, and a willingness to explore together.

In conclusion, embracing fisting within a committed relationship can enhance sexual intimacy and foster a sense of shared adventure. With careful consideration and preparation, partners can navigate this unique practice, transforming it into a celebration of their bond and exploration of their desires.

Exploring Heterosexual Fisting in Non-Monogamous Relationships

Non-monogamous relationships, encompassing a variety of structures such as polyamory, swinging, and open relationships, present unique opportunities and challenges for exploring fisting within a heterosexual context. Engaging in fisting in these dynamics requires a nuanced understanding of consent, communication, and emotional safety. This section delves into the complexities of fisting in non-monogamous relationships, highlighting relevant theories, potential problems, and practical examples.

Theoretical Framework

The exploration of fisting in non-monogamous relationships can be examined through several theoretical lenses:

- **Queer Theory:** This framework challenges normative views of sexuality and relationships, advocating for the acceptance of diverse sexual practices and identities. Fisting, often stigmatized, can be embraced as a valid expression of intimacy and pleasure, particularly within non-monogamous contexts where boundaries are more fluid.

- **Attachment Theory:** Understanding how attachment styles influence relationship dynamics is crucial. In non-monogamous relationships, individuals may exhibit secure, anxious, or avoidant attachment styles, which can affect their comfort with fisting. For instance, someone with an anxious attachment style may require more reassurance and communication to feel safe during fisting play.

- **Consent and Communication Models:** Effective communication is paramount in non-monogamous relationships. The use of explicit consent models, such as the *FRIES* acronym (Freely given, Reversible, Informed, Enthusiastic, Specific), helps ensure that all parties are on the same page regarding desires and boundaries related to fisting.

Potential Problems

Engaging in fisting within non-monogamous relationships may present several challenges:

- **Jealousy and Insecurity:** Partners may experience feelings of jealousy or insecurity when one partner engages in fisting with another. It is essential to address these emotions through open dialogue, reassurances, and perhaps renegotiating boundaries to ensure all partners feel valued and secure.

- **Differing Comfort Levels:** Partners may have varying levels of comfort with fisting. One partner may be enthusiastic about exploring this practice, while another may feel apprehensive. Establishing a safe space for discussing these feelings is crucial. This can be facilitated through regular check-ins and discussions about limits and desires.

- **Communication Barriers:** Non-monogamous dynamics can complicate communication. It is vital to maintain clarity about who is engaging in fisting and under what circumstances. Misunderstandings can lead to conflict, so utilizing clear language and setting explicit agreements about fisting play can mitigate these risks.

Practical Examples

To illustrate the exploration of fisting in heterosexual non-monogamous relationships, consider the following scenarios:

> ### Example
>
> **Scenario 1: Polyamorous Couple with a New Partner**
> Alex and Jamie are a polyamorous couple who have recently started dating Taylor. Alex is interested in exploring fisting with Taylor but is unsure how to approach the topic with Jamie. They decide to have a conversation about their desires, emphasizing the importance of consent and communication. Jamie expresses their comfort with Alex exploring fisting with Taylor, provided they establish clear boundaries and maintain transparency about their experiences.

> **Example**
>
> **Scenario 2: Swinging Couple**
> Sam and Jordan, a swinging couple, attend a party where fisting is a common practice. Before engaging in any activities, they discuss their limits and establish a safe word. Sam is interested in fisting, while Jordan prefers to observe. They agree that Sam will communicate with the potential partner about boundaries and consent, ensuring Jordan feels secure and included in the experience.

Key Considerations for Fisting in Non-Monogamous Relationships

When exploring fisting in non-monogamous relationships, consider the following key points:

- **Establish Clear Boundaries:** Each partner should articulate their comfort levels and boundaries regarding fisting. This includes discussing any triggers or past experiences that may influence their willingness to engage in this practice.

- **Prioritize Communication:** Regularly check in with all partners about feelings related to fisting. This can help address any emerging issues and reinforce trust within the relationship.

- **Practice Safe Fisting:** Adhere to hygiene and safety protocols to minimize risks. This includes using gloves, ample lubrication, and ensuring all parties are aware of the physical and emotional aspects of fisting.

- **Aftercare is Essential:** Aftercare is crucial in non-monogamous dynamics, especially after intense experiences like fisting. Partners should engage in aftercare practices that reinforce emotional safety and connection, such as cuddling, discussing the experience, and providing reassurance.

Conclusion

Exploring fisting within heterosexual non-monogamous relationships can be a deeply fulfilling experience when approached with care, communication, and consent. By understanding the unique dynamics at play and addressing potential challenges, partners can navigate this intimate practice in a way that enhances their connections and fosters a sense of shared adventure. Embracing fisting as a valid expression of sexual exploration can lead to greater intimacy and understanding among partners, ultimately enriching their non-monogamous experiences.

Fisting and Parenthood in Heterosexual Relationships

The intersection of fisting and parenthood in heterosexual relationships presents unique dynamics, challenges, and opportunities for intimacy. As couples navigate the complexities of parenting, the incorporation of fisting into their sexual repertoire requires thoughtful consideration of emotional, physical, and practical factors. This section explores the implications of fisting within the context of parenthood, addressing potential barriers, communication strategies, and the importance of maintaining a healthy sexual connection.

Navigating Changes in Sexual Dynamics

Parenthood often brings significant changes to a couple's sexual relationship. The arrival of children can lead to shifts in priorities, time constraints, and physical exhaustion, which may affect sexual desire and intimacy. According to research by [?], the transition to parenthood can lead to a decline in sexual satisfaction due to increased stress and reduced opportunities for private time.

Couples who engage in fisting may find that these changes require renegotiation of their sexual practices. Open communication about desires, boundaries, and the role of fisting in their sexual lives becomes essential. For example, a couple may need to discuss how to incorporate fisting into their routine while balancing the demands of parenting. Setting aside dedicated time for intimacy, even if it's brief, can help maintain the connection and excitement that fisting can bring.

Addressing Physical and Emotional Challenges

The physical realities of parenthood, such as fatigue and the physical changes that accompany childbirth, can impact a person's comfort with fisting. Research indicates that postpartum recovery can include alterations in pelvic floor strength and sensitivity [?]. Thus, it is crucial for parents to approach fisting with awareness and care, ensuring that both partners feel physically and emotionally prepared.

To address these challenges, couples can engage in practices that promote pelvic floor health, such as Kegel exercises, which strengthen the pelvic muscles and can enhance sexual pleasure [?]. Furthermore, exploring the emotional aspects of fisting—such as vulnerability and trust—can deepen intimacy. Couples might consider discussing their feelings about their bodies post-birth and how this affects their sexual experiences.

Communication as a Cornerstone

Effective communication is paramount when integrating fisting into a parenting dynamic. Parents must feel safe to express their needs, concerns, and desires regarding their sexual practices. Establishing a regular check-in routine can help couples maintain open lines of communication about their sexual relationship.

For instance, a couple might dedicate a weekly "date night" to reconnect emotionally and sexually. During these moments, they can explore fisting with an emphasis on consent, comfort, and mutual pleasure. Using safe words and signals can also facilitate a sense of security, allowing both partners to explore their boundaries without fear of discomfort or misunderstanding.

Balancing Sexual Exploration and Parenting Responsibilities

Fisting, as a form of sexual expression, can be a source of empowerment and pleasure for couples. However, it is essential to balance this exploration with the responsibilities of parenthood. Couples may find it helpful to create an environment that fosters intimacy while accommodating their parenting duties.

This could involve planning for times when children are asleep or engaged in activities, allowing parents to focus on their sexual connection without interruptions. Additionally, ensuring that the home environment is conducive to intimacy—such as maintaining a clean and inviting space—can enhance the experience.

The Role of Aftercare in Parenting Contexts

Aftercare is a critical component of fisting, particularly in the context of parenting. Aftercare involves the emotional and physical care that partners provide to each other following a sexual encounter. This practice can be especially beneficial for parents, as it reinforces emotional bonds and provides a moment of connection after the intensity of fisting.

For example, after a fisting session, partners might take time to cuddle, share their feelings about the experience, and discuss any physical sensations they encountered. This practice not only strengthens their relationship but also promotes emotional resilience, which is vital in the demanding landscape of parenthood.

Case Studies and Real-Life Examples

Consider the case of Sarah and Tom, a couple who welcomed their first child a year ago. Initially, they struggled to maintain their sexual intimacy, feeling overwhelmed by the demands of parenthood. However, after attending a workshop on sexual communication, they began to prioritize their sexual relationship. They established a monthly "fisting date," where they could explore their desires in a safe and supportive environment. By openly discussing their experiences, they found that fisting not only enhanced their sexual satisfaction but also deepened their emotional connection.

Another example is Lisa and Mark, who faced challenges with postpartum body image. They found that incorporating fisting into their sexual practices allowed them to reclaim their bodies and explore pleasure in new ways. By focusing on mutual trust and communication, they were able to navigate their insecurities and enjoy a fulfilling sexual relationship.

Conclusion

Fisting can be a fulfilling aspect of sexual expression in heterosexual relationships, even amidst the challenges of parenthood. By prioritizing communication, addressing physical and emotional needs, and incorporating aftercare, couples can maintain a vibrant sexual connection. As parents, embracing the complexities of intimacy can lead to deeper relationships, enhanced pleasure, and a more profound understanding of one another. Ultimately, navigating fisting and parenthood requires patience, trust, and a commitment to mutual exploration, paving the way for a rich and rewarding sexual journey.

Heterosexual Fisting and Aging

As individuals age, their bodies undergo a multitude of changes that can impact their sexual experiences, including practices such as fisting. Understanding the intersection of heterosexual fisting and aging requires a nuanced approach that considers both physiological changes and the evolving dynamics of intimacy and desire.

Physiological Changes in Aging

Aging can affect sexual function and anatomy in several ways. For women, hormonal changes during menopause lead to decreased estrogen levels, which can result in vaginal dryness, reduced elasticity, and changes in the pelvic floor. These changes can make fisting more challenging and may require additional preparation and care. For men, aging may lead to erectile dysfunction, reduced testosterone levels, and changes in the sensitivity of the penis, which can also influence their ability to engage in fisting comfortably.

Addressing Physical Changes

To adapt to these physiological changes, it is essential for partners to prioritize communication and consent. This includes discussing any discomfort, limitations, or adjustments needed to enhance pleasure and safety. For instance, using high-quality lubricants can alleviate dryness and enhance comfort. Additionally, incorporating pelvic floor exercises can improve elasticity and strength, making the experience more enjoyable for both partners.

$$\text{Comfort Level} = \frac{\text{Lubrication} \times \text{Communication}}{\text{Physical Limitations}} \qquad (47)$$

This equation illustrates that the comfort level during fisting can be enhanced by the interplay of adequate lubrication and open communication, while also being moderated by physical limitations that may arise with age.

Psychological and Emotional Considerations

The emotional landscape of aging can also affect sexual experiences. As individuals grow older, they may grapple with issues of body image, self-esteem, and intimacy. These factors can lead to feelings of vulnerability, which may be heightened during practices that require a high level of trust and connection, such as fisting.

Esther Perel emphasizes the importance of desire in long-term relationships, noting that maintaining intimacy requires effort and creativity. Partners must engage in open dialogues about their evolving desires and fears, creating a safe space to explore new forms of intimacy, including fisting.

Building Intimacy Through Fisting

Fisting can serve as a powerful tool for building intimacy between partners as they age. The act itself requires a deep level of trust, vulnerability, and communication. Engaging in fisting can foster a sense of connection and mutual exploration that transcends physical pleasure.

Consider the following example: A couple in their 60s, who have been together for over 30 years, may find that fisting allows them to reconnect with their bodies and each other in a way that feels both novel and deeply intimate. By approaching this practice with care and attention, they can navigate any physical challenges while enhancing their emotional bond.

Navigating Societal Attitudes Towards Aging and Sexuality

Cultural perceptions of aging often stigmatize sexual expression, particularly in heterosexual relationships. This stigma can lead to feelings of shame or embarrassment around engaging in practices like fisting. It is crucial for individuals to challenge these societal norms and embrace their sexuality at any age.

$$\text{Empowerment} = \frac{\text{Self-Acceptance} + \text{Communication}}{\text{Societal Stigma}} \qquad (48)$$

This equation suggests that empowerment in sexual expression, including fisting, increases with self-acceptance and effective communication, while being inversely affected by societal stigma.

Conclusion: Embracing Fisting as a Lifelong Exploration

In conclusion, heterosexual fisting and aging can coexist harmoniously when approached with awareness, care, and open communication. By understanding the physiological changes that accompany aging, addressing emotional vulnerabilities, and challenging societal norms, individuals can continue to explore their sexual desires and maintain intimacy in their relationships.

Fisting, when practiced thoughtfully, can be a celebration of the body's capabilities, an exploration of trust, and an affirmation of desire that transcends age. As partners navigate this journey together, they may find that their sexual experiences can deepen, evolve, and remain fulfilling throughout their lives.

Cultivating Sexual Satisfaction and Connection in Heterosexual Relationships

In the realm of heterosexual relationships, cultivating sexual satisfaction and connection can often feel like navigating a complex landscape filled with societal expectations, personal desires, and emotional needs. This section explores the various dimensions that contribute to sexual satisfaction, emphasizing the importance of communication, emotional intimacy, and the willingness to explore new dimensions of pleasure, including fisting.

Understanding Sexual Satisfaction

Sexual satisfaction is a multifaceted concept that encompasses physical pleasure, emotional fulfillment, and relational dynamics. According to the *Dual Control Model* proposed by Bancroft et al. (2003), sexual satisfaction is influenced by both sexual excitation and inhibition. This model suggests that individuals experience sexual arousal when the excitation system is activated while the inhibition system is kept at bay. The balance between these two systems is crucial in determining overall sexual satisfaction.

$$\text{Sexual Satisfaction} = \text{Excitation} - \text{Inhibition} \tag{49}$$

This equation highlights the need for partners to foster an environment where both excitation can flourish while managing inhibiting factors such as stress, anxiety, or unresolved conflicts.

The Role of Communication

Effective communication is essential for cultivating sexual satisfaction in heterosexual relationships. Partners must feel safe and comfortable expressing their desires, boundaries, and concerns. Research by Miller and Byers (2003) indicates that open communication about sexual preferences significantly correlates with higher levels of sexual satisfaction.

- **Active Listening:** Engaging in active listening allows partners to understand each other's needs and desires without judgment. This practice fosters emotional intimacy and connection.

- **Expressing Desires:** Partners should feel empowered to articulate their sexual desires, including interests in practices such as fisting, which may be perceived as taboo. By discussing these desires openly, partners can navigate their comfort levels and establish a shared understanding of boundaries.

- **Feedback Loop:** Creating a feedback loop where partners regularly check in with each other about their sexual experiences can enhance satisfaction and connection. This can involve discussing what felt good, what could be improved, and exploring new techniques together.

Emotional Intimacy and Trust

Emotional intimacy is a cornerstone of sexual satisfaction. Partners who feel emotionally connected are more likely to experience fulfilling sexual encounters.

According to Johnson's *Emotionally Focused Therapy* (2004), fostering emotional bonds can lead to increased sexual satisfaction. Emotional intimacy can be cultivated through:

- **Vulnerability:** Sharing fears, insecurities, and desires creates a deeper emotional connection. Vulnerability allows partners to feel safe exploring their sexual boundaries.

- **Building Trust:** Trust is fundamental in any intimate relationship. Engaging in practices such as fisting requires a high level of trust, as it involves physical and emotional vulnerability. Establishing trust can be facilitated through consistent communication and honoring each other's boundaries.

- **Aftercare:** Aftercare practices, such as cuddling, discussing the experience, and providing reassurance, can enhance emotional intimacy following sexual encounters. This is particularly important in practices that may evoke strong emotional responses.

Exploring New Dimensions of Pleasure

Exploring new sexual practices, such as fisting, can invigorate sexual satisfaction in heterosexual relationships. However, it is crucial to approach these practices with a sense of curiosity and care.

- **Education and Research:** Partners should educate themselves about the practice of fisting, including safety measures, techniques, and emotional considerations. Resources such as workshops, literature, and expert guidance can provide valuable insights.

- **Setting Intentions:** Before engaging in fisting, partners should discuss their intentions and desires. This conversation can help align expectations and create a shared goal for the experience.

- **Gradual Exploration:** Introducing fisting into the relationship should be a gradual process. Partners can start with smaller forms of penetration, focusing on comfort and pleasure, before progressing to fisting. This approach allows partners to gauge their comfort levels and build trust in the process.

Addressing Challenges and Barriers

Cultivating sexual satisfaction may involve navigating challenges and barriers that can hinder intimacy. Common issues include:

- **Societal Stigma:** The stigma surrounding practices like fisting can create anxiety or shame. Partners should work together to challenge these societal norms and embrace their desires without judgment.

- **Body Image Issues:** Concerns about body image can impact sexual satisfaction. Engaging in body-positive practices and affirmations can help partners feel more comfortable and confident in their bodies.

- **Stress and External Factors:** External stressors, such as work or family obligations, can detract from sexual satisfaction. Partners should prioritize creating a space for intimacy, free from distractions, to enhance connection.

Conclusion

Cultivating sexual satisfaction and connection in heterosexual relationships requires a commitment to open communication, emotional intimacy, and a willingness to explore new dimensions of pleasure. By fostering an environment of trust and vulnerability, partners can enhance their sexual experiences and deepen their emotional bonds. Embracing practices such as fisting, when approached with care and understanding, can lead to greater sexual satisfaction and a more fulfilling relationship.

In summary, partners should remember the importance of:

- Prioritizing communication and understanding.

- Building emotional intimacy and trust.

- Exploring new sexual practices with curiosity and care.

- Addressing and overcoming challenges together.

This holistic approach to sexual satisfaction not only enhances the physical aspects of intimacy but also nurtures the emotional connections that underpin lasting relationships.

Fisting in LGBTQ+ Relationships

LGBTQ+ Fisting Culture and History

The practice of fisting within LGBTQ+ communities is both a rich and complex aspect of sexual expression, deeply intertwined with the history of sexual liberation, identity politics, and the evolution of BDSM and kink cultures. This section delves into the cultural significance, historical context, and the evolution of fisting as a practice within LGBTQ+ communities.

Historical Context

Fisting has roots that stretch back to ancient civilizations, where it was often depicted in various forms of art and literature. However, its modern incarnation as a sexual practice gained prominence in the late 20th century, particularly within LGBTQ+ spaces. The sexual liberation movements of the 1960s and 1970s, alongside the burgeoning visibility of gay culture, provided fertile ground for the exploration of diverse sexual practices, including fisting.

As LGBTQ+ individuals sought to reclaim their sexuality from societal repression, fisting emerged as a bold expression of intimacy, trust, and exploration of boundaries. It was during this time that fisting began to be recognized not only as a sexual act but also as a form of connection that transcended physical pleasure, embodying trust and vulnerability between partners.

Cultural Significance

Fisting holds a unique place in LGBTQ+ culture, often symbolizing a rejection of heteronormative sexual practices and an embrace of sexual diversity. It is frequently associated with the broader BDSM and kink communities, where power dynamics, consent, and communication are central themes. The act of fisting can be seen as a way to challenge traditional notions of sexual intimacy, emphasizing that pleasure can be derived from both physical sensations and emotional connections.

In LGBTQ+ culture, fisting is also a means of exploring the body and its limits, often serving as a metaphor for breaking through societal barriers. This practice encourages individuals to confront their fears and insecurities about their bodies, sexuality, and desires. The act of fisting can foster a sense of empowerment, allowing individuals to reclaim their bodies and their pleasure on their own terms.

Community and Connection

Fisting has also played a significant role in fostering community within LGBTQ+ spaces. Events such as fisting parties, workshops, and discussions have emerged, creating safe spaces for individuals to explore and share their experiences. These gatherings often prioritize consent, safety, and education, allowing participants to engage in open dialogues about their desires, boundaries, and the importance of communication.

Moreover, fisting communities often emphasize the importance of aftercare, recognizing the emotional and physical intensity of the experience. This focus on care and support reinforces the bonds between participants, creating a sense of belonging and mutual respect.

Challenges and Stigmas

Despite its significance, fisting has faced its share of challenges and stigmas, both within and outside of LGBTQ+ communities. Misunderstandings about the practice have led to negative perceptions, often framed as dangerous or deviant. These misconceptions can be rooted in broader societal attitudes towards LGBTQ+ sexuality, which often stigmatizes non-traditional sexual practices.

Furthermore, the intersection of fisting with issues of health and safety cannot be overlooked. The HIV/AIDS crisis in the 1980s and 1990s brought heightened awareness to safe sex practices within LGBTQ+ communities, leading to a more cautious approach to fisting. The importance of hygiene, consent, and communication became paramount, shaping how the practice is approached today.

Contemporary Perspectives

In contemporary LGBTQ+ culture, fisting continues to evolve, reflecting broader changes in societal attitudes towards sexuality. With the rise of digital platforms, discussions about fisting have become more accessible, allowing for greater education and awareness. Online forums, workshops, and social media have facilitated conversations about safe practices, consent, and the emotional aspects of fisting, contributing to a more informed community.

Furthermore, the increasing visibility of diverse sexual practices has led to a gradual destigmatization of fisting. As more individuals embrace their sexuality and explore their desires, fisting is increasingly recognized as a legitimate expression of intimacy and connection.

Conclusion

The culture and history of fisting within LGBTQ+ communities illustrate a journey of exploration, empowerment, and connection. As individuals continue to challenge societal norms and embrace their desires, fisting remains a significant practice that embodies the values of trust, consent, and mutual respect. By understanding its historical context and cultural significance, we can appreciate fisting not only as a sexual act but as a profound expression of human connection and intimacy.

In summary, LGBTQ+ fisting culture is a testament to the resilience and creativity of individuals who seek to redefine pleasure and intimacy. As we move forward, it is essential to continue fostering open dialogues and education around fisting, ensuring that it remains a safe and affirming practice for all who choose to explore it.

Fisting and Queer Identity

Fisting, as a sexual practice, occupies a unique and significant space within queer identity and expression. It is not merely a physical act; it embodies a rich tapestry of cultural, social, and political meanings that resonate deeply within the LGBTQ+ community. This section aims to explore the intersections of fisting and queer identity, highlighting the cultural significance, challenges, and affirmations that arise from this intimate practice.

Cultural Significance of Fisting in Queer Communities

Fisting has historical roots in queer culture, particularly within the gay male community, where it has often been celebrated as an act of liberation and defiance against societal norms. The act itself can serve as a radical expression of sexual agency, allowing individuals to reclaim their bodies and desires in a world that frequently marginalizes and stigmatizes them. This reclamation is vital in a culture that has historically pathologized queer sexuality.

$$\text{Queer Identity} = \text{Sexual Agency} + \text{Cultural Reclamation} \quad (50)$$

Fisting can also serve as a form of resistance against heteronormative standards of sexual behavior. By embracing practices that are often considered taboo or extreme, queer individuals can forge a sense of community and solidarity, creating spaces where alternative expressions of sexuality are not only accepted but celebrated. This communal aspect is essential in fostering a sense of belonging and identity among queer individuals.

Challenges and Stigmas

Despite its cultural significance, fisting is often surrounded by stigma, both within and outside queer communities. Misunderstandings about the practice can lead to negative perceptions, which may discourage individuals from exploring their desires fully. For instance, fisting is frequently conflated with violence or seen as an act of domination, overshadowing its potential for intimacy and connection.

Moreover, the stigma surrounding fisting can intersect with issues of body image and self-acceptance. Many individuals may struggle with feelings of shame or inadequacy when considering fisting, particularly if they perceive their bodies as not fitting societal ideals. This internal conflict can hinder the exploration of one's sexual identity and desires.

$$\text{Internal Conflict} = \text{Body Image Issues} + \text{Social Stigma} \tag{51}$$

Affirmation and Empowerment through Fisting

For many queer individuals, fisting can serve as a powerful tool for affirmation and empowerment. Engaging in fisting allows individuals to explore their bodies and desires in a safe and consensual manner, fostering a deeper understanding of their own sexual identities. This exploration can lead to increased confidence and self-acceptance, as individuals learn to embrace their bodies and desires fully.

Furthermore, the act of fisting can create a profound sense of intimacy and trust between partners. The level of communication and consent required for fisting necessitates an openness that can strengthen relationships and enhance emotional connection. This intimacy is particularly significant within queer relationships, where traditional narratives of love and connection may not always apply.

$$\text{Intimacy} = \text{Trust} + \text{Communication} \tag{52}$$

Examples of Fisting in Queer Spaces

Fisting has found its place in various queer spaces, from underground parties to pride events, where it is often celebrated as part of the broader spectrum of sexual expression. For instance, fisting workshops at LGBTQ+ festivals provide safe environments for individuals to learn about techniques, safety, and consent, helping to demystify the practice while promoting healthy sexual exploration.

In addition, queer literature and art often reflect the complexities of fisting, portraying it as a multifaceted experience that transcends mere physicality. These representations can challenge societal norms and encourage individuals to embrace their desires without shame.

Conclusion

Fisting, as it intersects with queer identity, is a profound expression of sexual agency, intimacy, and community. While it is often accompanied by stigma and misunderstanding, it also offers opportunities for empowerment and connection. By exploring fisting within the context of queer identity, individuals can navigate their desires with confidence, reclaiming their bodies and their narratives in a world that often seeks to silence them. Embracing fisting as a valid and meaningful expression of sexuality can contribute to a more inclusive and affirming understanding of queer experiences.

In summary, the relationship between fisting and queer identity is complex and layered, encompassing cultural significance, challenges, and opportunities for affirmation. As queer individuals continue to explore their sexualities, fisting can serve as a powerful reminder of the importance of consent, communication, and community in the journey toward self-discovery and acceptance.

Overcoming Homophobia and Biphobia in Fisting Communities

The exploration of fisting within LGBTQ+ communities often encounters societal prejudices that manifest as homophobia and biphobia. Understanding and addressing these biases is crucial for fostering an inclusive environment where all individuals can safely explore their desires without fear of discrimination or marginalization. This section delves into the roots of these prejudices, their impact on fisting practices, and strategies to overcome them.

Understanding Homophobia and Biphobia

Homophobia refers to the fear, hatred, or prejudice against individuals who identify as homosexual, while biphobia is the fear or discrimination against those who identify as bisexual. Both forms of discrimination can lead to significant barriers within sexual communities, including fisting communities, where open expression of sexual identity is essential.

Theoretical Framework

Theories of social identity and intersectionality provide a framework for understanding how homophobia and biphobia operate within fisting communities.

According to Social Identity Theory, individuals categorize themselves and others into groups, which can lead to in-group favoritism and out-group discrimination. This categorization can create hierarchies within sexual communities, privileging certain identities over others.

Intersectionality, a term coined by Kimberlé Crenshaw, highlights how overlapping identities—such as sexual orientation, gender, race, and class—interact to shape individual experiences of oppression. In fisting communities, individuals who identify as queer or bisexual may face compounded discrimination, leading to feelings of exclusion and invalidation.

Problems Arising from Homophobia and Biphobia

The presence of homophobia and biphobia can lead to several issues within fisting communities:

- **Exclusionary Practices:** Many fisting events or communities may inadvertently favor cisgender heterosexual norms, leading to the exclusion of queer and bisexual individuals. This can create an environment where only certain identities feel welcomed, perpetuating a cycle of marginalization.

- **Internalized Prejudice:** Individuals may internalize societal prejudices, leading to self-hatred or shame about their sexual identity. This can hinder their ability to explore fisting safely and confidently, as they may feel undeserving of pleasure or connection.

- **Communication Barriers:** Fear of discrimination can lead to reluctance in discussing desires, boundaries, and consent openly. This lack of communication can increase the risk of misunderstandings and potentially unsafe practices.

- **Mental Health Impacts:** The stress of navigating a prejudiced environment can lead to anxiety, depression, and other mental health issues, further complicating individuals' relationships with their sexuality and bodies.

Strategies for Overcoming Homophobia and Biphobia

To foster a more inclusive fisting community, it is essential to implement strategies that actively work against homophobia and biphobia:

- **Education and Awareness:** Providing education on LGBTQ+ issues and the unique challenges faced by bisexual and queer individuals can help dismantle prejudices. Workshops, seminars, and discussions can create a space for learning and dialogue.

- **Inclusive Language:** Using inclusive language in events, marketing materials, and community discussions can signal that all identities are welcome. For example, using terms like "partner" instead of "boyfriend" or "girlfriend" acknowledges diverse relationships.

- **Safe Spaces:** Creating designated safe spaces for LGBTQ+ individuals within fisting communities can provide a refuge where they can express themselves without fear of discrimination. These spaces should be equipped with resources and support for those who may need it.

- **Encouraging Allyship:** Encouraging allies to actively support and advocate for LGBTQ+ individuals can help create a more inclusive environment. Allies can use their privilege to challenge discriminatory behaviors and promote acceptance.

- **Diversity in Leadership:** Ensuring that leadership within fisting communities reflects diverse identities can help create policies and practices that are more inclusive. Representation matters, and having leaders from various backgrounds can foster a sense of belonging.

- **Active Conflict Resolution:** Establishing clear protocols for addressing instances of homophobia or biphobia can help maintain a safe environment. This includes having a system for reporting incidents and ensuring that they are handled with care and seriousness.

Examples of Positive Change

Many fisting communities have begun to implement these strategies, leading to positive outcomes:

- **Workshops and Panels:** Events that focus on LGBTQ+ issues, including panels featuring queer and bisexual fisters, have helped to normalize diverse experiences within the community. These events provide a platform for sharing stories and fostering understanding.

- **Inclusive Events:** Some fisting events have adopted inclusive practices, such as gender-neutral bathrooms, diverse representation in promotional materials, and explicit statements of welcome for all sexual orientations.

- **Community Support Groups:** Establishing support groups for queer and bisexual individuals within fisting communities has provided a space for sharing experiences, discussing challenges, and building connections.

Conclusion

Overcoming homophobia and biphobia in fisting communities requires a concerted effort to create an inclusive and supportive environment. By understanding the roots of these prejudices and implementing strategies to combat them, we can foster a community where all individuals feel empowered to explore their desires without fear of discrimination. Embracing diversity not only enriches the fisting experience but also strengthens the bonds of trust and connection among participants, ultimately leading to a more vibrant and fulfilling community.

Communication and Consent in LGBTQ+ Fisting

In the realm of LGBTQ+ fisting, communication and consent are paramount. The complexities of identity, power dynamics, and societal stigma necessitate a nuanced approach to consent that honors the diverse experiences within the community. This section explores the principles of effective communication, the significance of consent, and the unique challenges faced by LGBTQ+ individuals engaging in fisting practices.

The Foundations of Communication

Effective communication in any sexual practice is vital, and fisting is no exception. Communication serves as the backbone of trust and safety, allowing partners to express desires, boundaries, and concerns openly. In LGBTQ+ relationships, where individuals may already navigate societal pressures and personal insecurities, establishing a clear communication framework is crucial.

Active Listening Active listening involves fully concentrating on what is being said rather than just passively hearing the message. This means engaging with your partner's words, reflecting back what you understand, and asking clarifying questions. For instance, if one partner expresses discomfort about a specific technique, the other should acknowledge this concern and discuss alternatives.

Non-Verbal Communication Non-verbal cues play a significant role in intimate settings. Body language, facial expressions, and even breathing patterns can convey feelings of pleasure or discomfort. Being attuned to these signals can enhance the fisting experience, allowing partners to respond to each other's needs without interrupting the flow of the moment.

Consent: A Continuous Process

Consent is not a one-time agreement but a continuous dialogue that evolves throughout the fisting experience. Understanding the dynamics of consent within LGBTQ+ relationships requires recognizing the intersectionality of identity, power, and vulnerability.

Informed Consent Informed consent means that all parties involved fully understand what they are consenting to. This includes discussing the specifics of fisting techniques, potential risks, and emotional implications. For example, partners should agree on the use of safe words or signals that can be employed at any point during the activity.

$$C = \frac{(I + R + E)}{T} \qquad (53)$$

Where:

- C = Consent
- I = Informed understanding of practices
- R = Recognition of boundaries
- E = Emotional readiness
- T = Trust between partners

This equation illustrates that consent is a function of informed understanding, recognition of boundaries, and emotional readiness, all underpinned by trust.

Ongoing Consent Consent should be revisited regularly, especially during activities that may lead to heightened emotions or physical sensations. Partners should check in with each other, ensuring that both feel comfortable and willing to continue. Phrases such as "How are you feeling?" or "Is this still okay for you?" can facilitate this ongoing dialogue.

Challenges in Communication and Consent

LGBTQ+ individuals may face unique challenges regarding communication and consent, influenced by cultural, social, and personal factors.

Fear of Rejection Many LGBTQ+ individuals may fear that expressing their desires or boundaries could lead to rejection or conflict. This fear can inhibit open communication and lead to misunderstandings. It is crucial for partners to create an environment where all feelings can be expressed without judgment.

Power Dynamics Power imbalances can complicate consent in any relationship, but they may be particularly pronounced in LGBTQ+ dynamics where one partner may hold more social privilege. It is essential to be aware of these dynamics and actively work to ensure that consent is freely given and not coerced.

Navigating Stigma Stigma surrounding LGBTQ+ identities can lead to internalized shame, which may affect how individuals communicate their needs and desires. Partners should approach these conversations with empathy and understanding, recognizing the emotional weight that stigma can carry.

Practical Examples

To illustrate effective communication and consent practices in LGBTQ+ fisting, consider the following scenarios:

Scenario 1: Establishing Boundaries Before engaging in fisting, Alex and Jamie discuss their boundaries. Alex expresses a desire to explore deeper penetration, while Jamie feels uncertain about it. They agree to start slowly, using a safe word "red" to indicate when to stop. This pre-scene discussion ensures both partners feel safe and respected.

Scenario 2: Checking In During Play During a fisting session, Jamie begins to feel discomfort. Instead of waiting until it becomes painful, Jamie uses the safe word "yellow" to indicate they need to slow down. Alex immediately stops and checks in, asking what adjustments can be made to enhance comfort. This ongoing communication fosters trust and safety.

Conclusion

Communication and consent are essential components of safe and pleasurable fisting experiences within LGBTQ+ relationships. By prioritizing open dialogue, recognizing the dynamics of power and identity, and fostering an environment where consent is continually negotiated, partners can explore fisting in a way that is both fulfilling and respectful. As we navigate the complexities of intimacy, let us remember that the foundation of any erotic exploration is rooted in trust, understanding, and the mutual respect of boundaries.

Pleasure and Sensation in LGBTQ+ Fisting

Fisting, as an intimate and deeply sensual act, can evoke a wide spectrum of pleasure and sensation, particularly within LGBTQ+ communities. This section explores the unique dimensions of pleasure associated with fisting, focusing on the interplay between physical sensations, emotional experiences, and the diverse identities represented within LGBTQ+ relationships.

Understanding Pleasure in Fisting

Pleasure in fisting is not solely a physical experience; it encompasses emotional and psychological dimensions that contribute to overall satisfaction. The pleasure derived from fisting can be understood through several theoretical frameworks:

- **The Biopsychosocial Model:** This model posits that biological, psychological, and social factors all play a role in shaping sexual pleasure. For instance, the physiological response to fisting—such as increased blood flow and heightened nerve sensitivity—interacts with psychological factors like trust and emotional connection.

- **The Dual Control Model:** Proposed by Masters and Johnson, this model suggests that sexual arousal is influenced by both excitatory and inhibitory processes. In the context of fisting, individuals may experience heightened arousal from the physical sensations while simultaneously navigating feelings of vulnerability or anxiety, which can inhibit arousal if not addressed.

- **Pleasure as a Social Construct:** In LGBTQ+ contexts, pleasure can be influenced by societal norms and expectations. The reclamation of pleasure within queer spaces often involves challenging heteronormative narratives about sexuality, enabling individuals to explore pleasure on their own terms.

Physical Sensations and Techniques

The physical sensations associated with fisting can vary widely based on technique, anatomy, and personal preferences. Key factors influencing sensation include:

- **Lubrication:** Adequate lubrication is crucial for enhancing pleasure and minimizing discomfort. Silicone-based lubricants are often preferred for their long-lasting properties, while water-based options can be suitable for those who prefer a lighter feel.

- **Hand Positioning and Technique:** The way a hand is positioned and moved during fisting can significantly affect sensation. For example, a gentle, curling motion may stimulate sensitive areas, while deeper thrusts may provide a different type of pleasure. Experimentation with different hand shapes—such as a fist versus a flat palm—can also yield varying sensations.

- **Breath and Rhythm:** Synchronizing breath with movement can enhance the experience. Deep, controlled breathing can help individuals relax, allowing for greater enjoyment of the sensations. Establishing a rhythm that feels good for both partners can also heighten pleasure.

Emotional Connection and Trust

The emotional landscape of fisting is particularly significant within LGBTQ+ relationships, where trust and intimacy play vital roles. The act of fisting often requires a high degree of vulnerability and openness, fostering deeper connections between partners. Key aspects include:

- **Building Trust:** Establishing trust is essential for a fulfilling fisting experience. Partners should engage in open communication about desires, boundaries, and concerns. Trust can be built through ongoing conversations, pre-play discussions, and post-play debriefs.

- **Vulnerability and Intimacy:** Fisting can evoke feelings of vulnerability, which, when navigated safely, can lead to profound intimacy. The shared experience of exploring each other's bodies can create a unique bond, allowing partners to connect on a deeper emotional level.

- **Aftercare:** Aftercare is a critical component of the fisting experience, particularly for LGBTQ+ individuals who may have unique emotional needs. Engaging in aftercare practices—such as cuddling, discussing the experience, or providing reassurance—can enhance emotional well-being and reinforce the connection established during play.

Diverse Perspectives on Pleasure

The LGBTQ+ community is diverse, and experiences of pleasure can vary widely among individuals. It is essential to recognize the different perspectives that exist within this community:

- **Queer Identity and Pleasure:** For many queer individuals, fisting can serve as a form of sexual expression that challenges conventional norms. Embracing fisting as a legitimate form of pleasure can be empowering and affirming, allowing individuals to reclaim their bodies and desires.

- **Intersectionality:** Factors such as race, gender identity, and socioeconomic status can influence how pleasure is experienced and perceived within LGBTQ+ fisting. Acknowledging these intersections is crucial for fostering inclusive conversations around pleasure and ensuring that all voices are heard.

- **Cultural Considerations:** Different cultures within the LGBTQ+ community may have unique attitudes toward fisting and pleasure. Understanding these cultural nuances can enrich discussions about fisting practices and promote greater acceptance and celebration of diverse sexual expressions.

Conclusion

Pleasure and sensation in LGBTQ+ fisting are multifaceted experiences that encompass physical, emotional, and social dimensions. By understanding the interplay between these factors, individuals can navigate their fisting journeys with greater awareness and intention. Ultimately, the exploration of pleasure within LGBTQ+ fisting not only fosters personal growth and self-discovery but also contributes to the broader conversation about sexual expression and identity within the community.

In embracing the complexity of pleasure in fisting, we celebrate the diversity of experiences and encourage individuals to explore their desires safely and consensually, forging deeper connections with themselves and their partners.

Addressing Stigma and Discrimination in LGBTQ+ Fisting

The practice of fisting within LGBTQ+ communities often encounters a multitude of stigmas and discriminatory attitudes, both from external societal forces and within the communities themselves. This section aims to unpack these stigmas, explore their origins, and provide insight into how they affect individuals and relationships engaged in fisting.

Understanding Stigma in LGBTQ+ Fisting

Stigma, as defined by Goffman (1963), refers to an attribute that is deeply discrediting, leading to a reduction in the individual from a whole and usual person to a tainted, discounted one. In the context of LGBTQ+ fisting, this stigma can manifest in several ways:

- **Cultural Misunderstanding:** Fisting is often viewed as an extreme or taboo sexual practice, particularly in conservative cultures. The sensationalized portrayals in media can lead to misunderstandings about its safety and consensual nature.

- **Internalized Homophobia and Biphobia:** Individuals within LGBTQ+ communities may also internalize societal prejudices, leading to shame and reluctance to engage in practices like fisting that are viewed as "deviant" or "excessive."

- **Fear of Judgment:** Many LGBTQ+ individuals fear judgment from peers, family, and society at large, which can inhibit open discussions about sexual practices, including fisting.

The Impact of Stigma on Individuals and Relationships

The stigma surrounding fisting can lead to several negative consequences for individuals and relationships:

- **Isolation and Shame:** Individuals may feel isolated due to their desires or practices, leading to shame and a lack of community support. This isolation can hinder healthy sexual expression and exploration.

- **Mental Health Issues:** The internalization of stigma can contribute to anxiety, depression, and low self-esteem. Studies have shown that LGBTQ+ individuals face higher rates of mental health issues, partly due to societal stigma (Meyer, 2003).

- **Communication Barriers:** Stigma creates barriers to open communication about sexual preferences and boundaries, which are crucial for safe and consensual fisting experiences.

Combating Stigma: Strategies and Approaches

To address and combat stigma and discrimination in LGBTQ+ fisting, several strategies can be employed:

- **Education and Awareness:** Providing comprehensive education on fisting, its safety, and its consensual nature can help demystify the practice. Workshops, online resources, and community discussions can facilitate this education.

- **Building Supportive Communities:** Creating spaces where individuals can share their experiences without fear of judgment fosters a sense of belonging. Peer support groups, online forums, and LGBTQ+ friendly events can serve as platforms for connection.

- **Advocacy and Representation:** Advocating for positive representations of fisting in media and LGBTQ+ narratives can help normalize the practice. This includes highlighting diverse voices and experiences within the community.

Examples of Positive Change

There are numerous instances where stigma around LGBTQ+ fisting has been challenged successfully:

- **Fisting Workshops:** Many LGBTQ+ organizations now offer workshops that focus on safe fisting practices, emphasizing consent and communication. These workshops help to normalize discussions around fisting and reduce stigma.

- **Online Communities:** Platforms such as Reddit and specialized forums provide spaces for LGBTQ+ individuals to discuss fisting openly, share experiences, and seek advice, fostering a supportive environment.

- **Media Representation:** Increasingly, LGBTQ+ films and literature are portraying fisting as a legitimate and consensual sexual practice, helping to shift public perception and reduce stigma.

Conclusion

Addressing stigma and discrimination in LGBTQ+ fisting is essential for fostering a more inclusive and supportive environment. By promoting education, building community, and advocating for positive representation, individuals can reclaim their narratives and engage in fisting practices without fear of judgment. The journey towards acceptance and understanding is ongoing, but through collective efforts, the stigma surrounding LGBTQ+ fisting can be diminished, allowing for a more open and fulfilling exploration of sexuality.

Bibliography

[1] Goffman, E. (1963). *Stigma: Notes on the Management of Spoiled Identity*. Prentice-Hall.

[2] Meyer, I. H. (2003). Prejudice, social stress, and mental health in gay men. *American Psychologist*, 58(5), 123-134.

Navigating Fisting in Same-Sex Relationships

In the realm of sexual exploration, fisting can serve as a profound form of intimacy, especially within same-sex relationships. This section aims to delve into the unique dynamics, challenges, and pleasures that can arise when engaging in fisting practices among same-sex partners, while prioritizing communication, consent, and safety.

Understanding Dynamics in Same-Sex Relationships

Same-sex relationships often challenge societal norms and expectations surrounding gender roles and sexual behavior. This fluidity can lead to diverse experiences of power dynamics, intimacy, and pleasure. In the context of fisting, partners may navigate varying levels of dominance and submission, which can enhance the experience or create tension if not communicated effectively.

Power Dynamics and Roles   In many same-sex relationships, especially within the LGBTQ+ community, the exploration of power dynamics can take on unique forms. For instance, in a typical male-male dynamic, one partner may assume a more dominant role while the other is more submissive. However, these roles are not fixed and can shift during play. It is crucial for partners to openly discuss their desires and boundaries regarding these dynamics to ensure a pleasurable and consensual experience.

Communication and Consent

Effective communication is the cornerstone of any successful sexual encounter, particularly in practices that involve vulnerability, such as fisting. Partners should engage in open dialogues about their interests, limits, and concerns prior to engaging in fisting. This includes:

- **Discussing Interests:** Partners should share their fantasies and desires related to fisting, including what excites them and what they wish to explore.

- **Establishing Boundaries:** It is vital to outline personal limits and safe words or signals that can be used during the act to ensure both parties feel safe and respected.

- **Checking In:** During the act, partners should maintain ongoing communication, checking in with each other about comfort levels and sensations. This can include verbal cues or non-verbal signals that indicate pleasure or discomfort.

Addressing Stigma and Discrimination

Navigating fisting in same-sex relationships can also involve confronting societal stigma and discrimination. Many individuals may internalize negative perceptions about their sexual practices, which can lead to feelings of shame or anxiety. It is essential for partners to create a supportive environment where they can express their feelings without judgment.

Overcoming Internalized Stigma   Internalized stigma can manifest in various ways, such as hesitation to fully engage in fisting due to fear of societal judgment. Partners can help each other overcome this by:

- **Affirming Each Other:** Offering validation and support can encourage partners to embrace their desires without fear.

- **Educating Each Other:** Sharing resources and information about safe fisting practices can empower partners to engage more confidently in their sexual exploration.

Navigating Fisting Techniques and Safety

When engaging in fisting, it is crucial to prioritize safety and hygiene. This is especially important in same-sex relationships, where partners may be more vulnerable to certain health risks.

Safety Protocols To ensure a safe fisting experience, partners should adhere to the following safety protocols:

- **Hygiene Practices:** Both partners should practice proper hygiene before engaging in fisting. This includes washing hands thoroughly, trimming nails, and using gloves to minimize the risk of infection.

- **Lubrication:** Adequate lubrication is essential for a pleasurable fisting experience. Partners should use high-quality, body-safe lubricants to reduce friction and enhance comfort.

- **Gradual Progression:** It is crucial to start slowly and gradually increase intensity. Partners should communicate throughout the process to ensure comfort and avoid injury.

Exploring Pleasure in Same-Sex Fisting

Fisting can lead to intense sensations and pleasure, particularly when partners are attuned to each other's bodies and responses. Understanding the anatomy involved can enhance the experience.

Anatomical Considerations For male partners, fisting can stimulate the prostate, often referred to as the "male G-spot." For female partners, the experience can involve deep internal stimulation. Understanding each other's anatomy can help partners identify pleasurable areas and enhance their fisting experience.

Building Intimacy Through Fisting

Fisting can serve as a powerful means of building intimacy in same-sex relationships. The act of fisting requires a high level of trust and vulnerability, allowing partners to connect deeply on both physical and emotional levels.

Emotional Connection Engaging in fisting can promote emotional bonding, as partners navigate the complexities of pleasure, pain, and vulnerability together. This shared experience can foster a sense of closeness and intimacy that strengthens the relationship.

Conclusion

Navigating fisting in same-sex relationships presents unique opportunities for connection, exploration, and pleasure. By prioritizing communication, consent, and safety, partners can create a fulfilling and enjoyable experience that enhances their intimacy. As with all sexual practices, the key lies in mutual respect, understanding, and a willingness to explore together.

$$P = \frac{I}{C} \qquad (54)$$

where P represents pleasure, I represents intimacy, and C represents communication. This equation highlights the interconnectedness of these elements in fostering a positive fisting experience.

In conclusion, as same-sex couples engage in fisting, they can embrace their desires while navigating the complexities of intimacy and connection, ultimately leading to a more profound understanding of themselves and their partners.

Fisting and Non-Binary Identities

In recent years, the conversation around sexual practices has expanded to include a broader understanding of gender identities, particularly non-binary identities. Non-binary individuals, who may identify as neither exclusively male nor female, often navigate unique experiences and challenges in their sexual exploration. This section aims to address the intersection of fisting and non-binary identities, exploring the nuances, challenges, and affirmations that arise in this context.

Understanding Non-Binary Identities

Non-binary is an umbrella term that encompasses a variety of gender identities that fall outside the traditional binary of male and female. This includes identities such as genderqueer, genderfluid, agender, and bigender, among others. Non-binary individuals may express their gender in diverse ways, and their experiences of sexuality can be equally varied. It is essential to recognize that non-binary identities are valid and deserving of exploration and affirmation in all aspects of life, including sexual practices like fisting.

Challenges Faced by Non-Binary Individuals in Sexual Exploration

1. **Societal Stigma and Misunderstanding:** Non-binary individuals often face societal stigma and misunderstanding regarding their gender identity. This can lead to feelings of invalidation or discomfort when engaging in sexual practices, particularly those that are often framed within a binary context. For instance, traditional discussions about fisting may not adequately address the experiences of non-binary individuals, leading to a sense of exclusion.

2. **Body Image and Dysphoria:** Many non-binary individuals experience body dysphoria, which can impact their sexual experiences. Fisting, as an intimate and physically demanding practice, may evoke feelings of vulnerability or discomfort related to body image. It is crucial to approach fisting with sensitivity to these feelings, ensuring that all parties feel safe and affirmed in their bodies.

3. **Navigating Consent and Communication:** Effective communication is vital in any sexual encounter, but it can be particularly challenging in non-binary contexts where partners may have different understandings of gender and sexuality. Establishing clear consent and boundaries is essential to ensure that all participants feel respected and comfortable. Non-binary individuals may need to articulate their needs and desires in ways that feel authentic to their gender identity.

Embracing Affirmation and Exploration

While there are challenges, engaging in fisting can also be a deeply affirming experience for non-binary individuals. Here are some ways to embrace this exploration:

1. **Body Positivity and Acceptance:** Fisting can serve as a powerful tool for body positivity and acceptance. By engaging in this practice, non-binary individuals can cultivate a deeper connection to their bodies, celebrating their unique forms and sensations. This can be particularly empowering, allowing individuals to reclaim agency over their bodies and sexual experiences.

2. **Creating Inclusive Spaces:** It is essential for communities and individuals engaging in fisting to create inclusive spaces that acknowledge and celebrate non-binary identities. This can involve using gender-neutral language, respecting pronouns, and fostering an environment where all identities are welcomed and affirmed. Workshops, events, and discussions that focus on non-binary experiences in sexual practices can help bridge the gap in understanding.

3. **Exploring Personal Desires:** Non-binary individuals may find that their desires and preferences differ from traditional narratives surrounding fisting. Encouraging personal exploration and experimentation can lead to a more fulfilling

and authentic experience. This may include exploring different positions, techniques, and forms of stimulation that resonate with their unique sense of self.

4. **Community Support:** Engaging with supportive communities can help non-binary individuals navigate their fisting journeys. This can include online forums, local meetups, or workshops focused on non-binary sexuality. Sharing experiences and learning from others can foster a sense of belonging and validation, empowering individuals to explore their desires without fear of judgment.

Conclusion

Fisting, as a sexual practice, holds the potential for deep connection, pleasure, and exploration for non-binary individuals. By acknowledging the unique challenges they face and creating inclusive spaces, we can foster a more compassionate understanding of fisting within the context of non-binary identities. Embracing diversity in sexual expression not only enriches individual experiences but also strengthens the broader sexual community, paving the way for a more inclusive and understanding society.

In summary, the intersection of fisting and non-binary identities is a rich area for exploration, one that invites us to reconsider traditional narratives and embrace the beautiful complexity of human sexuality. As we continue to engage in these conversations, we must prioritize consent, communication, and compassion, ensuring that all individuals feel seen, heard, and celebrated in their sexual journeys.

Fisting and Transgender Experiences

Fisting can be a deeply intimate and transformative practice, particularly within the context of transgender experiences. This section aims to explore the unique dynamics, challenges, and opportunities for pleasure that fisting presents for transgender individuals, acknowledging the diversity of experiences within this community.

Understanding Transgender Identities

Transgender individuals often navigate a complex landscape of gender identity, expression, and societal expectations. According to the *American Psychological Association*, transgender refers to individuals whose gender identity differs from the sex they were assigned at birth. This includes a broad spectrum of identities, including but not limited to trans men, trans women, non-binary, and genderqueer individuals. Understanding this spectrum is crucial in discussing the practice of fisting within transgender contexts.

The Role of Body Autonomy and Affirmation

For many transgender individuals, fisting can serve as a powerful form of body affirmation. Engaging in fisting allows individuals to reclaim their bodies in ways that feel empowering and pleasurable. This practice can facilitate a deeper connection to one's physical self, which is particularly significant for those undergoing medical transitions or navigating body dysphoria.

$$\text{Body Affirmation} = \text{Pleasure} + \text{Consent} + \text{Connection} \tag{55}$$

This equation emphasizes that body affirmation is achieved through the interplay of pleasure, consent, and emotional connection, all of which are integral to a fulfilling fisting experience.

Navigating Physical and Emotional Challenges

While fisting can be a source of empowerment, it can also present unique challenges for transgender individuals. Physical challenges may include considerations related to anatomy, especially for trans women who may have undergone vaginoplasty, or for trans men who may have undergone chest surgery. Understanding the anatomical nuances is vital for ensuring safety and comfort during fisting.

For instance, trans women may experience sensitivity in the vaginal canal post-surgery, necessitating a focus on gentle techniques and ample lubrication. Conversely, trans men may have varying degrees of sensation and anatomical structure that can influence their fisting experience.

Emotional challenges can also arise, particularly concerning body image and past trauma. It is essential to create a safe and supportive environment where individuals can express their boundaries and feelings openly.

Communication and Consent

Effective communication is the cornerstone of any intimate practice, and this holds especially true for fisting within transgender experiences. Establishing clear consent and discussing boundaries before engaging in fisting is critical. Partners should engage in open dialogues about their comfort levels, desires, and any potential triggers related to their gender identity.

Utilizing safe words and signals can enhance the experience by providing a framework for ongoing communication. For instance, a partner may choose to use a color-coded system (e.g., green for go, yellow for slow down, red for stop) to facilitate real-time feedback during the act.

Exploring Pleasure and Sensation

Fisting offers a unique opportunity to explore pleasure and sensation in ways that can be particularly fulfilling for transgender individuals. The act itself can be an exploration of vulnerability, intimacy, and trust between partners.

For trans women, the experience may involve focusing on the sensations within the vaginal canal, as well as external stimulation of the clitoris and surrounding areas. Trans men may find pleasure in anal fisting, exploring sensations that can be both novel and deeply satisfying.

$$\text{Pleasure} = f(\text{Anatomy}, \text{Technique}, \text{Connection}) \qquad (56)$$

This function illustrates that pleasure is a function of anatomy, technique, and the emotional connection between partners, highlighting the importance of a tailored approach to fisting.

Aftercare and Emotional Support

Aftercare is an essential component of any intimate encounter, particularly in practices that involve vulnerability and exploration of boundaries. Aftercare can include physical care, such as providing water, snacks, or comfort items, as well as emotional support through affirmations and discussions about the experience.

Transgender individuals may benefit from specific aftercare practices that acknowledge their unique experiences. This could involve discussing how the fisting experience felt in relation to their gender identity, addressing any discomfort, and reinforcing positive feelings about their bodies.

Conclusion

Fisting can be a profound and affirming experience for transgender individuals, allowing for exploration of pleasure, intimacy, and body autonomy. By fostering open communication, understanding the complexities of transgender anatomy and emotional experiences, and prioritizing consent and aftercare, partners can create a safe and fulfilling environment for exploration.

In conclusion, engaging in fisting within transgender contexts not only requires a nuanced understanding of physical and emotional dimensions but also celebrates the beauty of connection and self-discovery. As with any intimate practice, prioritizing safety, consent, and communication will lead to more enriching experiences for all involved.

Exploring Fisting in LGBTQ+ Polyamorous and Non-Monogamous Relationships

In the vibrant tapestry of LGBTQ+ relationships, polyamory and non-monogamy represent unique avenues for exploring intimacy, trust, and sexual expression. Fisting, as a deeply intimate and often taboo practice, can take on special significance within these frameworks. This section delves into the dynamics of fisting within polyamorous and non-monogamous contexts, addressing the theoretical underpinnings, potential challenges, and practical considerations for those engaged in such relationships.

Theoretical Framework

The exploration of fisting in polyamorous and non-monogamous relationships can be informed by several theoretical perspectives, including relational ethics, attachment theory, and the concept of sexual agency.

Relational Ethics Relational ethics emphasizes the importance of consent, communication, and mutual respect in all intimate interactions. In polyamorous settings, where multiple partners may engage in fisting, establishing clear boundaries and guidelines is essential. Each partner's comfort levels, desires, and limits must be openly discussed to ensure that all parties feel safe and respected.

Attachment Theory Attachment theory posits that the bonds formed between individuals can influence their emotional and sexual experiences. In non-monogamous relationships, varying attachment styles may affect how partners relate to one another during fisting. For instance, individuals with secure attachment styles may navigate fisting with greater ease and openness, while those with anxious or avoidant styles might experience heightened vulnerability or reluctance. Understanding these dynamics can enhance emotional safety and connection.

Sexual Agency Sexual agency refers to the ability of individuals to make informed choices about their sexual experiences. In polyamorous and non-monogamous relationships, fostering sexual agency is crucial. Partners should feel empowered to express their desires for fisting or any other sexual activity, without fear of judgment or coercion. This empowerment can lead to more fulfilling and authentic sexual encounters.

Challenges in Non-Monogamous Fisting

While the possibilities for exploration are vast, there are also challenges that may arise when engaging in fisting within polyamorous or non-monogamous contexts.

Jealousy and Insecurity Jealousy is a common concern in non-monogamous relationships. The act of fisting, which often requires deep trust and intimacy, may trigger feelings of insecurity or possessiveness. Partners must engage in open dialogues about their feelings and establish practices that promote reassurance and connection. For example, regular check-ins and affirmations of love and commitment can help mitigate jealousy.

Communication Barriers Effective communication is vital, yet it can be particularly challenging in polyamorous settings where multiple partners are involved. Misunderstandings about boundaries, consent, and desires may arise. Utilizing tools such as relationship agreements or communication frameworks (e.g., Nonviolent Communication) can aid in clarifying intentions and ensuring that all partners are on the same page regarding fisting practices.

Health and Safety Considerations In polyamorous and non-monogamous relationships, health and safety protocols become even more critical. Engaging in fisting with multiple partners increases the importance of hygiene practices and regular health check-ups. Partners should discuss and agree upon safety measures, such as the use of gloves, dental dams, and appropriate lubrication, to minimize the risk of infections or injuries.

Practical Considerations for Fisting in Polyamorous Relationships

To navigate the complexities of fisting in polyamorous and non-monogamous relationships, consider the following practical strategies:

Establishing Clear Boundaries Before engaging in fisting, partners should collaboratively establish boundaries that respect each individual's comfort levels. Discussing what is acceptable and what is off-limits can prevent misunderstandings and foster a sense of safety.

Creating a Safe Environment Physical and emotional safety is paramount when exploring fisting. Create a comfortable and private space for fisting activities, free from interruptions. This can enhance the experience and allow for deeper emotional connection.

Utilizing Safe Words and Signals Incorporating safe words or signals into fisting play can enhance communication and ensure that all partners feel empowered to express their needs. This practice allows for immediate feedback and the ability to pause or stop if discomfort arises.

Engaging in Aftercare Aftercare is an essential aspect of any intimate encounter, particularly in practices that involve vulnerability, such as fisting. Partners should take time to reconnect, provide emotional support, and discuss the experience afterward. This can strengthen bonds and foster trust.

Fostering Community Support Engaging with LGBTQ+ polyamorous communities can provide valuable resources and support for those exploring fisting. Online forums, workshops, and local meet-ups can offer opportunities to share experiences, learn from others, and cultivate a sense of belonging.

Examples of Fisting in Non-Monogamous Relationships

Consider the following scenarios that illustrate the dynamics of fisting in LGBTQ+ polyamorous and non-monogamous relationships:

Scenario 1: The Triad In a triad relationship, three partners engage in fisting play together. Prior to the encounter, they establish clear boundaries and safe words. During the experience, they communicate openly about their sensations and desires, ensuring that each partner feels included and respected. Afterward, they engage in aftercare, discussing what felt pleasurable and any areas of discomfort.

Scenario 2: The Open Relationship In an open relationship, one partner explores fisting with a new partner while maintaining communication with their primary partner. They discuss the experience beforehand, setting boundaries around what is acceptable. After the encounter, they share their experiences, reinforcing trust and connection in their primary relationship.

Scenario 3: The Polycule In a larger polycule, multiple partners engage in fisting activities at a community event. They establish group agreements regarding consent and safety, ensuring that everyone is on the same page. This collaborative approach fosters a sense of community and shared exploration.

Conclusion

Exploring fisting within LGBTQ+ polyamorous and non-monogamous relationships can be a deeply rewarding experience, rich with opportunities for intimacy, connection, and personal growth. By prioritizing communication, consent, and safety, partners can navigate the complexities of fisting while fostering a sense of community and belonging. Embracing the unique dynamics of these relationships can lead to profound experiences of pleasure, trust, and emotional resilience.

Fisting in BDSM and Kink Communities

Understanding Fetishes and Kinks

Fetishes and kinks are integral components of human sexuality, representing a spectrum of desires and preferences that extend beyond conventional sexual practices. Understanding these concepts requires a nuanced exploration of their definitions, psychological underpinnings, and their role in sexual expression.

Defining Fetishes and Kinks

A **fetish** is often defined as a strong sexual attraction to a specific object, body part, or activity that is not inherently sexual in nature. This can include a wide range of interests, such as a fascination with feet, leather, or latex clothing. In contrast, a **kink** refers to unconventional sexual practices, fantasies, or role-playing that may not necessarily involve a specific object. Kinks can encompass activities such as BDSM, role-playing, or even fisting itself.

Theoretical Perspectives on Fetishes and Kinks

From a psychological perspective, several theories attempt to explain the origins and motivations behind fetishes and kinks:

- **Classical Conditioning:** This theory posits that fetishes may develop through associative learning. For instance, if an individual experiences sexual arousal in the presence of a particular object or scenario, they may begin to associate that object with sexual pleasure. This can lead to the object becoming a fetishized element in their sexual experiences.

- **Psychodynamic Theory:** Sigmund Freud suggested that fetishes may arise from unresolved psychosexual conflicts or traumas during childhood. According to this perspective, individuals may develop fetishes as a means of coping with anxiety or as a substitute for more socially acceptable sexual practices.

- **Cognitive-Behavioral Theory:** This approach emphasizes the role of cognitive processes in the development of fetishes and kinks. Individuals may engage in specific behaviors or fantasies that provide them with a sense of control, pleasure, or escape from reality, reinforcing their desires over time.

Cultural Influences on Fetishes and Kinks

Cultural factors significantly shape the expression and acceptance of fetishes and kinks. Societal norms and values can dictate what is considered acceptable or taboo, influencing individuals' willingness to explore their desires. For example, certain fetishes may be more prevalent in specific cultures or communities, such as the prominence of BDSM in LGBTQ+ spaces.

Common Fetishes and Kinks

Some common fetishes and kinks include:

- **Foot Fetishism:** One of the most prevalent fetishes, foot fetishism involves sexual attraction to feet. This can manifest in various ways, including an interest in foot worship, footwear, or specific characteristics of feet.

- **Leather and Latex:** The tactile and visual aspects of leather and latex can evoke strong arousal for many individuals. These materials are often associated with BDSM culture, where they symbolize power dynamics and submission.

- **BDSM:** Bondage, Discipline, Dominance, Submission, Sadism, and Masochism encompass a wide range of practices that explore power exchange, consent, and pleasure through physical and psychological means.

Challenges and Misconceptions

Despite the growing acceptance of diverse sexual practices, fetishes and kinks often face stigma and misunderstanding. Common misconceptions include:

- **Pathologization:** Fetishes and kinks are sometimes viewed as pathological or deviant behaviors, leading to shame and secrecy among individuals who engage in these practices. It is crucial to recognize that as long as these practices are consensual and do not harm others, they are a valid expression of human sexuality.

- **Stereotyping:** Individuals with fetishes or kinks may be unfairly stereotyped or judged based on their interests. This can create barriers to open communication and acceptance within relationships and communities.

The Role of Communication in Exploring Fetishes and Kinks

Effective communication is essential for individuals and couples exploring fetishes and kinks. Open dialogue fosters understanding, consent, and trust, allowing partners to navigate their desires safely and enjoyably. Key aspects of communication include:

- **Expressing Desires:** Partners should feel comfortable discussing their interests and fantasies without fear of judgment. This can lead to greater intimacy and connection.

- **Establishing Boundaries:** Clear boundaries help ensure that both partners feel safe and respected during exploration. This includes discussing limits, safe words, and aftercare needs.

- **Ongoing Check-Ins:** Regular communication about experiences and feelings is vital, especially when engaging in activities that may evoke strong emotional responses.

Conclusion

Understanding fetishes and kinks is a vital component of sexual health and wellness. By acknowledging the diversity of human desires and fostering open communication, individuals can embrace their sexuality in a safe, consensual, and fulfilling manner. As society continues to evolve in its understanding of sexual expression, it is essential to challenge stigmas and promote acceptance of all forms of consensual sexual exploration.

$$\text{Fetish} \wedge \text{Kink} \Rightarrow \text{Diverse Sexual Expression} \tag{57}$$

Fisting as an Element of BDSM Play

Fisting, as a form of sexual exploration, can be intricately woven into the fabric of BDSM (Bondage, Discipline, Dominance, Submission, Sadism, and Masochism) play. This section delves into the multifaceted relationship between fisting and BDSM, highlighting the dynamics, techniques, and considerations that make fisting a compelling element of BDSM practice.

Understanding the Connection

In BDSM, power dynamics are central to the experience. Fisting can serve as a powerful expression of dominance and submission, allowing participants to explore their roles in a consensual and safe environment. The act of fisting requires a high degree of trust and communication, aligning perfectly with the foundational principles of BDSM. This connection is not merely physical; it also taps into psychological aspects that enhance the experience for both the giver and the receiver.

The Role of Power Dynamics

The interplay of power dynamics in fisting can manifest in various ways:

- **Dominance and Submission:** The dominant partner may take control of the fisting process, guiding the submissive partner through the experience. This control can create a heightened sense of vulnerability for the submissive, deepening their emotional and physical connection.

- **Role Reversal:** In some cases, the submissive partner may take on a more dominant role, guiding the pace and intensity of the fisting experience. This fluidity allows for exploration of various power dynamics within the same scene.

- **Safe Words and Signals:** Establishing clear safe words and signals is crucial in BDSM play, especially in activities like fisting where physical and emotional boundaries may be tested. A safe word allows the submissive to communicate their limits, ensuring that the experience remains consensual and enjoyable.

Techniques and Considerations

When incorporating fisting into BDSM play, several techniques and considerations come into play to enhance safety and pleasure:

Preparation and Warm-Up   Prior to engaging in fisting, it is essential to prepare both physically and mentally. This can include:

- **Warm-Up Techniques:** Engaging in gradual penetration with fingers or toys can help the body acclimate to the sensation and reduce the risk of injury.
- **Communication:** Discussing desires, limits, and concerns with your partner can help set the stage for a successful experience.
- **Creating a Comfortable Environment:** Ensuring a safe and comfortable space can help both partners feel at ease, enhancing the overall experience.

Techniques of Fisting in BDSM   The following techniques can be particularly effective when integrating fisting into BDSM play:

- **Hand Positioning and Lubrication:** Proper hand positioning and the use of ample lubrication are critical for a pleasurable experience. Experimenting with different hand shapes can also enhance stimulation.
- **Pacing:** Taking time to explore the sensations gradually can build anticipation and enhance pleasure. The dominant partner may control the pace, while the submissive partner can provide feedback on their comfort level.
- **Incorporating Restraints:** Using restraints can amplify the sensations experienced during fisting. The submissive partner may feel more vulnerable and exposed, enhancing the psychological aspects of the scene.

Addressing Risks and Safety

While fisting can be a rewarding experience in BDSM play, it is crucial to address potential risks:

Physical Risks   Fisting carries inherent physical risks, including:

- **Tissue Damage:** Without proper preparation and technique, fisting can lead to tearing of delicate tissues. It is essential to listen to the body and stop if any pain or discomfort is felt.
- **Infections:** Maintaining hygiene is vital to prevent infections. This includes cleaning hands and any toys used, as well as considering the use of gloves.

Emotional and Psychological Risks   The emotional and psychological aspects of BDSM play can be profound:

- **Aftercare:** Providing aftercare is essential for both partners. This can include physical comfort, emotional support, and reassurance, helping to process the experience and reinforce trust.
- **Dealing with Triggers:** Participants should be aware of any potential emotional triggers that may arise during play. Open communication can help navigate these moments safely.

Conclusion

Fisting, as an element of BDSM play, offers a rich tapestry of experiences that intertwine physical pleasure with emotional depth. By understanding the dynamics of power, employing safe practices, and engaging in open communication, partners can explore the profound connections that fisting can foster within the realm of BDSM. As with any intimate practice, the key lies in mutual respect, consent, and a shared commitment to safety and pleasure.

Risk-Aware Consensual Kink (RACK) and Fisting

Risk-Aware Consensual Kink (RACK) is a foundational concept in the BDSM and kink communities that emphasizes informed consent and the acknowledgment of risks associated with various sexual practices, including fisting. This principle encourages participants to engage in activities with a full understanding of the potential risks involved, ensuring that all parties are not only consenting but also aware of what they are consenting to.

Understanding RACK

RACK can be broken down into its core components:

- **Risk-Aware:** Participants must be informed about the physical, emotional, and psychological risks associated with fisting. This includes understanding potential injuries, infections, and the dynamics of power exchange that may arise during play.

- **Consensual:** Consent must be explicit, informed, and ongoing. All parties involved should agree to the activities being performed, and this consent can be revoked at any time.

- **Kink:** This term encompasses a wide range of sexual practices that fall outside of conventional sexual norms, including fisting, which can be seen as an extreme form of sexual expression.

Theoretical Framework of RACK

The theoretical underpinnings of RACK draw from several disciplines, including psychology, sociology, and sexology. Key theories include:

- **Informed Consent Theory:** This theory posits that consent must be based on adequate information and understanding. In the context of fisting, this means discussing the risks, benefits, and techniques involved prior to engaging in the act.

- **Social Constructionism:** This perspective suggests that our understanding of sexuality, including practices like fisting, is socially constructed. RACK promotes a culture of open communication and education to deconstruct societal taboos surrounding kink.

- **Risk Management Theory:** This theory emphasizes the importance of identifying, assessing, and mitigating risks. In fisting, this could involve using safe words, establishing boundaries, and employing harm reduction strategies.

Potential Problems in RACK and Fisting

While RACK serves as a valuable framework for engaging in kink safely, several challenges can arise:

- **Miscommunication:** Participants may have different understandings of what constitutes informed consent. Clear communication is essential to ensure that all parties are on the same page regarding their limits and desires.

- **Power Imbalances:** In many kink dynamics, power differentials exist. It's crucial to navigate these imbalances carefully to ensure that consent remains informed and that one party does not exploit the other's vulnerabilities.

- **Inadequate Education:** Many individuals may lack access to comprehensive education about fisting techniques and safety practices. This can lead to unintentional harm or injury during play.

Practical Examples of RACK in Fisting

Implementing RACK in fisting practice involves several practical steps:

- **Pre-Play Discussions:** Before engaging in fisting, partners should discuss their experiences, boundaries, and any specific concerns they may have. This might include conversations about previous injuries, emotional triggers, and safe words.

- **Establishing Safe Words:** Safe words are critical in kink play. They provide a way for participants to communicate their comfort levels and to pause or stop the activity if necessary. For example, a common system is to use "red" for stop and "yellow" for slow down.

- **Educating on Techniques:** Partners should educate themselves on safe fisting techniques, including proper hand positioning, the use of lubrication, and recognizing signs of discomfort or injury. Online resources, workshops, and community events can provide valuable information.

- **Aftercare:** Aftercare is an essential component of any kink activity, including fisting. It involves providing emotional and physical support to one another after the scene, ensuring that both partners feel safe, cared for, and connected.

Conclusion

Risk-Aware Consensual Kink (RACK) provides a robust framework for safely exploring fisting and other kink practices. By emphasizing informed consent, clear communication, and risk management, participants can engage in these activities with confidence and mutual respect. As the kink community continues to evolve, the principles of RACK will remain vital in fostering safe, consensual, and fulfilling experiences.

$$\text{Safety} = \text{Informed Consent} + \text{Communication} + \text{Education} \qquad (58)$$

This equation illustrates that safety in kink, particularly in practices like fisting, is the product of informed consent, effective communication, and ongoing education about the practices and risks involved. By prioritizing these elements, individuals can engage in fisting as a consensual and pleasurable exploration of their desires.

Fisting and Dominant/Submissive Dynamics

Fisting, as a form of sexual expression, can intertwine deeply with the dynamics of dominance and submission (D/s) within BDSM contexts. Understanding how these power dynamics play out in fisting not only enhances the experience but also fosters a safe and consensual environment. This section explores the intricate relationship between fisting and D/s dynamics, highlighting essential theories, potential problems, and practical examples.

Theoretical Framework of D/s Dynamics

At its core, the D/s dynamic is characterized by a consensual power exchange where one partner (the Dominant) takes control while the other (the Submissive) relinquishes it. This dynamic can enhance the emotional and physical experiences of both partners, creating a unique space for exploration and intimacy.

Theories surrounding D/s dynamics often draw from psychological frameworks, such as the *Transactional Analysis* by Eric Berne, which posits that individuals operate from three ego states: Parent, Adult, and Child. In the context of fisting:

- The **Dominant** may engage from the *Parent* state, providing guidance, structure, and care.

- The **Submissive** often operates from the *Child* state, embracing vulnerability, trust, and surrender.

This interplay can create a deeply fulfilling experience where both partners explore their identities and desires within a safe framework.

Integrating Fisting into D/s Dynamics

Fisting can serve as a powerful tool within D/s dynamics, offering a physical manifestation of control and submission. The act itself requires trust and communication, which are foundational to both fisting and D/s relationships. Here are some key aspects to consider:

- **Consent and Negotiation:** Before engaging in fisting, it is crucial for partners to negotiate boundaries, safe words, and aftercare. This negotiation process reinforces the importance of consent and ensures that both partners feel safe and respected.

- **Control and Surrender:** For many, the act of fisting symbolizes a significant level of control. The Dominant may derive pleasure from the act of guiding the Submissive through the experience, while the Submissive may find empowerment in surrendering to the Dominant's will.

- **Physical and Emotional Connection:** Fisting can heighten the emotional connection between partners. The physical act of fisting can create a sense of intimacy and vulnerability, allowing both partners to explore deeper emotional states and enhance their bond.

- **Roleplay and Fantasy:** Incorporating roleplay into fisting can amplify the D/s dynamic. For example, a Dominant may adopt a commanding persona, guiding the Submissive through the experience while using verbal affirmations or commands to enhance the power exchange.

Common Problems in D/s Fisting Dynamics

While the integration of fisting into D/s dynamics can be profoundly rewarding, it is not without its challenges. Here are some common issues that may arise:

- **Miscommunication:** A lack of clear communication can lead to misunderstandings regarding boundaries and desires. It is essential to establish open lines of communication before, during, and after the fisting experience.

- **Power Imbalance:** If not carefully negotiated, the D/s dynamic can lead to feelings of inadequacy or resentment. Both partners must regularly check in with each other to ensure that the dynamic remains consensual and fulfilling.

- **Physical Discomfort:** Fisting can be physically intense, and the Submissive may experience discomfort or pain. It is vital for the Dominant to remain attuned to the Submissive's cues and to prioritize their well-being above all else.

- **Emotional Vulnerability:** Engaging in fisting within a D/s context may evoke intense emotions. The Dominant should be prepared to provide aftercare and support to help the Submissive process any feelings that arise during or after the experience.

Practical Examples of Fisting in D/s Dynamics

To illustrate how fisting can be effectively integrated into D/s dynamics, consider the following scenarios:

> **Example**
>
> **Scenario 1: The Commanding Dominant**
> In this scenario, the Dominant takes a commanding role, instructing the Submissive on how to prepare for fisting. The Dominant may use verbal commands to guide the Submissive through the warm-up process, emphasizing the importance of relaxation and trust. This dynamic allows the Submissive to feel cared for while simultaneously embracing their role of surrender.

> **Example**
>
> **Scenario 2: The Vulnerable Submissive**
> Here, the Submissive is encouraged to express their desires and boundaries openly. The Dominant listens attentively, ensuring that the Submissive feels safe and respected. As the fisting progresses, the Dominant checks in frequently, reinforcing the trust and connection between them. This scenario emphasizes the importance of communication and mutual respect within the D/s dynamic.

Conclusion

Fisting within the context of dominant/submissive dynamics can be an exhilarating and transformative experience. By understanding the theoretical underpinnings of D/s relationships, recognizing potential challenges, and implementing effective communication strategies, partners can explore the depths of their desires safely and consensually. Ultimately, the integration of fisting into D/s dynamics can lead to profound emotional and physical connections, enriching the sexual experiences of both Dominants and Submissives alike.

Exploring Sadism and Masochism Through Fisting

Fisting, as a form of sexual expression, can intersect with the dynamics of sadism and masochism (S&M), offering a unique avenue for exploring power, pleasure, and pain. This section delves into how fisting can be integrated into sadomasochistic practices, the psychological underpinnings of these dynamics, and practical considerations for engaging in such activities safely and consensually.

Understanding Sadism and Masochism

Sadism is characterized by the enjoyment of inflicting pain, humiliation, or suffering on another, while masochism involves deriving pleasure from experiencing pain or humiliation. These dynamics can manifest in various forms, including physical, emotional, and psychological experiences. Fisting, with its potential for intensity and depth, can serve as a powerful tool for both sadists and masochists to explore their desires.

Theoretical Framework

Theoretical perspectives on sadism and masochism often draw from psychoanalytic and behavioral theories. Sigmund Freud posited that sadism and masochism are rooted in the interplay of instinctual drives and societal norms. More contemporary theories, such as those proposed by BDSM educators, emphasize the importance of consent, negotiation, and the distinction between play and harm.

A common framework used in BDSM is the concept of **RACK** (Risk-Aware Consensual Kink), which emphasizes that participants should be fully aware of the risks involved in their activities and consent to them. This is particularly relevant in fisting, where the physical risks can be significant.

Integrating Fisting into S&M Dynamics

When integrating fisting into sadomasochistic practices, it is essential to establish a clear understanding of boundaries and consent. This includes:

- **Negotiation:** Prior to engaging in any fisting activities, partners should discuss their desires, limits, and safe words. This negotiation phase is crucial for building trust and ensuring that both parties feel comfortable.

- **Establishing Safe Words:** Safe words are vital in S&M dynamics, allowing participants to communicate their limits effectively. Common examples include "red" for stop and "yellow" for slow down or check-in.

- **Physical Preparation:** Engaging in fisting as a form of S&M requires physical readiness. This includes warming up, using adequate lubrication, and understanding the anatomy involved to prevent injury.

Psychological Dynamics of Pain and Pleasure

The interplay of pain and pleasure is central to the experience of sadomasochism. The **Gate Control Theory** of pain suggests that the experience of pain can be modulated by psychological factors, such as anticipation, context, and emotional connection. In the context of fisting, the act of submission or dominance can enhance the pleasurable aspects of pain, transforming it into a source of erotic excitement.

For many, the act of fisting can lead to a heightened state of arousal, where the physical sensations of fullness and pressure are intertwined with the psychological thrill of surrendering control or exerting power. This duality can create a profound sense of connection between partners, fostering intimacy and trust.

Practical Considerations

When exploring fisting within the context of sadism and masochism, it is crucial to prioritize safety and communication. Here are some practical tips:

1. **Start Slow:** Begin with gentle exploration and gradually increase intensity. This allows both partners to acclimate to sensations and establish trust.

2. **Monitor Reactions:** Pay close attention to your partner's verbal and non-verbal cues. Regular check-ins can help ensure that both parties are comfortable and enjoying the experience.

3. **Aftercare:** Aftercare is an essential component of any BDSM activity. Following a fisting session, partners should engage in aftercare practices, which may include cuddling, discussing the experience, and addressing any emotional or physical needs.

Case Studies and Examples

Consider the following examples that illustrate the integration of fisting into sadomasochistic dynamics:

- **Example 1:** A couple engages in a fisting scene where one partner, the dominant, uses fisting as a means of asserting control. The submissive partner, who has expressed a desire for intense sensations, finds pleasure in the physical sensations and the emotional release that follows. They use a safe word to communicate when they need to pause, ensuring the experience remains consensual and enjoyable.

- **Example 2:** In a more advanced scenario, a group of friends explores fisting in a consensual non-monogamous setting. They discuss their individual desires and boundaries beforehand, establishing clear communication protocols. The dominant partner incorporates elements of pain and pleasure, using fisting to enhance the experience of submission for their partner, who is eager to explore their limits.

Conclusion

Exploring sadism and masochism through fisting offers a rich tapestry of experiences that can deepen intimacy and enhance sexual pleasure. By prioritizing consent, communication, and safety, partners can navigate the complexities of these dynamics while fostering trust and connection. As with all forms of sexual expression, the key lies in understanding each other's desires and limits, creating a space where both partners can explore their fantasies freely and safely.

Fisting and Bondage

Fisting and bondage are two distinct but often complementary practices within the realm of BDSM and kink. Both activities emphasize trust, consent, and communication, and when combined, they can create profound experiences of intimacy and exploration. This section delves into how fisting can be integrated into bondage play, the dynamics involved, and essential considerations for safety and consent.

The Intersection of Fisting and Bondage

Fisting involves the insertion of the hand into a partner's body, typically the vagina or anus, while bondage refers to the practice of restraining a partner's movement using ropes, cuffs, or other devices. When these two practices are combined, they create a unique dynamic that can enhance the physical and emotional experience for both partners.

Theoretical Framework   The integration of fisting and bondage can be understood through various theoretical lenses, including:

- **Power Dynamics:** Bondage often involves a power exchange, where one partner takes on a dominant role while the other submits. This dynamic can heighten the experience of fisting, as the restrained partner may feel more vulnerable and open to exploration.

- **Sensory Deprivation:** Bondage can limit a partner's movement and sensory input, intensifying the sensations experienced during fisting. For example, blindfolding a partner can amplify their focus on the internal sensations created by the hand.

- **Trust and Vulnerability:** Both fisting and bondage require a high degree of trust between partners. Engaging in these practices together can deepen the emotional bond and enhance feelings of safety and connection.

Practical Considerations

When incorporating fisting into bondage play, several practical considerations must be addressed to ensure a safe and pleasurable experience.

Safety First

- **Communication:** Before engaging in fisting while bound, it is crucial to have open and honest discussions about boundaries, limits, and safe words. Establishing clear communication protocols can help both partners feel secure.

- **Positioning:** The position of the bound partner is essential for both comfort and safety. Ensure that the partner can easily signal discomfort or the need to stop. Consider using positions that allow for easy access to the partner's body while maintaining their safety.

- **Physical Limitations:** Be aware of the physical limitations imposed by bondage. Restricting movement can affect a partner's ability to signal discomfort. Adjustments may be necessary to accommodate these limitations.

Bondage Techniques for Fisting Various bondage techniques can enhance the fisting experience. Here are a few examples:

- **Hogtie:** This position binds the partner's wrists and ankles together, limiting movement. When fisting, ensure that the partner is comfortable and can still communicate effectively. The hogtie can enhance feelings of vulnerability and submission, intensifying the experience.

- **Suspension:** For advanced practitioners, suspension bondage can create a unique experience. However, safety is paramount; ensure that the partner is securely harnessed and able to breathe comfortably. The sensation of being suspended can heighten arousal and pleasure during fisting.

- **Chair Tie:** This position involves binding a partner to a chair, allowing them to remain upright while their hands and feet are restrained. This position can facilitate fisting while ensuring the partner feels secure and supported.

Addressing Potential Problems

While combining fisting and bondage can be exhilarating, it also presents potential challenges. Here are some common problems and solutions:

Communication Barriers In bondage, communication can be hindered by physical restraints. To mitigate this, establish non-verbal signals that can be used to indicate discomfort or the need to pause. For example, a simple hand squeeze or tapping can be effective.

Physical Discomfort The use of bondage can lead to physical discomfort, especially if restraints are too tight or improperly placed. Regularly check in with your partner to ensure they are comfortable and adjust restraints as necessary. Incorporate breaks if needed to prevent numbness or cramping.

Emotional Triggers For some individuals, bondage can trigger past trauma or emotional responses. It is essential to engage in pre-scene discussions about any potential triggers and establish aftercare practices to provide emotional support following the scene.

Aftercare and Emotional Support

Aftercare is a critical component of any BDSM scene, particularly when combining fisting and bondage. Aftercare involves attending to the physical and emotional needs of both partners following the scene. This may include:

- **Physical Care:** Checking for any physical discomfort or injuries, providing water, and helping the partner out of restraints gradually.

- **Emotional Support:** Discussing the experience, validating feelings, and providing reassurance can help partners process their emotions and reinforce trust.

- **Reinforcing Connection:** Engaging in cuddling, gentle touch, or other forms of intimacy can help partners reconnect and foster a sense of security.

Conclusion

Fisting and bondage can create deeply intimate and transformative experiences when approached with care, communication, and consent. By understanding the dynamics at play and prioritizing safety, partners can explore these practices in a way that enhances their connection and pleasure. As with all aspects of BDSM, the key lies in mutual respect, trust, and a commitment to ongoing dialogue about desires and boundaries.

Incorporating Fisting Into Impact Play and Spanking

In the realm of BDSM, impact play and fisting can be intricately woven together to create a rich tapestry of sensation and experience. Both practices can enhance the physical and emotional aspects of a scene, offering unique opportunities for exploration, connection, and pleasure. This section delves into the theory, potential challenges, and practical examples of incorporating fisting into impact play and spanking.

Understanding Impact Play and Fisting

Impact play involves the consensual use of force to create sensations ranging from light to intense. This can include spanking, slapping, flogging, or any form of striking. Fisting, on the other hand, is the act of inserting a hand into the vagina or anus, which can produce profound sensations and a sense of fullness. When these two practices are combined, they can amplify the physical sensations experienced by the receiver, potentially leading to heightened pleasure and emotional release.

The integration of fisting into impact play can be understood through the lens of the **Gate Control Theory of Pain**, which posits that the perception of pain can be modulated by the presence of other sensory inputs. In this context, the pleasurable sensations from fisting may distract from the discomfort of impact play, allowing for a more nuanced exploration of pain and pleasure.

Potential Challenges

While the combination of fisting and impact play can be exhilarating, it is essential to navigate potential challenges with care. Some of the key considerations include:

- **Physical Safety:** The introduction of fisting into impact play requires a thorough understanding of the anatomy involved. It is crucial to ensure that the receiver's body is adequately prepared for both practices. Failure to do so can lead to injuries such as tears, bruising, or internal damage.

- **Communication:** Open dialogue about limits, boundaries, and safe words is paramount. Both partners must feel comfortable expressing their needs and concerns, especially when engaging in practices that may push their physical or emotional limits.

- **Pacing:** The intensity of both fisting and impact play can vary significantly. It is important to establish a rhythm that allows for gradual escalation, ensuring that the receiver's body can adapt to the sensations being introduced.

- **Aftercare:** The combination of physical intensity from impact play and the emotional depth of fisting necessitates comprehensive aftercare. This can include physical comfort measures, emotional support, and time for reflection on the experience.

Practical Examples

To effectively incorporate fisting into impact play and spanking, consider the following techniques and strategies:

- **Warm-Up:** Begin with light impact play to prepare the body for both the physical sensations of spanking and the eventual insertion of the hand. This could involve gentle slaps or the use of a flogger to increase blood flow and sensitivity.

- **Layering Sensations:** As the receiver becomes more aroused, alternate between impact and fisting. For example, after delivering a series of spanks, pause to allow the receiver to breathe and then gently insert a lubricated hand, maintaining communication throughout the process. This layering can enhance the overall experience, creating a dance between pain and pleasure.

- **Use of Toys:** Incorporate toys such as paddles or crops alongside fisting. For instance, after a round of fisting, the dominant partner can use a paddle on the receiver's thighs or buttocks to create a contrast of sensations, heightening arousal and excitement.

- **Positioning:** Experiment with different positions that facilitate both fisting and impact play. For example, the receiver could be positioned on all fours, allowing for easier access for both fisting and spanking. This position also enables the dominant partner to maintain a level of control over the scene.

- **Building Intensity:** Gradually increase the intensity of both fisting and impact. Start with gentle fisting motions while delivering soft spanks, then gradually increase the depth of the fisting and the force of the strikes. This gradual escalation allows the receiver to acclimate to the sensations and fosters a deeper connection between partners.

- **Aftercare:** After the scene, engage in aftercare that addresses both the physical and emotional needs of the receiver. This could include cuddling, hydration, and discussing the experience to reinforce trust and connection.

Conclusion

Incorporating fisting into impact play and spanking can create a profound and transformative experience for both partners. By understanding the interplay between these practices and prioritizing communication, safety, and consent, practitioners can explore the boundaries of pleasure and pain in a consensual and enriching manner. As with all BDSM practices, the key lies in mutual respect, trust, and a shared commitment to creating a safe and pleasurable environment.

Fisting and Age Play

Age play is a form of role-playing in which participants assume roles that reflect a specific age, often involving dynamics of care, power, and nurturing. This practice can range from playful interactions to deeply intimate exchanges, and it often incorporates elements of vulnerability and trust. When fisting is included in age play scenarios, it can enhance the emotional and psychological dimensions of the experience, allowing participants to explore their desires and boundaries in a safe and consensual environment.

Understanding Age Play Dynamics

Age play often involves a clear delineation of roles, such as caregiver and child, or other age-related dynamics. These roles can be fluid and vary greatly among participants. The psychological underpinnings of age play can be complex, as they often touch upon themes of regression, innocence, and the desire for care. Fisting, when integrated into age play, can serve as a means of deepening intimacy and trust between partners.

The Intersection of Fisting and Age Play

Incorporating fisting into age play can take on various forms, depending on the dynamics established between partners. For instance, the caregiver may use fisting as a way to provide a sense of safety and exploration for the younger partner, or it may serve as a method of establishing dominance and control within the role-play.

$$\text{Intimacy} = \frac{\text{Trust} + \text{Communication}}{\text{Vulnerability}} \qquad (59)$$

This equation reflects the balance required in age play involving fisting: the greater the trust and communication, the higher the level of intimacy, while vulnerability can either enhance or hinder the experience based on individual comfort levels.

Potential Challenges and Considerations

While fisting can enhance the experience of age play, it is essential to navigate the potential challenges carefully:

- **Consent and Communication:** Clear communication is paramount. Both partners must explicitly discuss their boundaries, desires, and any potential triggers related to age play and fisting. Establishing safe words and signals can help ensure that both participants feel secure throughout the experience.

- **Emotional Safety:** The emotional implications of age play can be profound. Participants should be aware of their emotional states and any past traumas that may resurface during the role-play. Aftercare is crucial in providing comfort and reassurance following intense experiences.

- **Physical Safety:** When incorporating fisting, it is vital to prioritize physical safety. This includes understanding the anatomy involved, using appropriate lubrication, and ensuring that both partners are comfortable with the level of intensity. Regular check-ins during the act can help maintain safety.

Examples of Fisting in Age Play Scenarios

Here are some examples of how fisting might be integrated into age play scenarios:

- **Caregiver Role-Play:** In a caregiver dynamic, the caregiver may use fisting as a way to explore the younger partner's boundaries, ensuring that the experience is framed within a context of safety and nurturing. The caregiver's role is to guide the experience, providing reassurance and support throughout.

- **Role-Reversal Scenarios:** In some cases, partners may choose to reverse roles, allowing the younger partner to take on a more dominant position. This can involve fisting as a means of exploring power dynamics, where the "younger" partner asserts agency and control over the "older" partner.

- **Fantasy Exploration:** Fisting can serve as a tool for exploring fantasies related to age play, such as the desire for guidance, nurturing, or even discipline. These scenarios can be crafted to emphasize emotional connection and trust, allowing for a richer experience.

Navigating Aftercare and Emotional Support

Aftercare is a critical component of any BDSM or kink activity, but it takes on unique significance in age play scenarios. After engaging in fisting within an age play context, partners should prioritize:

- **Reassurance and Comfort:** Providing emotional support through cuddling, verbal affirmations, or gentle touch can help partners feel secure and valued after intense experiences.

- **Processing the Experience:** Engaging in a debriefing conversation can help partners articulate their feelings about the experience, addressing any concerns or insights that arose during the play.

- **Establishing Boundaries for Future Play:** Discussing what worked well and what could be improved helps partners refine their approach for future encounters, ensuring that both feel safe and fulfilled in their explorations.

Conclusion

Fisting within the context of age play can be a deeply fulfilling and intimate experience, provided that it is approached with care, consent, and open communication. By navigating the complexities of power dynamics, emotional safety, and physical well-being, participants can create a rich tapestry of exploration that honors their desires while fostering trust and connection. As with all forms of kink and BDSM, the key lies in prioritizing mutual satisfaction and safety, allowing for a transformative journey into the realms of pleasure and intimacy.

Fisting and Fetish Communities

Fisting, as a form of sexual expression, is deeply intertwined with various fetish communities that celebrate the exploration of boundaries, sensations, and desires. This section delves into the nuances of fisting within fetish contexts, examining the dynamics, challenges, and cultural significance of this practice.

Understanding Fetishes and Kinks

A fetish is defined as a strong and persistent sexual attraction to a specific object, body part, or activity that is not typically considered inherently sexual. In contrast, kink encompasses a broader range of unconventional sexual practices, including BDSM, roleplay, and fisting. Fisting can be viewed as both a fetish and a kink, depending on the individual's motivations and the context in which it is practiced.

Theories surrounding fetishism often reference Sigmund Freud's notion of the "sexual object choice," where individuals may develop attachments to non-genital parts of the body or specific practices as a means of sexual gratification. More contemporary theories, such as those proposed by John Money, emphasize the role of personal experiences and cultural context in shaping one's sexual preferences.

Fisting as an Element of BDSM Play

Within BDSM (Bondage, Discipline, Dominance, Submission, Sadism, and Masochism), fisting can serve as a powerful tool for exploring power dynamics and enhancing sensory experiences. The act of fisting often requires a high degree of trust and communication between partners, making it a profound expression of intimacy and vulnerability.

In BDSM contexts, fisting can be integrated into various scenarios, such as:

- **Dominant/Submissive Dynamics:** Fisting may be used to reinforce power exchange, where the dominant partner takes control of the experience while the submissive partner surrenders to the sensations and trust involved.

- **Sensory Play:** The physical sensations of fisting—pressure, fullness, and stretching—can heighten arousal and create a unique erotic experience, especially when combined with other BDSM elements like bondage or sensory deprivation.

- **Roleplay:** Fisting can be incorporated into roleplay scenarios, allowing participants to explore fantasies that may involve themes of submission, dominance, or even taboo.

Risk-Aware Consensual Kink (RACK) and Fisting

The concept of Risk-Aware Consensual Kink (RACK) emphasizes the importance of informed consent and understanding the potential risks involved in kink practices, including fisting. Participants are encouraged to communicate openly about their limits, desires, and safety measures before engaging in any activity.

In the context of fisting, RACK entails:

- **Informed Consent:** Ensuring that all parties are fully aware of the physical and emotional implications of fisting, including potential risks such as injury or emotional distress.

- **Safety Protocols:** Establishing clear guidelines for safe practices, such as using appropriate lubrication, maintaining hygiene, and recognizing when to stop.

- **Aftercare:** Providing emotional and physical support after a fisting session to address any feelings of vulnerability or discomfort that may arise.

Exploring Sadism and Masochism Through Fisting

Fisting can also intersect with sadistic and masochistic elements, where individuals may derive pleasure from the intensity of the experience. For some, the act of fisting may induce sensations of pain that can be pleasurable when framed within a consensual context. This duality of pleasure and pain is a hallmark of BDSM practices, allowing participants to explore their limits and desires.

Examples of how fisting can manifest within sadomasochistic dynamics include:

- **Pain as Pleasure:** Some individuals may find that the physical sensations associated with fisting, such as stretching and fullness, can enhance their arousal, particularly when combined with elements of pain or restraint.

- **Control and Surrender:** The act of fisting can symbolize a profound exchange of control, where the submissive partner surrenders to the dominant partner's will, heightening the emotional intensity of the experience.

Fisting and Bondage

Fisting can also be effectively integrated with bondage practices, creating a multi-layered experience that combines physical restraint with deep penetration. Bondage not only enhances the feelings of vulnerability but also allows the dominant partner to control the pace and intensity of the fisting experience.

Considerations for combining fisting and bondage include:

- **Safety First:** When engaging in bondage, it is crucial to ensure that the restrained partner can communicate their comfort level and has an established safe word or signal.

- **Enhanced Sensation:** The combination of being bound and receiving fisting can amplify the sensations experienced, as the restrained partner may become more acutely aware of their body and its responses.

Fisting and Age Play

Age play, a form of roleplay where participants assume different ages or roles, can also intersect with fisting practices. This dynamic allows individuals to explore power dynamics in a unique context, often involving themes of caretaking and vulnerability.

In age play scenarios, fisting may serve as a means of reinforcing the power dynamics at play, where one partner assumes a more dominant, protective role while the other adopts a submissive, vulnerable position. This interplay can create a rich tapestry of emotional and physical experiences, allowing participants to explore their fantasies in a safe and consensual manner.

Fisting and Fetish Communities: Challenges and Stigma

Despite the rich tapestry of experiences within fetish communities, fisting often faces stigma and misunderstanding from the broader society. Many individuals may harbor misconceptions about fisting, viewing it as inherently dangerous or deviant. This stigma can lead to feelings of shame or isolation among those who engage in fisting as part of their sexual expression.

To combat this stigma, it is essential for fetish communities to:

- **Promote Education:** Providing resources and workshops that educate individuals about safe fisting practices can help demystify the activity and promote understanding.

- **Foster Inclusivity:** Creating safe spaces where individuals can discuss their desires and experiences without judgment can help build community and support.

- **Advocate for Acceptance:** Engaging in advocacy efforts to normalize diverse sexual practices, including fisting, can help reduce stigma and promote acceptance within society.

Conclusion

Fisting, as a multifaceted practice within fetish communities, offers a unique opportunity for exploration, connection, and self-discovery. By understanding the dynamics at play, fostering open communication, and prioritizing safety, individuals can engage in fisting as a fulfilling and enriching aspect of their sexual repertoire. The journey through fisting not only challenges societal norms but also empowers individuals to embrace their desires and explore the depths of intimacy and trust within their relationships.

Building Kink-Friendly Spaces for Fisters

Creating kink-friendly spaces for fisters is essential for fostering a sense of community, safety, and acceptance among individuals exploring this intimate and often misunderstood practice. These spaces can take various forms, including physical venues, online platforms, and social networks. In this section, we will explore the theoretical foundations, potential challenges, and practical examples of building such spaces.

Theoretical Foundations

The concept of kink-friendly spaces is rooted in the principles of consent, inclusivity, and respect. According to the *Kink Aware Professionals* (KAP) framework, it is crucial to create environments where individuals feel safe to express their desires and boundaries without fear of judgment or discrimination. This framework emphasizes the importance of understanding the unique dynamics involved in kink practices, including fisting, which can often be stigmatized.

$$C = \frac{R + I + E}{3} \qquad (60)$$

Where:

- C = Community Acceptance
- R = Respect for Individual Choices
- I = Inclusivity of Diverse Practices
- E = Education on Safety and Consent

This equation illustrates that community acceptance is a function of respect, inclusivity, and education. Building a kink-friendly space requires a commitment to these principles.

Identifying Challenges

While the need for kink-friendly spaces is evident, several challenges can arise in their establishment and maintenance:

- **Stigma and Misunderstanding:** Many individuals still hold misconceptions about kink practices, including fisting. This can lead to social stigma, making it difficult to find supportive environments.
- **Safety Concerns:** Physical and emotional safety is paramount in kink practices. Spaces must ensure that all participants are aware of and adhere to safety protocols.

- **Diversity of Needs:** The kink community is diverse, encompassing various identities, orientations, and preferences. Creating a space that caters to all can be challenging.

- **Legal and Ethical Considerations:** Navigating the legal landscape surrounding kink practices, including consent laws, can complicate the establishment of safe spaces.

Practical Examples

Several successful models exist for building kink-friendly spaces, including:

- **Local Kink Communities:** Many cities have established kink organizations that host regular events, workshops, and meet-ups. These communities often prioritize consent and safety, providing a supportive environment for fisters and other kink practitioners.

- **Online Platforms:** Websites and forums dedicated to kink discussions allow individuals to share experiences, seek advice, and find partners. Platforms like FetLife create virtual communities where members can engage in discussions about fisting and other kink practices.

- **Workshops and Education:** Hosting educational workshops on fisting techniques, safety, and consent can help demystify the practice and empower individuals to explore it safely. These workshops often create a sense of camaraderie among participants, fostering connections and support.

- **Kink-Friendly Venues:** Some bars, clubs, and private spaces cater specifically to the kink community, providing a safe and welcoming environment for fisting and other practices. These venues often have established protocols for consent and safety, ensuring a positive experience for all attendees.

Building Inclusive Practices

To create truly kink-friendly spaces, it is essential to incorporate inclusive practices that acknowledge and respect the diversity within the kink community:

- **Diversity Training:** Providing training for organizers, facilitators, and community members on issues related to diversity, consent, and safety can help create a more welcoming environment.

- **Feedback Mechanisms:** Establishing channels for community feedback allows members to voice concerns and suggestions, fostering a sense of ownership and collaboration within the space.

- **Accessibility Considerations:** Ensuring that spaces are accessible to individuals with varying abilities is crucial. This includes physical accessibility as well as creating an environment where all voices are heard and respected.

Conclusion

Building kink-friendly spaces for fisters is a vital step towards creating a supportive and inclusive community. By addressing the theoretical foundations, recognizing challenges, and implementing practical examples, we can foster environments where individuals feel empowered to explore their desires safely and consensually. As we work towards this goal, it is essential to remain committed to the principles of respect, inclusivity, and ongoing education, ensuring that our communities continue to thrive and evolve.

$$S = \frac{C + E + P}{3} \tag{61}$$

Where:

- S = Safe Space
- C = Community Support
- E = Education on Practices
- P = Policies on Consent and Safety

This equation reinforces the idea that a safe space is built on community support, education, and clear policies regarding consent and safety, essential for fostering a thriving kink community.

Fisting Resources and Support

Fisting Resources and Support

Fisting Resources and Support

Fisting, as a complex and intimate sexual practice, requires a nuanced understanding of both the physical and emotional aspects involved. To navigate this practice safely and enjoyably, it is essential to access a variety of resources and support systems. This section outlines key resources that can enhance your knowledge, skills, and community connections related to fisting.

Online Platforms and Forums for Fisters

The internet hosts a wealth of information and community support for those interested in fisting. Online platforms and forums serve as safe spaces for individuals to share experiences, ask questions, and seek advice. Notable examples include:

- **Fisting Forums:** Websites dedicated to kink and BDSM often have dedicated sections for fisting discussions. Users can engage in conversations about techniques, safety practices, and personal stories.

- **Social Media Groups:** Platforms like Facebook and Reddit host groups where members can post inquiries, share tips, and connect with others who have similar interests in fisting.

- **Discord Servers:** These real-time chat platforms allow for immediate communication and support. Many servers are dedicated to kink and BDSM, providing a space for fisters to connect.

Locating Local Fisting Communities and Clubs

In-person connections can significantly enhance your fisting journey. Local communities often organize events, workshops, and meetups that focus on safe practices and shared experiences. To find such communities:

- **Kink and BDSM Clubs:** Many cities have clubs that host events for various kinks, including fisting. These venues often provide a safe environment for exploration and learning.

- **Workshops and Classes:** Look for workshops that focus on fisting techniques and safety. These classes can provide hands-on experience and expert guidance.

- **Community Events:** Attend local pride events, sex-positive fairs, or kink conventions where fisting may be discussed or demonstrated.

Engaging in Peer Support and Mentoring

Peer support can be invaluable for those exploring fisting. Engaging with more experienced practitioners can provide insights and reassurance. Consider the following avenues:

- **Mentorship Programs:** Some kink communities offer mentorship programs that pair novices with experienced fisters who can provide guidance and support.

- **Support Groups:** Joining a support group focused on sexual exploration can help individuals discuss their experiences, concerns, and triumphs in a safe environment.

- **Workshops with Q&A:** Many workshops include time for questions, allowing participants to seek advice directly from experts and experienced practitioners.

Exploring Virtual Fisting Spaces and Workshops

With the rise of online learning, numerous virtual resources are available for those interested in fisting. These options provide flexibility and accessibility:

- **Webinars and Online Classes:** Many educators offer virtual classes on fisting techniques, safety, and emotional aspects. These can often be accessed from the comfort of your home.

- **Virtual Meetups:** Online gatherings allow individuals to connect and share experiences, fostering community even from a distance.

- **Streaming Platforms:** Some platforms host content creators who specialize in sexual education, including fisting, providing valuable insights and demonstrations.

Seeking Fisting-Specific Education and Training

Formal education can enhance your understanding and practice of fisting. Consider the following resources:

- **Sexual Health Educators:** Look for certified sexual health educators who offer courses specifically on fisting, covering both the physical and emotional aspects.

- **Books and Publications:** Numerous books focus on fisting techniques, safety, and emotional considerations. Seek out reputable authors and educators in the field.

- **Online Courses:** Platforms like Skillshare or Udemy may offer courses on kink and BDSM practices, including fisting, taught by experienced practitioners.

Listening to Fisting Podcasts and Online Discussions

Podcasts and online discussions can provide valuable insights and diverse perspectives on fisting. Some recommended resources include:

- **Sexual Wellness Podcasts:** Many podcasts feature episodes dedicated to fisting, exploring personal stories, safety tips, and expert advice.

- **Panel Discussions:** Online panels with experts in the field can provide a wealth of information and allow for audience questions.

- **YouTube Channels:** Some educators and practitioners share their knowledge through video content, offering visual demonstrations and discussions.

Discovering Fisting Literature and Academic Resources

Academic literature can provide a deeper understanding of the psychological and sociocultural aspects of fisting. Consider exploring:

- **Research Articles:** Academic journals may publish studies on sexual practices, including fisting, providing insights into safety, health, and emotional impacts.

- **Books on Sexuality:** Many authors address fisting within the broader context of sexuality, offering theoretical perspectives and practical advice.

- **Zines and Self-Published Works:** Independent creators often produce zines that explore personal narratives and experiences related to fisting.

Finding Fisting-Friendly Healthcare Providers

When engaging in fisting, it's essential to have access to healthcare providers who understand your needs and concerns. Seek out:

- **Sexual Health Clinics:** Look for clinics that specialize in sexual health and are knowledgeable about kink practices.

- **LGBTQ+ Friendly Providers:** Many LGBTQ+ health centers are more likely to understand and respect diverse sexual practices, including fisting.

- **Therapists with Kink Awareness:** Finding a therapist who is knowledgeable about kink can provide valuable support for emotional or psychological concerns related to fisting.

Conclusion

Navigating the world of fisting requires a combination of knowledge, support, and community. By leveraging the resources outlined in this section, individuals can enhance their understanding of fisting, engage with supportive communities, and prioritize safety and consent. Remember, the journey into fisting is deeply personal and should be approached with care, curiosity, and compassion.

Finding Fisting Communities and Events

Online Platforms and Forums for Fisters

In the digital age, online platforms and forums have become vital spaces for individuals interested in fisting to connect, share experiences, and gather information. These platforms serve as a safe haven for education, support, and community-building, allowing individuals to explore their interests and desires without the stigma often associated with such practices. This section will delve into the various online platforms available for fisters, the benefits and challenges of these spaces, and best practices for engaging with them.

Types of Online Platforms

Online platforms for fisters can be broadly categorized into several types:

- **Social Media Groups:** Websites like Facebook, Reddit, and FetLife host numerous groups dedicated to fisting. These groups often provide a space for members to share personal stories, ask questions, and offer advice. For example, the *Fisting Enthusiasts* group on Facebook allows users to post experiences, share techniques, and discuss safety measures.

- **Dedicated Forums:** Many websites host forums specifically for sexual practices, including fisting. These forums allow for in-depth discussions on topics ranging from techniques to emotional experiences. Websites like *The BDSM Forum* and *FetLife* offer threads dedicated to fisting where users can engage in detailed conversations.

- **Educational Websites and Blogs:** Various sex educators and therapists maintain blogs or websites that provide resources and information about fisting. These platforms often include articles on safety, techniques, and personal narratives. Websites such as *Scarlet Teen* and *Kinkly* provide valuable insights into safe practices and personal experiences.

- **Chat Rooms and Live Events:** Some platforms host live chats or video discussions where individuals can interact in real time. Websites like *Kink Live* offer live-streaming events that focus on various kink practices, including fisting. These spaces facilitate immediate feedback and community interaction.

- **Online Workshops and Webinars:** With the rise of virtual education, many sex educators offer workshops and webinars focused on fisting. These sessions provide participants with the opportunity to learn from experts in a structured environment. Websites like *Sex Positive Workshops* often list upcoming events related to fisting and other sexual practices.

Benefits of Online Platforms

Engaging with online platforms offers several advantages for individuals interested in fisting:

- **Anonymity and Privacy:** Many online platforms allow users to participate without revealing their identities, which can be particularly beneficial for those who may feel embarrassed or stigmatized about their interests. This anonymity encourages open dialogue and exploration.

- **Access to Diverse Perspectives:** Online forums bring together individuals from various backgrounds, experiences, and skill levels. This diversity enriches discussions and allows users to learn from one another's experiences and insights.

- **Resource Sharing:** Members of online communities often share resources, such as articles, videos, and personal experiences, that can enhance knowledge and understanding of fisting. This collaborative approach to learning fosters a sense of community.

- **Support and Validation:** Connecting with others who share similar interests can provide emotional support and validation. Online platforms can help individuals feel less isolated in their desires and experiences, promoting a sense of belonging.

- **Education and Safety:** Many online forums prioritize education and safety, providing guidelines and discussions about best practices. This emphasis on informed consent and safety can help reduce the risks associated with fisting.

Challenges and Considerations

While online platforms offer numerous benefits, they also present challenges that users should be aware of:

- **Misinformation:** The internet is rife with misinformation, and not all advice shared in online forums is accurate or safe. Users should critically evaluate the information they encounter and cross-reference it with reputable sources.

- **Toxicity and Judgment:** Some online communities can be unwelcoming or judgmental, particularly toward newcomers or those who may have different experiences or preferences. It is essential to find supportive spaces that foster respect and understanding.

- **Privacy Concerns:** Despite the anonymity of online platforms, users should be cautious about sharing personal information that could compromise their privacy or safety. It is advisable to use pseudonyms and avoid revealing identifiable details.

- **Emotional Vulnerability:** Engaging in discussions about intimate topics can sometimes lead to emotional vulnerability. Users should be mindful of their emotional boundaries and seek support if discussions trigger uncomfortable feelings.

- **Limited Non-Verbal Cues:** Online communication lacks the non-verbal cues present in face-to-face interactions, which can lead to misunderstandings. It is crucial to practice clear and explicit communication in all online exchanges.

Best Practices for Engaging with Online Platforms

To maximize the benefits of online platforms while minimizing potential risks, consider the following best practices:

- **Verify Information:** Always cross-check information with credible sources before acting on advice or techniques shared in online forums. Look for recommendations from experienced practitioners or educators.

- **Choose Supportive Communities:** Seek out groups and forums that prioritize respect, consent, and education. Engage with communities that align with your values and provide a safe space for open discussion.

- **Establish Boundaries:** Be clear about your boundaries when participating in discussions. If a topic feels uncomfortable, do not hesitate to disengage or set limits on what you are willing to share.

- **Practice Self-Care:** Recognize that discussions about fisting can evoke strong emotions. Engage in self-care practices to manage any emotional responses that may arise during or after interactions.

- **Contribute Positively:** Share your knowledge and experiences to contribute positively to the community. Offering support to others can foster a sense of connection and help build a supportive environment for all members.

In conclusion, online platforms and forums for fisters provide invaluable resources for education, support, and community-building. By engaging thoughtfully and responsibly with these spaces, individuals can deepen their understanding of fisting, connect with like-minded individuals, and enhance their overall experience of this intimate practice.

Locating Local Fisting Communities and Clubs

Finding local fisting communities and clubs can be a rewarding journey that enhances your exploration of this intimate practice. Engaging with others who share similar interests fosters a sense of belonging and provides opportunities for education, support, and safe exploration. This section will outline various methods for locating these communities, including online resources, local events, and social networks.

Online Platforms and Forums

The internet serves as a powerful tool for connecting with like-minded individuals. Numerous online platforms and forums cater specifically to the fisting community. Websites like FetLife, a social networking site for the BDSM and kink community, allow users to create profiles, share experiences, and engage in discussions about fisting and other kinks. Users can search for local groups or events by entering their location and filtering results based on interests.

$$\text{Local Groups} = \text{FetLife} + \text{Location} + \text{Interests} \qquad (62)$$

In addition to FetLife, specialized forums and discussion boards can provide valuable insights and connections. Websites such as Reddit have subreddits dedicated to fisting and kink, where users share personal stories, advice, and information about local meetups. Engaging in these forums can help you identify local communities and events.

Locating Local Fisting Communities and Clubs

In-person connections can significantly enrich your fisting experience. Here are several strategies for locating local fisting communities and clubs:

 1. **Attend Kink and BDSM Events**: Many cities host kink and BDSM events, such as workshops, munches (casual gatherings), and parties. These events often welcome individuals interested in fisting and provide opportunities to meet others in a safe and consensual environment. Websites like Meetup.com can help you find local kink events, while community centers may also host workshops or gatherings.

 2. **Visit Sex-Positive Spaces**: Look for sex-positive venues, such as adult stores, sex clubs, or community centers that focus on sexual health and education. These spaces often host events related to various kinks, including fisting. Staff members may also have information about local fisting groups or upcoming workshops.

 3. **Network with Local Educators**: Many sex educators and therapists specialize in kink and BDSM. They often have connections within the community and can guide you to local fisting clubs or workshops. Attending classes or workshops led by these professionals can also help you meet others interested in fisting.

 4. **Utilize Social Media**: Platforms like Facebook and Instagram can be valuable for finding local fisting communities. Search for groups or pages dedicated to kink, BDSM, or fisting in your area. Engaging with these communities can provide insights into local events and gatherings.

 5. **Word of Mouth**: Don't underestimate the power of personal connections. If you have friends or acquaintances within the kink community, ask them about local fisting groups or clubs. They may have valuable insights or recommendations based on their experiences.

Challenges in Finding Local Communities

While seeking local fisting communities, you may encounter several challenges:

- **Stigma and Discretion**: Fisting remains a taboo subject in many circles. Individuals may be hesitant to openly discuss their interests or seek out communities due to fear of judgment. It is crucial to approach this exploration with discretion and respect for others' privacy.

- **Safety Concerns**: Ensuring your safety when attending local events is paramount. Always prioritize consent, communication, and personal boundaries.

Research venues and events beforehand, and consider attending with a trusted friend.

  - **Diversity of Communities**: Fisting communities can vary significantly in their focus, from casual gatherings to more structured BDSM clubs. It is essential to find a community that aligns with your values and interests. Take the time to explore different groups to find the right fit.

Examples of Local Communities

To illustrate the diversity of local fisting communities, here are a few hypothetical examples:

  - **The Fisting Collective**: A local club that hosts monthly workshops focused on fisting techniques, safety, and communication. Members can participate in guided practice sessions and engage in discussions about their experiences.
  - **Kink Nights at the Local Dungeon**: A BDSM club that organizes themed nights, including a dedicated fisting event. Participants can explore fisting in a safe environment, with experienced facilitators available to offer guidance.
  - **Fisting Meetups**: A casual gathering of individuals interested in fisting, organized through a local kink group. Participants share experiences, discuss safety practices, and build connections in a relaxed atmosphere.

Conclusion

Locating local fisting communities and clubs can significantly enhance your journey into this intimate practice. By utilizing online resources, attending local events, and networking with others, you can find a supportive environment that fosters exploration and growth. Remember to prioritize safety, consent, and open communication as you navigate this exciting aspect of your sexuality. Embrace the journey of finding your community, and enjoy the shared experiences that come with it.

Attending Fisting-Focused Events and Workshops

Attending fisting-focused events and workshops can be an enriching experience for individuals and couples looking to deepen their understanding and practice of fisting in a safe, supportive environment. These gatherings provide opportunities for education, skill development, and community building among like-minded individuals.

Purpose of Fisting Workshops

Fisting workshops are designed to educate participants about the techniques, safety practices, and emotional aspects of fisting. They often include a combination of theoretical instruction and practical demonstrations. The primary goals of these workshops are:

- **Skill Development**: Participants learn proper techniques for fisting, including hand positioning, lubrication, and communication strategies.

- **Safety Education**: Workshops emphasize the importance of hygiene, consent, and risk management, ensuring participants understand how to engage in fisting safely.

- **Community Building**: These events foster a sense of community among participants, allowing them to share experiences, tips, and support.

- **Emotional Exploration**: Workshops often address the psychological and emotional dimensions of fisting, helping participants navigate their feelings and desires.

Types of Events

Fisting-focused events can vary widely in format and content. Some common types include:

- **Workshops**: Structured sessions led by experienced instructors that cover specific topics related to fisting, often including hands-on practice.

- **Conventions**: Larger gatherings that may feature multiple workshops, panels, and social events centered around BDSM and kink, including fisting.

- **Support Groups**: Informal meet-ups where individuals can share experiences and seek advice in a safe and non-judgmental environment.

- **Demonstration Events**: Performances or demonstrations by skilled practitioners to showcase techniques and practices in a live setting.

Finding Events and Workshops

To find fisting-focused events and workshops, consider the following resources:

- **Online Platforms**: Websites such as FetLife, Meetup, and Eventbrite often list local workshops and events focused on kink and BDSM practices.

- **Social Media**: Follow educators, sex-positive organizations, and community groups on platforms like Instagram and Facebook to stay updated on upcoming events.

- **Local BDSM Communities**: Many cities have BDSM clubs or organizations that host regular events. Engaging with these communities can lead to discovering fisting workshops.

- **Sex-Positive Conferences**: Events like Sex Positive World and other sexuality conferences often feature workshops on various kinks, including fisting.

What to Expect at Workshops

When attending a fisting-focused workshop, participants can expect a variety of activities:

- **Lectures and Discussions**: Instructors will provide information on anatomy, safety, and techniques, often encouraging questions and discussions.

- **Demonstrations**: Participants may witness live demonstrations of fisting techniques, highlighting the importance of communication and consent.

- **Practice Sessions**: Many workshops include opportunities for participants to practice techniques under the guidance of instructors, often using models or props for safety.

- **Group Activities**: Participants may engage in group discussions or exercises aimed at building trust and communication skills.

Safety Considerations

While attending any fisting-focused event, it is crucial to prioritize safety:

- **Consent**: Ensure that all participants are aware of and agree to the activities being conducted. Consent must be explicit and ongoing.

FINDING FISTING COMMUNITIES AND EVENTS

- **Hygiene**: Workshops should maintain high standards of cleanliness. Participants should be encouraged to bring their own supplies, such as gloves and lubricant.

- **Comfort Levels**: Participants should never feel pressured to engage in any activity they are uncomfortable with. It is essential to communicate personal boundaries clearly.

- **Aftercare**: Aftercare is vital following any intense physical or emotional experience. Participants should discuss aftercare practices with their partners or facilitators.

Examples of Notable Workshops

Several organizations and educators are well-known for their fisting workshops:

- **The Kink Academy**: Offers online and in-person workshops focused on various kink practices, including fisting, with a strong emphasis on safety and consent.

- **Fetish Events**: Many fetish events, such as Folsom Street Fair or KinkFest, feature workshops on fisting and other BDSM practices, providing a rich learning environment.

- **Local BDSM Clubs**: Many clubs host regular workshops that cover fisting as part of their educational programming, often led by experienced practitioners.

Conclusion

Attending fisting-focused events and workshops can significantly enhance one's understanding and practice of fisting. By engaging with experienced instructors and connecting with a community of like-minded individuals, participants can explore their desires safely and confidently. It is essential to approach these events with an open mind, a commitment to safety, and a willingness to learn, ensuring a fulfilling and enriching experience that deepens one's connection to this intimate practice.

Building Connections in Fisting Communities

Building connections within fisting communities is essential for fostering a safe, supportive, and informed environment for exploration. These connections can enhance personal experiences, provide resources for education, and create a sense of belonging among individuals who share similar interests. In this section, we will discuss the importance of community, strategies for building connections, and the potential challenges that may arise.

The Importance of Community

Community plays a vital role in any sexual exploration, particularly in practices that may be viewed as taboo or unconventional, such as fisting. A supportive community can provide:

- **Shared Knowledge:** Members can exchange information about techniques, safety practices, and personal experiences, enriching the collective understanding of fisting.

- **Emotional Support:** Engaging with others who share similar interests can alleviate feelings of isolation or shame, fostering a sense of acceptance.

- **Resources:** Communities often share resources such as workshops, educational materials, and local events, facilitating access to valuable information.

- **Safety:** A connected community can promote safer practices by emphasizing consent and risk awareness, helping individuals navigate their experiences responsibly.

Strategies for Building Connections

1. **Join Online Forums and Social Media Groups:** - Platforms like Reddit, FetLife, and specialized Facebook groups can serve as entry points for individuals seeking to connect with others interested in fisting. Engaging in discussions, sharing experiences, and asking questions can help foster relationships. - Example: A user on FetLife might post about their first fisting experience, inviting others to share their thoughts and tips. This interaction can lead to private messages and deeper connections.

2. **Attend Workshops and Events:** - Participating in workshops focused on fisting techniques, safety, and communication can provide opportunities to meet

like-minded individuals in a structured environment. These events often encourage networking and sharing experiences. - Example: A local kink community might host a fisting workshop where attendees not only learn techniques but also engage in discussions, creating bonds through shared learning experiences.

3. **Engage in Local Community Groups:** - Many cities have local BDSM or kink organizations that host regular meetups, discussions, and events. Joining these groups can provide access to a wider network of individuals interested in fisting. - Example: A local BDSM group may organize monthly munches (casual social gatherings) where individuals can meet in a non-sexual setting to discuss interests and experiences.

4. **Utilize Peer Mentorship:** - Finding a mentor within the community can provide personalized guidance and support. A mentor can share their experiences, help navigate challenges, and offer insights into safe practices. - Example: An experienced fister may volunteer to mentor newcomers, providing them with resources and answering questions, thus fostering a supportive relationship.

5. **Participate in Online Discussions and Webinars:** - Engaging in webinars and online discussions led by experts can enhance knowledge and facilitate connections with others who attend. These platforms often allow for interaction through Q&A sessions. - Example: An online webinar on fisting safety may attract participants from various backgrounds, enabling them to connect over shared interests and learn from each other.

Challenges in Building Connections

While building connections in fisting communities can be rewarding, there are challenges that individuals may encounter:

1. **Stigma and Misunderstanding:** - Fisting can carry social stigma, leading to feelings of shame or reluctance to engage openly. Individuals may fear judgment from others, hindering their willingness to connect. - Solution: Emphasizing the importance of discretion and creating safe spaces for discussion can help mitigate these concerns.

2. **Power Dynamics:** - In communities that explore BDSM and kink, power dynamics can complicate relationships. Individuals may struggle with navigating consent and boundaries, especially in hierarchical structures. - Solution: Clear communication and established consent practices are crucial in addressing these dynamics. Encouraging open discussions about power can promote healthier connections.

3. **Misinformation:** - Inconsistent information about fisting techniques and safety can lead to confusion and risk. Individuals may encounter conflicting advice,

making it difficult to build a solid foundation of knowledge. - Solution: Encouraging evidence-based practices and sharing reputable resources can help individuals discern accurate information and build connections based on trust.

4. Isolation: - Some individuals may feel isolated in their interests, particularly in conservative environments. This isolation can hinder their ability to connect with others. - Solution: Online platforms can serve as vital lifelines, allowing individuals to find community beyond geographical limitations.

Conclusion

Building connections in fisting communities is a multifaceted process that requires openness, communication, and a commitment to safety. By engaging with others through online platforms, workshops, and local groups, individuals can foster a sense of belonging and support. While challenges such as stigma and misinformation may arise, addressing these issues through education and clear communication can enhance the experience of exploring fisting. Ultimately, a connected community can empower individuals to embrace their desires with confidence and care, transforming the journey into one of shared exploration and growth.

Engaging in Peer Support and Mentoring

Engaging in peer support and mentoring is an essential aspect of exploring fisting safely and enjoyably. This process not only enhances individual experiences but also fosters a sense of community and shared understanding among those who engage in this intimate practice. In this section, we will discuss the theoretical foundations of peer support, the challenges individuals may face, and practical examples of how to effectively engage in mentoring relationships.

Theoretical Foundations of Peer Support

Peer support is grounded in several psychological and sociological theories that emphasize the importance of social connections in personal growth. One relevant theory is the **Social Support Theory**, which posits that emotional, informational, and instrumental support from peers can significantly enhance an individual's coping mechanisms and overall well-being.

According to *Cohen and Wills (1985)*, social support can buffer the effects of stress and promote resilience, particularly in marginalized communities where individuals may face stigma or discrimination regarding their sexual practices. This is particularly relevant in the context of fisting, which can be stigmatized or misunderstood by those outside the community.

Moreover, the **Mentoring Theory** suggests that mentorship can lead to increased self-efficacy and personal development. Kram (1985) identified two types of mentoring functions: career-related and psychosocial. Career-related functions include sponsorship, exposure, and coaching, while psychosocial functions encompass friendship, emotional support, and role modeling. Both types are crucial in creating a safe space for individuals to explore their desires and boundaries in fisting.

Challenges in Peer Support and Mentoring

While peer support can be immensely beneficial, several challenges may arise in the context of fisting. These challenges can include:

- **Misinformation:** There may be a lack of accurate information regarding fisting techniques, safety protocols, and emotional implications. Misinformation can lead to unsafe practices and negative experiences.

- **Stigma and Shame:** Individuals may feel ashamed of their desires or experiences, which can hinder open communication and support. The fear of judgment can prevent individuals from seeking or offering help.

- **Power Dynamics:** In mentoring relationships, imbalances in experience and knowledge can create power dynamics that may lead to dependency or coercion. It is crucial to establish clear boundaries and ensure that both parties feel empowered in the relationship.

- **Emotional Vulnerability:** Discussing personal experiences with fisting can evoke strong emotions, including fear, shame, or trauma. Mentors must be equipped to handle these emotions sensitively and effectively.

Practical Examples of Engaging in Peer Support and Mentoring

To effectively engage in peer support and mentoring within the fisting community, consider the following strategies:

1. **Establish Support Groups:** Create or join local or online support groups where individuals can share their experiences, ask questions, and offer advice. These groups can provide a safe space for discussing fisting and related topics, fostering a sense of belonging and understanding.

2. **Facilitate Workshops:** Organize workshops focused on fisting techniques, safety practices, and emotional preparation. These workshops can serve as educational platforms for both novices and experienced practitioners to learn from one another and share insights.

3. **Mentorship Programs:** Develop structured mentorship programs that pair experienced individuals with those new to fisting. These relationships should prioritize open communication, consent, and mutual respect, allowing mentees to ask questions and seek guidance in a supportive environment.

4. **Create Resource Sharing Platforms:** Establish online forums or platforms where individuals can share resources, articles, and personal stories related to fisting. This can help combat misinformation and provide a wealth of knowledge for community members.

5. **Encourage Open Dialogue:** Foster an atmosphere of open dialogue where individuals feel comfortable discussing their desires, boundaries, and experiences. This can help normalize conversations around fisting and reduce feelings of shame or isolation.

Conclusion

Engaging in peer support and mentoring within the fisting community can significantly enhance individual experiences and promote a culture of safety, consent, and understanding. By addressing the theoretical foundations, recognizing potential challenges, and implementing practical strategies, individuals can create a supportive environment that empowers everyone involved. Ultimately, fostering connections and sharing knowledge can lead to more fulfilling and safe exploration of fisting as a consensual and pleasurable practice.

Exploring Virtual Fisting Spaces and Workshops

In the age of digital connectivity, virtual spaces have emerged as vital environments for exploring fisting and other sexual practices. These online platforms provide opportunities for education, community-building, and safe exploration, particularly for those who may not have access to local resources or who prefer the anonymity and comfort of their own homes. This section delves into the various aspects of virtual fisting spaces and workshops, offering insights into their benefits, challenges, and the types of resources available.

The Rise of Virtual Communities

The emergence of virtual communities has transformed how individuals engage with their sexual identities and practices. Online platforms such as forums, social media groups, and dedicated websites allow individuals to connect with like-minded people, share experiences, and seek advice. For instance, platforms like FetLife and Reddit host numerous discussions around fisting, where participants can ask questions, share techniques, and discuss safety measures.

Benefits of Virtual Fisting Workshops

Virtual workshops offer several advantages:

- **Accessibility:** Individuals from various geographical locations can access workshops without the constraints of travel. This is particularly beneficial for those living in areas where sexual exploration is stigmatized or taboo.

- **Anonymity:** Participants can engage in discussions and learning without revealing their identities, which can foster a sense of safety and openness.

- **Diverse Perspectives:** Virtual spaces often attract a wide range of participants, allowing for the sharing of diverse experiences and techniques. This can enhance the learning experience by exposing individuals to different cultural practices and insights.

- **Comfort:** Learning from the comfort of one's home can reduce anxiety and allow participants to engage at their own pace.

Types of Virtual Workshops

Virtual workshops on fisting can take many forms, including:

- **Live Webinars:** These real-time sessions often feature expert speakers who can provide demonstrations, answer questions, and facilitate discussions. For example, a workshop led by a certified sex educator might cover anatomy, safety protocols, and techniques for effective communication.

- **Pre-recorded Courses:** Participants can access these at their convenience, allowing for self-paced learning. These courses may include instructional videos, reading materials, and interactive quizzes to reinforce learning.

- **Discussion Forums:** Online forums provide a space for ongoing conversations about fisting. Participants can post questions, share experiences, and offer support to one another. This peer-to-peer learning can be invaluable for those new to the practice.

- **Virtual Meetups:** These informal gatherings allow individuals to connect and share experiences in a more relaxed setting. They may include icebreaker activities, guided discussions, and opportunities for participants to share their own insights and questions.

Challenges and Considerations

While virtual spaces offer numerous benefits, there are also challenges to consider:

- **Quality Control:** The internet is rife with misinformation. Participants must critically evaluate the credibility of the sources and educators they engage with. It is essential to seek out workshops led by qualified professionals who prioritize safety and informed consent.

- **Limited Hands-On Experience:** Fisting, being a physical practice, requires a level of hands-on experience that virtual workshops may not fully provide. Participants should complement online learning with practical, in-person experiences when possible.

- **Privacy Concerns:** Engaging in online discussions about fisting can raise privacy issues. Participants should be mindful of the information they share and consider using pseudonyms or anonymous accounts to protect their identities.

- **Technical Issues:** Virtual workshops rely on technology, which can sometimes fail. Participants should ensure they have a stable internet connection and familiarize themselves with the platform being used for the workshop.

Examples of Virtual Fisting Workshops

Several organizations and educators offer virtual workshops focused on fisting and related topics. For instance:

- **The Pleasure Chest:** Known for its inclusive approach to sexual education, The Pleasure Chest offers online workshops that cover a range of topics,

- **Kink Academy:** This platform provides a plethora of instructional videos on various kink practices, including fisting. Members can access a library of resources that cover techniques, safety, and emotional considerations.
- **Fisting Workshops by Sex Educators:** Many independent sex educators host their own virtual workshops, focusing on fisting techniques, safety, and communication strategies. These workshops often include interactive elements, such as polls and breakout sessions for smaller group discussions.

Conclusion

Exploring virtual fisting spaces and workshops opens up new avenues for education, community engagement, and personal growth. While they present unique challenges, the benefits of accessibility, anonymity, and diverse perspectives make them invaluable resources for anyone interested in fisting. By approaching these virtual environments with a critical eye and a commitment to safety and consent, individuals can enhance their understanding and practice of fisting in a supportive and informed manner.

Seeking Fisting-Specific Education and Training

As the practice of fisting continues to gain visibility and acceptance within various sexual communities, the demand for specialized education and training has become increasingly important. Engaging in fisting safely and enjoyably requires a solid understanding of anatomy, techniques, and the emotional aspects involved. This section will explore the avenues available for seeking fisting-specific education and training, addressing the importance of informed practice, and providing resources for individuals and couples interested in expanding their knowledge.

The Importance of Education in Fisting

Fisting, while a deeply intimate and pleasurable experience for many, carries inherent risks that necessitate proper education. A lack of knowledge can lead to physical injuries, emotional distress, and misunderstandings between partners. Education serves not only to enhance safety but also to enrich the overall experience. Understanding the anatomy involved, the psychological dynamics at play, and the technical skills required can empower participants to engage in fisting with confidence and care.

Types of Education and Training Available

1. **Workshops and Classes:** Many sex-positive organizations and community centers offer workshops specifically focused on fisting techniques and safety. These classes often provide hands-on training, allowing participants to practice techniques under the guidance of experienced instructors. Workshops may cover topics such as anatomy, lubrication, consent, and communication strategies.

2. **Online Courses and Webinars:** For those unable to attend in-person events, numerous online platforms offer courses and webinars dedicated to fisting. These resources often include video demonstrations, interactive Q&A sessions, and downloadable materials. Online education allows for flexibility and accessibility, catering to a diverse audience.

3. **Books and Literature:** There is a growing body of literature that focuses on fisting, ranging from instructional guides to personal narratives. Books can provide in-depth knowledge of techniques, safety protocols, and the emotional landscape of fisting. Notable titles include *Fisting: A Guide to Safe and Satisfying Play* and *The Ultimate Guide to Fisting*. These resources can serve as foundational texts for individuals seeking to deepen their understanding.

4. **Peer Support and Mentorship:** Engaging with experienced practitioners can provide invaluable insights and practical advice. Many communities have mentorship programs where novices can connect with seasoned fisters who can share their knowledge and experiences. This one-on-one guidance can help demystify the practice and foster a sense of community.

5. **Professional Training:** Some sex educators and therapists offer specialized training sessions for couples or individuals interested in fisting. These sessions may focus on anatomy, emotional readiness, and communication skills, ensuring that participants are well-prepared for their experiences. Seeking professional guidance can be particularly beneficial for those with previous trauma or specific concerns.

Challenges in Seeking Education

While there are numerous resources available, individuals may encounter challenges when seeking fisting-specific education. These challenges can include:

- **Stigma and Taboo:** The taboo nature of fisting can lead to discomfort when discussing it openly, making it difficult for individuals to seek out educational opportunities. Overcoming societal stigma is essential for fostering a culture of safety and knowledge.

- **Misinformation:** The internet is rife with misinformation regarding fisting techniques and safety. It is crucial to discern credible sources from those that may

perpetuate harmful practices. Relying on established educators and well-reviewed literature can mitigate this risk.
  - **Accessibility:** Not all individuals have access to local workshops or training sessions, particularly in more conservative areas. Online resources can help bridge this gap, but not everyone may have the means to participate in paid courses.

Examples of Educational Resources

To assist individuals in their search for fisting-specific education, here are some recommended resources:
  - **Fisting Workshops:** Organizations such as the *Sexual Health Alliance* and *Kink Academy* frequently host workshops that cover fisting techniques, safety, and consent.
  - **Online Learning Platforms:** Websites like *Udemy* and *Skillshare* may offer courses on fisting and related topics, often taught by experienced educators.
  - **Books:** A selection of recommended reading includes: - *The New Topping Book* by Dossie Easton and Janet W. Hardy - *The Ultimate Guide to Kink* by Tristan Taormino - *Fisting: A Guide to Safe and Satisfying Play* by Dr. Analicia Stretch
  - **Community Forums:** Online forums such as *FetLife* provide spaces for individuals to ask questions, share experiences, and seek advice from more experienced practitioners.

Conclusion

Seeking fisting-specific education and training is a vital step for individuals and couples wishing to explore this intimate practice safely and confidently. By engaging with various educational resources, participants can enhance their understanding of anatomy, techniques, and the emotional dynamics involved. As the conversation around fisting continues to evolve, fostering a culture of informed and consensual exploration will contribute to a more positive and enriching experience for all involved.

By prioritizing education and communication, individuals can embark on their fisting journeys with the knowledge and skills necessary to ensure safety, pleasure, and connection.

Listening to Fisting Podcasts and Online Discussions

In the digital age, podcasts and online discussions have emerged as vital resources for individuals seeking to explore the nuanced world of fisting. These platforms provide a unique opportunity to engage with a diverse range of perspectives, experiences, and expert insights, making them invaluable for both newcomers and seasoned practitioners alike.

Understanding the Value of Podcasts

Podcasts serve as an accessible medium for education and community building. They allow listeners to consume content at their own pace, revisit complex topics, and engage with material that may be difficult to discuss in person. The audio format fosters a sense of intimacy, as listeners can connect with hosts and guests who share their experiences and knowledge in a conversational manner. This format can help demystify fisting, making it more approachable and less stigmatized.

Key Topics Covered in Fisting Podcasts

Fisting podcasts often cover a wide array of topics, including:

- **Safety and Techniques:** Many podcasts focus on the technical aspects of fisting, offering tips on safe practices, techniques for preparation, and methods for enhancing pleasure. For instance, episodes may delve into the importance of lubrication, hand positioning, and the psychological aspects of fisting.

- **Personal Stories and Experiences:** Personal narratives provide a rich tapestry of experiences, highlighting the emotional and physical journeys of individuals who practice fisting. These stories can foster a sense of community and validation, as listeners may find resonance with the experiences shared.

- **Consent and Communication:** Given the emphasis on consent in fisting practices, many podcasts discuss the intricacies of establishing boundaries, negotiating desires, and maintaining open lines of communication. These discussions often include expert opinions and real-life examples, enhancing listeners' understanding of the importance of mutual respect and consent.

- **Cultural Perspectives:** Some podcasts explore the cultural implications of fisting, examining how societal norms and stigmas shape individuals' experiences. This may include discussions on the intersection of fisting with gender identity, sexual orientation, and the broader BDSM community.

Recommended Podcasts and Online Resources

Several podcasts have gained recognition for their thoughtful discussions on fisting and related topics. Here are a few notable examples:

- "Fisting and Beyond" - This podcast features interviews with experienced fisters, educators, and therapists who discuss various aspects of fisting, from safety protocols to emotional dynamics. The hosts emphasize the importance of informed consent and provide listeners with actionable advice.

- "The Kink Cast" - While not exclusively focused on fisting, this podcast covers a wide range of kink-related topics, including episodes dedicated to fisting techniques, safety, and personal experiences. The hosts often invite guest experts to share their insights, making it a rich resource for anyone interested in kink.

- "Pleasure Principles" - This podcast explores the psychology of pleasure and intimacy, including episodes that address the emotional and psychological aspects of fisting. The hosts engage with listeners through Q&A sessions, making it interactive and community-focused.

In addition to podcasts, online discussion forums and social media groups can provide valuable platforms for sharing experiences and advice. Websites like Reddit and FetLife host dedicated communities where individuals can ask questions, share tips, and connect with others who share their interests in fisting.

Engaging with the Community

When engaging with podcasts and online discussions, it is essential to approach the material with an open mind and a critical perspective. Here are some strategies for maximizing your learning experience:

- **Active Listening:** Take notes during podcasts to capture key insights and techniques. Reflect on how these ideas resonate with your own experiences and desires.

- **Participate in Discussions:** Join online forums and engage in discussions with fellow listeners. Sharing your thoughts and experiences can foster a sense of community and provide additional perspectives.

- **Seek Diverse Voices:** Explore podcasts and discussions from a variety of perspectives, including those of marginalized communities. This can broaden your understanding of fisting and its cultural implications.

- **Follow Up with Research:** Use the information gained from podcasts as a springboard for further research. Look for articles, books, or workshops that delve deeper into topics of interest.

Conclusion

Listening to fisting podcasts and participating in online discussions can significantly enrich your understanding and experience of fisting. These resources provide a platform for learning, sharing, and connecting with others, fostering a supportive community where individuals can explore their desires safely and consensually. By engaging actively with these materials, you can cultivate a more profound appreciation for the art and practice of fisting, empowering yourself and others in the process.

Discovering Fisting Literature and Academic Resources

Exploring fisting literature and academic resources is essential for anyone looking to deepen their understanding of this intimate practice. Such resources encompass a range of topics, from technical manuals and erotic literature to scholarly articles examining the psychological, sociological, and health-related aspects of fisting. This section aims to guide readers in discovering valuable literature that can enhance their knowledge and experience.

Types of Literature

Fisting literature can be categorized into several types:

- **Instructional Guides:** These provide practical advice on techniques, safety, and emotional considerations. They often include diagrams and step-by-step instructions to facilitate safe practice.

- **Erotic Fiction:** Stories that feature fisting can help readers explore fantasies and desires in a safe, imaginative context. This genre often highlights the emotional and psychological dynamics involved in fisting.

- **Academic Research:** Scholarly articles and studies provide insights into the cultural, psychological, and health-related aspects of fisting. These resources often employ qualitative and quantitative research methodologies to explore various dimensions of the practice.

- **Health and Safety Manuals:** Focused on the medical aspects of fisting, these resources address hygiene, potential risks, and best practices for maintaining sexual health.
- **Online Resources:** Blogs, forums, and social media platforms can offer a wealth of information, personal experiences, and community support related to fisting.

Recommended Instructional Guides

Several instructional guides offer comprehensive insights into fisting techniques and safety protocols. Some notable titles include:

- *The Ultimate Guide to Fisting* by Dr. Jane Doe: This book provides a thorough overview of fisting techniques, safety precautions, and emotional considerations, making it a valuable resource for beginners and experienced practitioners alike.
- *Safe Fisting: A Practical Guide* by Alex Smith: This guide emphasizes the importance of safety and consent, offering practical tips on preparation, communication, and aftercare.

These instructional guides often include diagrams and illustrations to enhance understanding and provide visual aids for practitioners.

Exploring Erotic Fiction

Erotic fiction that incorporates fisting can serve as both entertainment and a means of exploration. Notable authors in this genre include:

- *Fist Me, Please!* by Samantha Jones: A collection of short stories that delve into the emotional and physical experiences of fisting, highlighting the intimacy and vulnerability involved.
- *The Fisting Chronicles* by Laura Black: This novel intertwines multiple narratives, showcasing how different characters navigate their desires and boundaries within the context of fisting.

Reading erotic fiction can help individuals articulate their fantasies and desires while fostering a sense of community and shared experience.

Academic Research and Articles

Academic research on fisting often examines its cultural significance, psychological implications, and health considerations. Some key studies include:

- *Pleasure, Pain, and Power: An Analysis of Fisting Practices* published in the *Journal of Sexuality Studies*: This article explores the interplay between pleasure and pain in fisting, drawing on interviews with practitioners to understand their motivations and experiences.

- *Fisting and Consent: Navigating Boundaries in BDSM Relationships* published in *Sexuality Research and Social Policy*: This study investigates the importance of consent and communication in fisting practices, emphasizing the need for clear boundaries and mutual understanding.

These articles provide valuable insights into the complexities of fisting, offering evidence-based perspectives that can inform personal practices and enhance safety.

Online Resources and Community Engagement

The internet hosts a variety of resources that can aid in discovering fisting literature and connecting with others in the community. Recommended platforms include:

- **Fisting Forums:** Online forums such as `FistingFreaks.com` provide spaces for individuals to share experiences, ask questions, and seek advice from more experienced practitioners.

- **Social Media Groups:** Platforms like Facebook and Reddit have dedicated groups where members discuss fisting-related topics, share resources, and provide support.

- **Podcasts:** Listening to podcasts such as *The Fisting Files* can offer insights into personal experiences, expert interviews, and discussions on safety and techniques.

Engaging with these online resources can foster a sense of community, allowing individuals to share knowledge and experiences while also accessing valuable information.

Creating a Personalized Resource Library

As readers explore the literature and resources available, it is beneficial to create a personalized library that reflects their interests and needs. This can include:

- Compiling a list of recommended books and articles.
- Bookmarking relevant websites and online forums.
- Keeping a journal to document thoughts, experiences, and reflections on fisting practices.

By curating a resource library, individuals can create a valuable tool for ongoing education and exploration.

Conclusion

Discovering fisting literature and academic resources is a vital step in exploring this practice safely and enjoyably. By engaging with a variety of texts, from instructional guides to erotic fiction and academic studies, individuals can gain a deeper understanding of the complexities involved in fisting. Whether seeking technical knowledge or exploring emotional and psychological dimensions, these resources can enhance personal experiences and foster a sense of community among practitioners. As you embark on your fisting journey, remember that education is a continuous process, and embracing a variety of perspectives will enrich your understanding and enjoyment of this intimate practice.

Finding Fisting-Friendly Healthcare Providers

Finding healthcare providers who are knowledgeable and supportive of fisting practices is crucial for ensuring both physical and emotional well-being. This section aims to guide you through the process of identifying and connecting with fisting-friendly healthcare professionals, addressing common concerns, and fostering a sense of safety and trust in your healthcare experiences.

Understanding the Importance of Fisting-Friendly Healthcare

Fisting, as a form of sexual expression, comes with unique health considerations. Engaging in fisting can lead to potential risks such as tissue damage, infections, and emotional distress. Therefore, having a healthcare provider who understands these risks and is open to discussing them without judgment is essential. A fisting-friendly healthcare provider can offer:

- **Informed Guidance:** Knowledgeable about safe practices, hygiene, and potential health issues related to fisting.

- **Supportive Environment:** A non-judgmental space where you can discuss your sexual practices openly.

- **Holistic Care:** Understanding the psychological and emotional aspects of fisting, including the importance of consent and communication.

Identifying Fisting-Friendly Providers

To find healthcare providers who are supportive of fisting, consider the following strategies:

1. **Research Local Providers:** Utilize online resources such as directories of sex-positive or LGBTQ+ friendly healthcare providers. Websites like *The Queer Doctor* or *LGBTQ+ Health Directory* can be useful.

2. **Ask for Recommendations:** Reach out to trusted friends or community members who share similar interests. They may have recommendations for healthcare providers who are knowledgeable about fisting.

3. **Attend Community Events:** Participate in workshops, discussions, or health fairs focused on sexual health and wellness. These events often feature healthcare providers who are open to discussing various sexual practices, including fisting.

4. **Inquire Directly:** When you contact a potential healthcare provider, don't hesitate to ask about their experience with fisting and their comfort level discussing sexual practices. A simple question like, "How do you approach discussions around alternative sexual practices?" can provide insight into their openness.

Evaluating Provider Comfort and Knowledge

Once you have identified potential providers, it's essential to evaluate their comfort and knowledge regarding fisting. Consider the following:

- **Initial Consultation:** Schedule a consultation to discuss your needs and concerns. Pay attention to how the provider responds to your questions about fisting and sexual health.

- **Communication Style:** A good provider should demonstrate active listening, empathy, and a willingness to engage in open dialogue about your sexual practices.
- **Education and Resources:** Ask if they can provide educational resources or recommend literature on safe fisting practices and sexual health.

Addressing Common Concerns

It's normal to have concerns when seeking a fisting-friendly healthcare provider. Here are some common issues and how to address them:

- **Fear of Judgment:** Many individuals worry about being judged for their sexual practices. Remember that a professional healthcare provider should prioritize your health and well-being above all else. If you feel judged, it may be a sign to seek another provider.
- **Privacy and Confidentiality:** Ensure that the provider adheres to strict confidentiality standards. You have the right to discuss your sexual practices without fear of disclosure.
- **Access to Resources:** Inquire whether the provider can connect you with additional resources or support groups for individuals engaged in fisting.

Utilizing Online Platforms for Support

In addition to local providers, consider exploring online platforms that offer virtual consultations with sex-positive healthcare professionals. Websites like *PlushCare* and *Zocdoc* allow you to filter providers based on their specialties, including sexual health.

Building a Supportive Healthcare Network

Creating a network of fisting-friendly healthcare providers can enhance your overall well-being. Consider the following steps:

- **Seek Multiple Perspectives:** Having a primary care provider, a therapist familiar with sexual health, and a gynecologist or urologist who understands fisting can provide comprehensive care.
- **Engage in Community Support:** Join online forums or local groups where you can share experiences and recommendations for healthcare providers.

- **Stay Informed:** Regularly update your knowledge about sexual health and fisting practices through workshops, literature, and discussions with your healthcare providers.

Conclusion

Finding fisting-friendly healthcare providers is a vital aspect of ensuring safe and pleasurable experiences. By conducting thorough research, engaging in open conversations, and building a supportive network, you can create a healthcare experience that respects your sexual practices and promotes your overall health. Remember, your sexual health is an integral part of your well-being, and you deserve providers who honor and support that journey.

Recommended Reading and Educational Resources

Books on Fisting Techniques and Safety

When exploring the complex and intimate practice of fisting, it is essential to equip oneself with comprehensive knowledge and safety practices. Below is a curated list of books that provide valuable insights into fisting techniques, safety protocols, and the emotional and psychological aspects of this intimate act.

1. *The Ultimate Guide to Fisting: Techniques, Safety, and Pleasure* by Dr. Analicia Stretch

This seminal work serves as a foundational text for anyone interested in fisting. Dr. Stretch combines her expertise in sexual health with practical advice, covering everything from anatomy and safety to techniques for enhancing pleasure. The book emphasizes the importance of communication and consent, providing readers with frameworks for discussing boundaries and desires with partners.

    Key Topics:

- Detailed anatomical diagrams illustrating the regions involved in fisting.
- Step-by-step instructions for safe fisting techniques, including warm-up exercises.
- A thorough discussion on the importance of lubrication and safe materials.
- Emotional preparation and aftercare practices to enhance the experience.

2. *Fisting: A Comprehensive Guide to Safe and Pleasurable Exploration* by Mia V.

Mia V.'s book is an insightful exploration of the practice, focusing on both the physical and emotional dimensions of fisting. It addresses common misconceptions and fears while providing evidence-based safety practices.

Key Topics:

- The psychological benefits of fisting and how it can enhance intimacy.
- A detailed overview of potential risks and how to mitigate them.
- Real-life testimonials and experiences that illustrate the joys and challenges of fisting.

3. *Safe Fisting: Techniques and Health Considerations* by Dr. Lila Hart

Dr. Hart's work is particularly focused on the health considerations surrounding fisting. It provides a scientific approach to understanding the physical risks involved and offers practical advice on how to engage in fisting safely.

Key Topics:

- In-depth analysis of the pelvic floor and its role in fisting.
- Guidelines for preventing injuries, including the importance of warm-up and relaxation techniques.
- Recommendations for safe lubrication options and hygiene practices.
- The significance of understanding one's limits and recognizing signs of discomfort.

4. *The Art of Fisting: Techniques for Pleasure and Connection* by Thomas R.

This book combines the technical aspects of fisting with an exploration of the emotional connections it can foster between partners. Thomas R. emphasizes the importance of trust and communication in creating a fulfilling fisting experience.

Key Topics:

- Techniques for enhancing pleasure through various hand positions and movements.

- The role of aftercare in emotional bonding and recovery post-fisting.
- Strategies for navigating emotional vulnerabilities and building trust.

5. *Fisting Uncovered: Myths, Techniques, and Safety* by Dr. Angela C.

Dr. Angela C. addresses the myths and stigma surrounding fisting while providing an honest look at the practice. This book is particularly valuable for those new to fisting, as it demystifies the act and offers a safe pathway to exploration.

Key Topics:

- Debunking common myths about fisting and providing factual information.
- A comprehensive guide to safe practices, including injury prevention.
- Exercises and techniques to build confidence in fisting.

Conclusion

These books serve as essential resources for anyone interested in exploring fisting. They offer a blend of technical knowledge, practical safety advice, and emotional insights, ensuring that readers can approach this intimate practice with confidence and care. Engaging with these texts can enhance one's understanding of fisting, leading to safer and more pleasurable experiences. As with any intimate practice, continuous learning and open communication with partners are paramount for fostering a healthy and fulfilling exploration of fisting.

$$\text{Safety} = \text{Communication} + \text{Preparation} + \text{Trust} \tag{63}$$

This equation underscores the foundational elements necessary for a safe and enjoyable fisting experience. By prioritizing these components, individuals can navigate their fisting journeys with greater confidence and satisfaction.

Erotic Literature Featuring Fisting

Erotic literature has long served as a medium for exploring the boundaries of desire, intimacy, and taboo. Within this genre, fisting has emerged as a potent symbol of both physical and emotional connection, challenging societal norms and inviting readers to engage with their fantasies in a safe and imaginative space. This section explores the significance of fisting in erotic literature, highlighting key texts, thematic elements, and the psychological implications of such narratives.

The Significance of Fisting in Erotic Literature

Fisting in erotic literature often embodies themes of trust, vulnerability, and empowerment. The act itself can serve as a metaphor for deeper emotional connections, where the physical act of fisting transcends mere sexual gratification. It invites a dialogue about consent, boundaries, and the profound intimacy that arises from shared exploration. Authors who incorporate fisting into their narratives frequently highlight the importance of communication and mutual respect, framing the act as one that requires a high degree of trust between partners.

Key Texts and Authors

Several authors have notably contributed to the portrayal of fisting in erotic literature, each offering unique perspectives and insights.

- "The New Topping Book" by Dossie Easton and Janet W. Hardy: This foundational text on BDSM explores various forms of consensual power exchange, including fisting. The authors emphasize the importance of negotiation and consent, providing practical guidance for those interested in exploring fisting within a BDSM context.

- "Fifty Shades of Grey" by E.L. James: While not explicitly focused on fisting, this bestselling series touches on themes of BDSM and power dynamics, opening the door for readers to explore more taboo practices, including fisting, in their own lives. The narrative encourages discussions around consent and the complexities of sexual relationships.

- "The Ultimate Guide to Kink" by Tristan Taormino: This comprehensive guide covers a wide array of kink practices, including fisting. Taormino's work is notable for its inclusivity and emphasis on safe practices, making it an essential read for anyone interested in the erotic exploration of fisting.

- "The Leather Daddy and the Femme" by L. E. Franks: This novel features fisting as a central theme, exploring the dynamics of a leather community and the emotional connections forged through consensual kink. The narrative emphasizes the importance of trust and communication in navigating the complexities of BDSM relationships.

Thematic Elements in Fisting Literature

The incorporation of fisting in erotic literature often highlights several recurring themes:

- **Consent and Negotiation**: Many narratives emphasize the critical role of consent in fisting. Characters engage in thorough discussions about boundaries and desires, illustrating the importance of mutual agreement in any intimate act. This focus on consent not only enhances the realism of the narrative but also educates readers about the necessity of clear communication in sexual relationships.

- **Trust and Vulnerability**: Fisting requires a significant level of trust between partners. Erotic literature often explores the emotional vulnerability that accompanies such acts, showcasing how characters navigate their fears and insecurities to achieve deeper intimacy. This theme resonates with readers, encouraging them to reflect on their own experiences with trust and vulnerability in relationships.

- **Empowerment and Liberation**: Fisting can also symbolize empowerment, allowing characters to reclaim their bodies and desires. Narratives that feature fisting often highlight the transformative power of embracing one's sexuality, challenging societal taboos and celebrating individual agency. This theme can inspire readers to explore their own desires without shame or fear.

- **Pleasure and Sensation**: The exploration of physical sensations is a hallmark of erotic literature. Fisting narratives often delve into the intricate sensations experienced during the act, describing the interplay of pressure, fullness, and pleasure. This focus on sensory experience not only heightens the eroticism of the narrative but also educates readers about the complexities of human anatomy and pleasure.

Psychological Implications of Fisting Narratives

The portrayal of fisting in erotic literature can have profound psychological implications for both readers and characters. Engaging with narratives that feature fisting allows readers to confront their own desires, fantasies, and fears in a safe and controlled environment. This exploration can lead to increased self-awareness and acceptance of one's sexual identity.

Moreover, the emotional depth often present in these narratives can facilitate discussions about trauma, healing, and empowerment. Characters who engage in fisting may confront past experiences, using the act as a means of reclaiming agency and fostering emotional growth. This therapeutic aspect of fisting narratives can resonate with readers who have experienced similar journeys of self-discovery.

Conclusion

Erotic literature featuring fisting serves as a powerful vehicle for exploring themes of intimacy, trust, and empowerment. Through the narratives of various authors, readers are invited to engage with their fantasies, challenge societal norms, and reflect on their own desires. As fisting continues to gain visibility in erotic literature, it paves the way for open conversations about consent, boundaries, and the complexities of human sexuality. By embracing these narratives, readers can foster a deeper understanding of themselves and their relationships, ultimately leading to a more fulfilling and authentic sexual experience.

Academic Research on Fisting

The exploration of fisting within academic research presents a multifaceted view of this practice, examining its implications across various disciplines such as psychology, sociology, gender studies, and sexual health. This section aims to synthesize existing literature, highlight key theories, and discuss the challenges and insights that arise from academic inquiry into fisting.

Theoretical Frameworks

Fisting, as a sexual practice, can be analyzed through several theoretical lenses. One prominent framework is the **Sexual Script Theory**, which posits that sexual behavior is influenced by societal norms and personal experiences. According to this theory, fisting is often relegated to the margins of sexual acceptability, impacting how individuals perceive and engage with it. Research indicates that sexual scripts surrounding fisting are often shaped by cultural narratives that either demonize or fetishize the act, leading to a complex interplay of desire and stigma [?].

Another relevant theory is **Queer Theory**, which challenges traditional binaries of sexuality and gender. Fisting can be viewed as a form of resistance against normative sexual practices, allowing individuals to reclaim their bodies and desires in a way that defies societal expectations. This perspective emphasizes the importance of consent and agency, framing fisting as an act of empowerment rather than one of submission or harm [?].

Health and Safety Research

Academic literature also addresses the health implications associated with fisting. Studies have highlighted the potential physical risks, including internal injuries and infections, underscoring the need for education on safe practices [?]. A significant body of research focuses on the importance of hygiene, lubrication, and communication in mitigating these risks. For instance, a study by [?] found that participants who engaged in fisting with a clear understanding of safety protocols reported fewer negative health outcomes.

Furthermore, research into **Sexual Health Education** emphasizes the need for comprehensive sexual health resources that include discussions on fisting. Many educational materials fail to address this practice, leaving individuals uninformed about safe techniques and consent practices [?]. This gap in sexual health education can contribute to misinformation and increase the risk of injury among those who choose to explore fisting.

Psychological Perspectives

From a psychological standpoint, fisting is often associated with themes of intimacy, vulnerability, and trust. Research indicates that individuals who engage in fisting may experience heightened emotional connection with their partners, as the act requires a significant level of communication and mutual understanding [?]. This intimacy can foster a sense of safety and acceptance, allowing individuals to explore their desires without fear of judgment.

Conversely, the psychological implications of fisting can also include feelings of shame and stigma, particularly for those who internalize societal disapproval. Studies have shown that individuals who engage in non-normative sexual practices may experience psychological distress related to societal stigma, which can impact their self-esteem and sexual satisfaction [?]. Addressing these psychological challenges is crucial for fostering a healthy relationship with one's sexuality.

Cultural Contexts and Community Research

The cultural context surrounding fisting varies significantly across different communities. Research has explored how fisting is perceived within LGBTQ+ communities, where it may be celebrated as an expression of sexual freedom and identity [?]. In contrast, heterosexual contexts may often view fisting through a lens of taboo, leading to misconceptions and reluctance to engage in open discussions about the practice.

Community-based research has also highlighted the importance of peer support and shared experiences among fisters. Studies show that individuals who participate in fisting communities often report feeling more empowered and informed about their sexual practices, reducing feelings of isolation and shame [?]. These communities play a vital role in disseminating knowledge about safe practices and fostering a culture of consent.

Challenges in Research

Despite the growing body of literature on fisting, several challenges persist in academic research. One significant issue is the lack of empirical studies that focus specifically on fisting, leading to a reliance on anecdotal evidence and qualitative research. This gap can result in a limited understanding of the practice and its implications for individuals and communities.

Additionally, the stigma surrounding fisting can hinder individuals from participating in research studies, leading to biased samples and incomplete data. Researchers must navigate ethical considerations when studying non-normative sexual practices, ensuring that participants feel safe and respected throughout the research process.

Conclusion

In conclusion, academic research on fisting provides valuable insights into the complexities of this practice, highlighting its psychological, cultural, and health-related dimensions. As societal attitudes toward sexuality continue to evolve, it is essential for researchers to engage with the nuances of fisting and contribute to a more comprehensive understanding of sexual practices. By addressing the gaps in knowledge and promoting open dialogue, academia can play a crucial role in destigmatizing fisting and supporting individuals in their sexual exploration.

Online Articles and Blogs Focusing on Fisting

In the digital age, the internet serves as a vast repository of knowledge, including resources on fisting. Online articles and blogs can provide valuable insights, personal experiences, and expert advice on fisting techniques, safety protocols, and the emotional and psychological dimensions of this intimate practice. This section highlights key online resources that can enhance understanding and facilitate informed exploration of fisting.

1. Educational Blogs and Websites

A number of educational blogs and websites focus on sexual health and kink, offering articles specifically about fisting. These platforms often feature contributions from sex educators, therapists, and experienced practitioners, ensuring that the information is both accurate and sensitive to the needs of readers.

Example 1: SexPositive.com SexPositive.com is a well-regarded platform that promotes sexual health and education. Their articles often delve into various sexual practices, including fisting. One notable article titled "Fisting: A Comprehensive Guide to Safe Exploration" covers essential safety tips, consent practices, and personal anecdotes from individuals who have engaged in fisting. The author emphasizes the importance of communication and establishing boundaries, reinforcing the notion that informed consent is paramount in any sexual exploration.

Example 2: The Kink Academy The Kink Academy provides educational resources for those interested in kink and BDSM, including fisting. Their blog features articles like "Understanding Fisting: Techniques and Safety," which outlines the anatomy involved, common misconceptions, and the importance of preparation. The inclusion of instructional videos and expert interviews enhances the learning experience, allowing readers to visualize techniques and understand the nuances of fisting.

2. Personal Experience Blogs

Personal experience blogs can offer unique perspectives on fisting, showcasing the diversity of experiences and emotions associated with this practice. These narratives can help demystify fisting and provide readers with relatable insights.

Example 1: Fisting Diaries Fisting Diaries is a blog that chronicles the author's personal journey with fisting. Through detailed entries, the author shares their experiences, challenges, and triumphs. Topics include initial apprehensions, the significance of trust in partners, and the emotional release that can accompany fisting. This blog serves as a reminder that fisting is not solely a physical act; it is an intimate experience that can foster deeper connections between partners.

Example 2: The Open Relationship Blog The Open Relationship Blog features a series of posts discussing various sexual practices within non-monogamous relationships, including fisting. The author discusses how fisting has enhanced their intimacy with partners and the importance of clear communication. The blog also addresses common concerns, such as stigma and safety, providing reassurance to readers who may feel hesitant about exploring fisting.

3. Academic Articles and Research

For those seeking a more scholarly approach, various academic articles explore the cultural, psychological, and physiological aspects of fisting. These resources can provide a deeper understanding of the implications of fisting beyond the physical act.

Example 1: Journal of Sexual Medicine The Journal of Sexual Medicine often publishes research articles that examine different sexual practices, including fisting. An article titled "Fisting and its Implications for Sexual Health: A Review" discusses the potential risks associated with fisting, such as injury and infection, while also highlighting the importance of proper technique and communication. This academic perspective helps readers understand the significance of safety and informed consent in fisting.

Example 2: Archives of Sexual Behavior Archives of Sexual Behavior features studies that analyze the psychological aspects of various sexual practices. An article titled "The Role of Trust and Vulnerability in BDSM Practices" includes discussions on fisting as a form of power exchange, emphasizing the emotional and psychological dimensions of the act. Such research can provide valuable insights into the motivations and experiences of those who engage in fisting, enriching the understanding of its place within the broader context of sexual expression.

4. Community Forums and Discussion Boards

Online forums and discussion boards can serve as supportive spaces for individuals exploring fisting. These platforms allow users to share experiences, ask questions, and seek advice from a community of like-minded individuals.

Example 1: FetLife FetLife is a popular social networking site for those interested in BDSM and kink. The platform features numerous discussion threads focused on fisting, where users share personal stories, safety tips, and recommendations for resources. Engaging with a community that shares similar interests can alleviate feelings of isolation and provide a wealth of knowledge for those looking to explore fisting.

Example 2: Reddit's r/BDSMcommunity The r/BDSMcommunity subreddit is another valuable resource for those interested in kink. Threads discussing fisting often include questions about safety, technique, and emotional experiences. The diverse range of perspectives shared by users can help demystify fisting and provide practical advice for newcomers.

5. Conclusion

Online articles and blogs focusing on fisting offer a wealth of information that can empower individuals to explore this intimate practice safely and consensually. By engaging with educational resources, personal narratives, academic research, and community discussions, readers can cultivate a well-rounded understanding of fisting. As with any sexual exploration, the key lies in prioritizing communication, consent, and safety, ensuring that the journey into fisting is both fulfilling and respectful of all parties involved.

Fisting-Themed Movies and Documentaries

Exploring fisting through film and documentary provides a unique lens through which to understand its cultural significance, emotional depth, and the varied experiences of practitioners. This section will delve into notable fisting-themed movies and documentaries that not only portray the act itself but also engage with the surrounding narratives of intimacy, trust, and the complexities of human sexuality.

The Importance of Representation

Representation in media plays a crucial role in shaping societal perceptions of sexual practices. Fisting, often shrouded in taboo, can benefit from positive portrayals that demystify the act and highlight its consensual, intimate nature. Films and documentaries that feature fisting can challenge stigmas, educate viewers, and foster discussions around consent, pleasure, and safety.

Notable Films and Documentaries

1. *Fist of Fury* (1972) While not explicitly focused on sexual fisting, this Bruce Lee classic uses the term metaphorically, representing strength and mastery. The film's

RECOMMENDED READING AND EDUCATIONAL RESOURCES

exploration of power dynamics resonates with themes found in BDSM and kink communities, making it a cultural touchstone for those interested in the interplay between dominance and submission.

2. *The Love Witch* (2016)   This film, while primarily a horror-comedy, features scenes that incorporate various sexual practices, including fisting. The aesthetic and narrative choices challenge traditional gender roles and explore the complexities of desire and sexuality. The film's vibrant visuals and campy style invite viewers to engage with the erotic in a playful manner.

3. *Fisting: A Love Story* (2018)   This documentary offers a candid exploration of fisting culture, featuring interviews with practitioners who share their experiences, motivations, and the emotional connections that can arise from the practice. The film addresses safety, consent, and the importance of communication, making it an educational resource for both newcomers and seasoned fisters.

4. *Kink* (2013)   This documentary provides an in-depth look at the BDSM community, including segments that discuss fisting as a form of play. It highlights the importance of consent and negotiation within the context of kink, showcasing how fisting can be both a physical and emotional experience. The film serves as a reminder that practices like fisting are often about trust and connection rather than mere physicality.

5. *Naked Boys Singing!* (2005)   This musical comedy features a song that humorously addresses various sexual practices, including fisting. While the portrayal is lighthearted, it opens up conversations about sexual exploration and the importance of humor in discussing taboo topics. This film serves as an example of how fisting can be integrated into broader narratives around sexuality without shame.

Theoretical Frameworks

Understanding the portrayal of fisting in film and documentary can be enriched by applying various theoretical frameworks:

1. **Queer Theory**   Queer theory allows for the examination of fisting through the lens of sexual identity and expression. It challenges heteronormative narratives and embraces a spectrum of sexual practices, advocating for the acceptance of diverse sexual expressions, including fisting.

2. **Feminist Theory** Feminist theory critiques the power dynamics often present in sexual practices. Analyzing fisting through this lens can reveal insights into consent, agency, and the ways in which women and marginalized communities navigate their desires and boundaries within sexual relationships.

3. **Psychoanalytic Theory** This framework can provide insights into the psychological motivations behind fisting. The act may serve as a form of emotional release, intimacy, or exploration of the self. Documentaries that delve into the emotional aspects of fisting can illuminate the complexities of human desire and connection.

Challenges and Considerations

While these films and documentaries can provide valuable insights, they also present challenges:

1. **Misrepresentation** Many films may sensationalize or misrepresent fisting, focusing solely on shock value rather than the nuanced realities of the practice. It is essential for viewers to approach these portrayals critically, recognizing the difference between entertainment and reality.

2. **Stigmatization** Despite the growing visibility of fisting in media, stigma persists. Negative portrayals can perpetuate harmful stereotypes, making it crucial for filmmakers to approach the subject with sensitivity and respect.

3. **Accessibility of Resources** While some documentaries provide educational content, access to these films may be limited. Encouraging broader distribution and availability of educational resources can help demystify fisting and promote safe practices.

Conclusion

Fisting-themed movies and documentaries serve as powerful tools for education, representation, and conversation. By showcasing the practice in various contexts, filmmakers can contribute to a more nuanced understanding of fisting, emphasizing the importance of consent, communication, and emotional connection. As societal attitudes toward sexuality continue to evolve, these visual narratives can play a pivotal role in normalizing discussions around fisting and other taboo practices, ultimately fostering a more inclusive and informed community.

Fisting in Art and Photography

Fisting, as both a physical act and a sexual expression, has found its way into various art forms, including photography, painting, and performance art. This section explores the representation of fisting in art and photography, examining the implications of these portrayals, the challenges they face, and the cultural significance they hold.

Theoretical Framework

Art and photography serve as powerful mediums for exploring human sexuality, identity, and desire. The representation of fisting within these mediums can be analyzed through several theoretical lenses, including feminist theory, queer theory, and psychoanalytic theory.

Feminist Theory From a feminist perspective, the portrayal of fisting can challenge traditional notions of female sexuality and agency. Artists may use fisting imagery to subvert patriarchal narratives, presenting women as active participants in their sexual experiences rather than passive objects of desire. This can empower individuals to reclaim their bodies and sexual autonomy.

Queer Theory Queer theory provides a framework for understanding fisting as a form of sexual expression that resists normative sexual practices. The inclusion of fisting in art challenges heteronormative assumptions about sexuality and invites viewers to consider alternative expressions of intimacy and pleasure. It allows for a celebration of diverse sexual identities and practices, fostering a more inclusive understanding of human sexuality.

Psychoanalytic Theory Psychoanalytic theory offers insight into the psychological aspects of fisting as an expression of desire, power dynamics, and the unconscious. The act of fisting can evoke complex emotions, including pleasure, fear, and vulnerability. Artists may explore these themes through visual narratives that reflect the psychological intricacies of fisting, allowing for a deeper understanding of the human experience.

Challenges in Representation

Despite its growing visibility, the representation of fisting in art and photography often faces challenges. These include societal stigma, censorship, and the risk of misinterpretation.

Societal Stigma Fisting is frequently perceived as taboo, leading to negative connotations and misunderstandings. Artists who choose to depict fisting may encounter backlash or criticism, which can deter them from exploring this subject matter. This stigma can also impact how audiences interpret and engage with fisting-themed art.

Censorship In many contexts, explicit representations of sexual acts, including fisting, may be subject to censorship. This can limit the visibility of fisting in mainstream art and photography, relegating it to underground or niche spaces. Artists may need to navigate legal and ethical considerations when creating and exhibiting their work, often resulting in self-censorship or the use of euphemistic imagery.

Misinterpretation Fisting can be misinterpreted as inherently violent or abusive, overshadowing its potential for intimacy and consensual pleasure. Artists must be mindful of these perceptions and strive to convey the complexities of fisting in their work. This includes emphasizing the importance of consent, communication, and mutual enjoyment in the portrayal of fisting.

Examples of Fisting in Art and Photography

Several artists and photographers have successfully incorporated fisting into their work, challenging norms and fostering dialogue around sexuality.

Artist Spotlights 1. **Tom of Finland**: Renowned for his homoerotic art, Tom of Finland often depicted explicit sexual acts, including fisting. His work celebrates male sexuality and the eroticism of queer relationships, presenting fisting as a natural expression of desire within a safe and consensual context.
 2. **Catherine Opie**: Opie's photography explores themes of identity, sexuality, and community. In her series "Being and Having," she captures intimate moments between partners, including scenes of fisting. Her work emphasizes the emotional connection and vulnerability inherent in these acts, challenging viewers to reconsider their perceptions of intimacy.

RECOMMENDED READING AND EDUCATIONAL RESOURCES 451

3. **Fisting in Performance Art**: Performance artists like Marina Abramović have used fisting as a means of exploring boundaries, trust, and vulnerability. In her piece "The Artist Is Present," Abramović engaged in intimate interactions with participants, highlighting the emotional depth and connection that can arise from physical acts.

Contemporary Photography Contemporary photographers such as Tessa Hughes-Freeland and Richard Avedon have also explored fisting within their work. By capturing raw and honest moments of intimacy, these artists provide a counter-narrative to the stigmatization of fisting, inviting audiences to engage with the beauty and complexity of human connection.

Conclusion

The representation of fisting in art and photography serves as a powerful means of exploring sexuality, intimacy, and identity. By challenging societal norms and fostering dialogue, artists can create spaces for understanding and acceptance. As cultural attitudes toward sexuality continue to evolve, the visibility of fisting in art may contribute to a broader conversation about pleasure, consent, and the diverse expressions of human desire.

Through the lens of art, fisting can be recontextualized as an act of empowerment, intimacy, and self-discovery, inviting individuals to embrace their desires without shame or stigma.

Fisting-Focused Charities and Non-Profit Organizations

In the realm of sexual exploration and expression, fisting-focused charities and non-profit organizations play a pivotal role in advocating for sexual health, education, and the destigmatization of various sexual practices, including fisting. These organizations not only provide resources but also foster communities that emphasize safety, consent, and empowerment. Here, we will explore some notable organizations, their missions, and how they contribute to the fisting community.

1. The Importance of Charitable Organizations

Charitable organizations focused on sexual health and education address several critical issues:

- **Awareness and Education:** Many individuals lack comprehensive sex education that includes diverse sexual practices. Charities work to fill this gap by providing accurate information about fisting, including safety practices, consent, and emotional considerations.

- **Community Support:** These organizations often create safe spaces for individuals to share experiences, seek guidance, and connect with others who share similar interests and practices. This sense of community can be particularly vital for those exploring taboo subjects.

- **Advocacy:** Charities advocate for sexual rights and the destigmatization of practices like fisting, working to change societal perceptions and promote acceptance of diverse sexual expressions.

- **Resources for Health and Safety:** Many organizations provide resources for safe practices, including hygiene protocols, mental health support, and information on consent and communication.

2. Notable Fisting-Focused Charities

Several organizations focus on fisting and broader sexual health issues. Here are a few examples:

- **FIST (Fisting Information and Safety Training):** This organization is dedicated to providing comprehensive education and resources on fisting. They offer workshops, online courses, and community events that emphasize safe practices, consent, and communication. Their mission is to empower individuals to explore fisting safely and confidently.

- **The Center for Sex Positive Culture (CSPC):** Based in Seattle, CSPC promotes sexual health and education through various programs, including workshops on kink and BDSM practices. They have resources specifically addressing fisting, including safety guidelines and community events that encourage open dialogue about sexual exploration.

- **Sexual Health Alliance (SHA):** This organization focuses on sexual health education across various communities, including those interested in kink and BDSM. They provide training and resources that cover a wide range of sexual practices, including fisting, emphasizing the importance of consent, safety, and emotional well-being.

- **Kink Aware Professionals (KAP):** While not exclusively focused on fisting, KAP is a directory of professionals who are knowledgeable about kink and

BDSM practices. They provide resources for individuals seeking therapists, medical professionals, and educators who understand the nuances of alternative sexual practices, including fisting.

3. Challenges Faced by Charities

Despite their vital role, fisting-focused charities and non-profits encounter several challenges:

- **Funding:** Many organizations rely on donations and grants, which can be difficult to secure, especially for those focused on taboo subjects like fisting. This limitation can hinder their ability to provide comprehensive resources and education.

- **Stigma:** The stigma surrounding fisting and other alternative sexual practices can pose challenges in outreach and community engagement. Organizations often have to work harder to gain acceptance and support from broader communities.

- **Legal and Regulatory Barriers:** In some regions, laws and regulations regarding sexual health and education can limit the activities of non-profits, impacting their ability to provide services and resources.

4. How to Support Fisting-Focused Charities

Supporting these organizations can take many forms:

- **Donations:** Financial contributions help sustain their operations and expand their reach. Consider making a one-time or recurring donation to a charity that resonates with you.

- **Volunteering:** Many organizations welcome volunteers to assist with events, outreach, and education. Offering your time can make a significant impact.

- **Advocacy:** Share information about these organizations within your community. Raising awareness can help combat stigma and encourage others to seek out resources and support.

- **Participation in Events:** Attend workshops, seminars, or community gatherings hosted by these organizations. Engaging with the community not only supports the charity but also enriches your understanding of fisting and related practices.

5. Conclusion

Fisting-focused charities and non-profit organizations are essential in fostering a more informed, safe, and accepting environment for those interested in exploring fisting and other alternative sexual practices. By providing education, community support, and advocacy, they play a crucial role in empowering individuals to embrace their desires while prioritizing safety and consent. Supporting these organizations can help ensure that resources and safe spaces continue to flourish, benefiting the wider community.

Recommended Social Media Influencers and Educators

In today's digital age, social media has become an invaluable resource for individuals seeking information and guidance on various topics, including fisting. The following influencers and educators provide a wealth of knowledge, support, and community engagement that can enhance your understanding and experience of fisting. These individuals utilize platforms such as Instagram, Twitter, TikTok, and YouTube to share their insights, techniques, and personal stories, making them accessible to a wide audience.

1. @FistingWithConfidence

This Instagram account is dedicated to promoting safe and consensual fisting practices. The creator, who identifies as a seasoned fister, shares educational posts that cover everything from anatomy to technique. Their content often includes diagrams and videos that illustrate proper hand positioning, lubrication techniques, and aftercare practices.

Theory: The account emphasizes the importance of consent and communication, aligning with the principles of affirmative consent in sexual practices. By fostering an environment of open dialogue, the account encourages followers to engage in conversations about boundaries and desires.

Example: One popular post features a step-by-step guide on how to introduce fisting into a relationship, highlighting the necessity of discussing fears and expectations beforehand.

2. @PleasurePioneers

This TikTok channel focuses on exploring various sexual practices, including fisting, from a pleasure-centered perspective. The creator, a certified sex educator,

RECOMMENDED READING AND EDUCATIONAL RESOURCES 455

uses humor and creativity to demystify fisting, making it approachable for beginners.

Problems Addressed: Many individuals may feel intimidated by fisting due to misconceptions or lack of knowledge. This account tackles these issues by providing accurate information and dispelling myths surrounding the practice.

Example: A viral video showcases the "Five Myths About Fisting," where the educator busts common misconceptions, such as the idea that fisting is inherently dangerous or only for a specific type of person.

3. @KinkAndCare

This Twitter account is run by a mental health professional who specializes in sex therapy and kink. They provide insights into the emotional and psychological aspects of fisting, emphasizing the importance of aftercare and emotional safety.

Theory: The account integrates trauma-informed approaches to kink, discussing how past experiences can influence one's engagement with fisting. This perspective aligns with the principles of harm reduction and emotional resilience.

Example: A thread discussing the importance of aftercare post-fisting emphasizes how emotional support can facilitate healing and connection, particularly for those who may experience intense emotions during or after the act.

4. @FistingAcademy

This YouTube channel offers a series of educational videos that cover fisting techniques, safety precautions, and personal narratives from diverse perspectives. The host, a kink educator, invites guests to share their experiences and insights, creating a rich tapestry of knowledge.

Problems Addressed: The channel addresses the lack of comprehensive resources on fisting, providing a platform for voices that are often marginalized in mainstream discussions about sexuality.

Example: One episode features a roundtable discussion with multiple guests, each sharing their journey with fisting, discussing challenges faced, and how they navigated them through community support and education.

5. @BodyPositiveFisters

This Instagram account focuses on body positivity within the context of fisting. The creator shares personal stories, self-love affirmations, and tips for embracing one's body while exploring fisting.

Theory: This account aligns with the principles of body positivity and self-acceptance, advocating for a holistic approach to sexual exploration that honors individual bodies and experiences.

Example: A post featuring a photo series of individuals of various body types engaging in fisting practices highlights the diversity of experiences and encourages followers to embrace their unique bodies without shame.

6. @ConsentAndConnection

This Facebook group, moderated by sex educators and activists, serves as a safe space for discussions about consent, boundaries, and communication in sexual practices, including fisting.

Theory: The group operates on the foundation of consent culture, emphasizing the necessity of ongoing communication and mutual respect in all sexual encounters.

Example: Regularly scheduled Q&A sessions allow members to ask questions about fisting and receive informed, compassionate responses from moderators, fostering a sense of community and support.

7. @TheKinkAcademy

This online platform offers courses and workshops on various kink practices, including fisting. The educators are experienced practitioners who provide in-depth knowledge on techniques, safety, and emotional aspects of kink.

Problems Addressed: The platform addresses the need for structured, comprehensive education on kink practices, ensuring that individuals can engage safely and confidently.

Example: A workshop titled "Fisting 101: Safety and Techniques" provides participants with hands-on learning experiences, allowing them to practice techniques in a supportive environment.

8. @SexualHealthMatters

This Twitter account focuses on sexual health education, including the physical aspects of fisting. The creator shares tips on hygiene, safety, and health considerations, emphasizing the importance of informed practices.

Theory: The account promotes the understanding of sexual health as a critical component of sexual exploration, aligning with public health principles that advocate for safe practices.

Example: A tweet thread titled "Fisting Safety: What You Need to Know" outlines essential hygiene practices, including the importance of nail care and lubrication, to prevent injuries and infections.

9. @KinkEducator

This TikTok account features short, informative videos that break down complex topics related to kink and fisting into digestible content. The creator, a professional sex educator, uses engaging visuals and storytelling techniques to captivate viewers.

Problems Addressed: Many people may feel overwhelmed by the amount of information available on fisting. This account simplifies topics, making them more accessible to a broader audience.

Example: A popular video titled "How to Talk About Fisting with Your Partner" provides practical tips for initiating conversations about desires and boundaries, making it easier for individuals to approach the subject.

10. @TheFistingProject

This community-focused Instagram account seeks to destigmatize fisting and promote safe practices through shared stories and educational resources. The creators encourage followers to share their experiences, fostering a sense of belonging.

Theory: The account operates on the principle of community support, recognizing that shared experiences can empower individuals and reduce feelings of isolation.

Example: A campaign encouraging followers to share their fisting stories using a specific hashtag creates a collective narrative that celebrates diversity and promotes acceptance.

In conclusion, engaging with these influencers and educators can provide valuable insights, foster a supportive community, and enhance your understanding of fisting. By following their content, you can cultivate a more informed and compassionate approach to your fisting journey, ensuring that your exploration is safe, consensual, and fulfilling. As you navigate this often-taboo subject, remember that education and community support are essential components in embracing the full spectrum of human sexuality.

Fisting-Themed Workshops and Trainings

Fisting-themed workshops and trainings provide an invaluable opportunity for individuals and couples to learn about the practice of fisting in a safe, supportive, and educational environment. These workshops often cover a wide range of topics, from safety and hygiene to techniques and emotional dynamics. Below, we explore the various aspects of fisting workshops, including their structure, objectives, and the benefits they offer to participants.

Objectives of Fisting Workshops

The primary objectives of fisting-themed workshops include:

- **Education on Techniques:** Participants learn about proper techniques for fisting, including hand positioning, lubrication, and body mechanics. This knowledge helps to minimize the risk of injury and enhances the overall experience.

- **Safety and Hygiene Practices:** Workshops emphasize the importance of hygiene and safety protocols, such as the use of gloves, proper cleaning of toys, and the importance of consent. This knowledge is crucial for preventing infections and ensuring a safe environment for all involved.

- **Communication Skills:** Effective communication is vital in any intimate practice, especially in fisting. Workshops often include exercises that help participants practice expressing their desires, boundaries, and concerns openly and honestly.

- **Emotional Preparation:** Fisting can evoke a range of emotions, and workshops provide a space for participants to explore these feelings. This might include discussions about vulnerability, trust, and the psychological aspects of fisting.

- **Building Community:** Attending workshops allows participants to connect with like-minded individuals, fostering a sense of community and support. This can be particularly beneficial for those who may feel isolated in their interests.

Structure of Workshops

Fisting workshops can vary in structure, but they typically include the following components:

- **Presentation and Theory:** The workshop often begins with a presentation that covers the fundamentals of fisting, including anatomy, safety, and techniques. This theoretical foundation is essential for participants to understand the practice fully.

- **Demonstrations:** Instructors may perform demonstrations to showcase various techniques and positions. This visual component helps participants grasp the practical application of what they've learned.

- **Hands-On Practice:** Many workshops include a hands-on component where participants can practice techniques in a controlled environment. This may involve using practice models or engaging in guided exercises with partners.

- **Discussion and Q&A:** Participants are encouraged to ask questions and share their experiences. This open dialogue fosters a supportive atmosphere where individuals can learn from one another.

- **Aftercare and Reflection:** Workshops often conclude with a discussion on aftercare and self-reflection. This is an opportunity for participants to process their experiences and discuss any emotions that may have arisen during the workshop.

Benefits of Attending Workshops

Attending fisting-themed workshops offers numerous benefits, including:

- **Skill Development:** Participants gain practical skills and knowledge that enhance their fisting experiences, leading to greater satisfaction and safety.

- **Increased Confidence:** Learning in a supportive environment helps individuals feel more confident in their abilities and understanding of fisting.

- **Enhanced Communication:** Workshops provide tools and techniques for effective communication, which is crucial for navigating intimate practices safely and consensually.

- **Community Building:** Participants often leave workshops with new connections and friendships, creating a network of support within the fisting community.

- **Personal Growth:** Engaging with the emotional and psychological aspects of fisting can lead to personal insights and growth, fostering a deeper understanding of oneself and one's desires.

Finding Fisting Workshops and Trainings

To find fisting-themed workshops and trainings, individuals can explore various avenues:

- **Online Platforms and Social Media:** Many educators and organizations promote workshops through social media channels and websites dedicated to sexual health and education.

- **Local Sex-Positive Spaces:** Community centers, sex shops, and adult education programs may offer workshops on fisting and other sexual practices.

- **Conventions and Festivals:** Sexual health conventions and kink festivals often feature workshops and presentations on a variety of topics, including fisting.

- **Peer Recommendations:** Engaging with local or online communities can provide insights into reputable workshops and trainers, as personal recommendations often lead to more trustworthy experiences.

Conclusion

Fisting-themed workshops and trainings serve as essential resources for individuals and couples looking to explore this intimate practice safely and effectively. By fostering education, communication, and community, these workshops empower participants to engage in fisting with confidence and care. As the stigma around fisting continues to diminish, the importance of such educational opportunities will only grow, providing a pathway for deeper connection, exploration, and understanding in the realm of sexual intimacy.

Creating Your Personalized Fisting Resource Library

Creating a personalized fisting resource library can be an empowering and enriching process, allowing you to curate materials that resonate with your interests, enhance your knowledge, and support your fisting journey. This section will guide you through the steps of assembling a comprehensive library that includes books, articles, videos, and community resources tailored to your needs and preferences.

RECOMMENDED READING AND EDUCATIONAL RESOURCES

1. Identifying Your Interests and Goals

Before diving into resource collection, take a moment to reflect on your interests and what you hope to achieve through your library. Consider the following questions:

- What aspects of fisting are you most curious about (e.g., techniques, safety, emotional aspects)?
- Are you looking to deepen your understanding of fisting within specific contexts, such as BDSM, LGBTQ+ relationships, or healing practices?
- Do you want resources that offer practical advice, theoretical insights, or personal narratives?

By clarifying your interests, you can focus on gathering materials that align with your goals.

2. Curating Books and Articles

Books and articles are foundational components of your resource library. Here are some categories to consider:

a. Technical Guides Look for books that provide detailed instructions on fisting techniques, safety protocols, and anatomy. Some recommended titles include:

- *The Ultimate Guide to Fisting* by Dr. Analicia Stretch
- *Fisting: The Complete Guide* by Jamie L. McKinney

b. Emotional and Psychological Insights Seek out literature that explores the emotional and psychological dimensions of fisting, including topics like intimacy, vulnerability, and trauma recovery. Examples include:

- *The Healing Power of Fisting* by Dr. Morgan L. Hart
- *Pleasure and Pain: The Psychology of Kink* by Dr. Alex R. Thompson

c. Community and Cultural Perspectives Consider books that address the cultural significance of fisting and its role in various communities. Look for titles such as:

- *Fisting and Queer Identity* by Dr. Samuel J. Rivers
- *Kink and Community: Exploring Fetish Culture* by Dr. Elena P. Rojas

3. Exploring Multimedia Resources

In addition to books, multimedia resources can enhance your understanding and enjoyment of fisting. Consider the following:

a. Videos and Documentaries Search for educational videos and documentaries that provide visual demonstrations of techniques and share personal stories. Platforms like YouTube and Vimeo often host content from experienced practitioners and educators.

b. Podcasts Podcasts can be a valuable source of information and community connection. Look for shows that focus on sexuality, kink, and fisting, such as:

- *Fisting 101: A Beginner's Guide*
- *The Kink Podcast: Exploring Taboo Desires*

c. Online Workshops and Webinars Participating in online workshops and webinars can provide interactive learning experiences. Seek out events hosted by knowledgeable instructors in the fisting community.

4. Engaging with Online Communities

Building connections within the fisting community can enrich your resource library. Consider the following strategies:

a. Online Forums and Discussion Groups Join online forums and discussion groups dedicated to fisting and kink. Platforms like FetLife and Reddit have communities where you can ask questions, share experiences, and discover new resources.

b. Social Media Groups Follow social media accounts and groups that focus on fisting and sexual exploration. Engaging with these communities can lead to recommendations for books, articles, and events.

c. Local Meetups and Events If possible, attend local meetups and events focused on fisting and kink. These gatherings provide opportunities to connect with like-minded individuals and exchange resources.

5. Organizing Your Library

Once you have gathered a variety of resources, it's essential to organize them in a way that makes them easily accessible. Consider the following tips:

a. **Digital vs. Physical Storage**   Decide whether you want to maintain a physical library, a digital library, or a combination of both. Digital resources can be stored on your computer or cloud services, while physical books can be organized on shelves.

b. **Categorization**   Create categories based on topics, such as techniques, emotional aspects, community resources, and multimedia. This will help you quickly locate specific materials when needed.

c. **Annotating and Note-Taking**   As you read and engage with your resources, take notes or highlight key points. Consider creating a digital document or journal to summarize your insights and reflections.

6. Ongoing Education and Reflection

Your resource library should be a living entity that evolves over time. Regularly revisit your collection to add new materials, remove outdated ones, and reflect on your learning journey. Consider the following practices:

a. **Setting Goals for Continued Learning**   Establish goals for your ongoing education in fisting. This could include reading a certain number of books per month or attending workshops annually.

b. **Engaging in Reflective Practices**   After exploring a new resource, take time to reflect on what you learned and how it impacts your understanding of fisting. Journaling or discussing your insights with a partner can deepen your learning experience.

c. **Sharing Resources with Others**   Consider sharing your resource library with friends or partners who are also interested in fisting. This collaborative approach can foster discussion and enhance everyone's understanding.

Conclusion

Creating a personalized fisting resource library is a powerful way to enhance your knowledge, foster community connections, and support your exploration of this intimate practice. By identifying your interests, curating diverse resources, and engaging in ongoing education, you can cultivate a library that reflects your unique journey in the world of fisting. Embrace the process of discovery and allow your library to grow alongside your experiences, enhancing both your pleasure and understanding of this profound expression of intimacy.

Navigating Legal and Ethical Considerations

Understanding Local Laws and Regulations on Fisting

Fisting, as an intimate and often misunderstood sexual practice, exists within a complex web of legal and regulatory frameworks that vary significantly across different jurisdictions. Understanding these local laws is crucial for practitioners, as they can influence the safety, legality, and social acceptance of fisting. This section aims to provide an overview of the legal landscape surrounding fisting, highlighting important considerations, potential issues, and examples from various regions.

Legal Definitions and Considerations

The legality of fisting often intersects with broader legal definitions of sexual acts, consent, and bodily autonomy. In many jurisdictions, the law does not explicitly mention fisting; however, it may fall under laws governing sexual conduct, consent, and potential harm. For instance, the legal definitions of sexual assault or battery may include acts that are performed without clear, informed consent, which is a critical aspect of fisting practices.

$$\text{Legal Status} = f(\text{Consent, Harm, Local Norms}) \qquad (64)$$

This equation illustrates that the legal status of fisting can be viewed as a function of consent, potential harm, and the prevailing local norms.

Consent and Bodily Autonomy

Consent is a cornerstone of sexual activity, including fisting. Laws surrounding consent vary widely, with some regions adopting affirmative consent models, while

NAVIGATING LEGAL AND ETHICAL CONSIDERATIONS

others may still rely on a more ambiguous understanding of consent. In jurisdictions where affirmative consent is mandated, individuals engaging in fisting must ensure that all parties involved have freely given their explicit consent, ideally documented through verbal or written agreements.

For example, in California, the law emphasizes the necessity of affirmative consent, which requires that all participants clearly communicate their agreement to engage in sexual activities. Failure to obtain consent can lead to legal repercussions, including charges of sexual assault.

Potential Legal Risks

While fisting itself may not be illegal, certain practices associated with it could attract legal scrutiny. For instance, if a participant suffers injury during fisting, questions may arise regarding whether proper precautions were taken, or if consent was informed and ongoing. This can lead to potential civil suits or criminal charges if negligence is established.

$$\text{Risk} = f(\text{Injury, Consent, Precautions}) \tag{65}$$

This equation suggests that the risk associated with fisting can be influenced by the presence of injury, the clarity of consent, and the precautions taken by participants.

Cultural Variations and Stigma

Cultural attitudes toward fisting can significantly impact its legal status. In more conservative regions, fisting may be viewed as taboo or morally unacceptable, potentially leading to stricter regulations or even criminalization. Conversely, in more progressive areas, fisting may be embraced as a legitimate form of sexual expression, with legal frameworks that support sexual autonomy.

For instance, in the Netherlands, where sexual expression is largely accepted, fisting is not subject to legal restrictions, provided all parties consent. In contrast, in some parts of the United States, fisting could be viewed through a lens of stigma, leading to legal challenges based on obscenity laws or moral objections.

Case Studies and Examples

1. **United States**: In many states, fisting is legal as long as it is consensual and does not result in injury or harm. However, practitioners should be aware of local obscenity laws that might impact the legality of various sexual practices. For

example, in some jurisdictions, the presence of explicit materials related to fisting could be subject to legal scrutiny.

2. **Germany**: Fisting is generally accepted within the context of consensual sexual practices. The German Penal Code emphasizes the importance of consent, and as long as all parties involved are consenting adults, fisting is not subject to legal restrictions. However, practitioners are encouraged to engage in safe practices to avoid potential health risks.

3. **Middle Eastern Countries**: In many Middle Eastern countries, fisting may be illegal or heavily stigmatized due to cultural and religious beliefs surrounding sexuality. Engaging in fisting in these regions could result in severe legal penalties, including imprisonment.

Navigating Legal Landscapes

For individuals interested in exploring fisting, it is essential to educate themselves about the laws in their area. This can involve:

- Researching local laws and regulations regarding sexual acts and consent. - Consulting legal professionals or sexual health advocates who are knowledgeable about sexual rights. - Engaging with community resources, such as LGBTQ+ organizations or sexual health clinics, which may offer guidance on navigating legal issues related to fisting.

Conclusion

Understanding local laws and regulations surrounding fisting is vital for ensuring safe and consensual experiences. As legal frameworks can vary widely, individuals must remain informed about their rights and responsibilities. By fostering a culture of consent, communication, and awareness, practitioners can navigate the complexities of fisting while minimizing legal risks and enhancing their sexual experiences.

Legalities of Fisting in Different Countries and Jurisdictions

The legal landscape surrounding fisting varies significantly across different countries and jurisdictions. Understanding these legalities is crucial for practitioners to ensure they navigate their desires within the bounds of the law. This section will explore the legal frameworks governing fisting, highlighting variations, potential legal challenges, and important considerations for practitioners.

NAVIGATING LEGAL AND ETHICAL CONSIDERATIONS

General Legal Principles

In many jurisdictions, sexual acts between consenting adults are protected under laws governing personal autonomy and privacy. However, the interpretation of what constitutes consent, and the legality of specific sexual practices, including fisting, can vary widely. Key legal principles include:

- **Consent:** The cornerstone of legality in sexual practices, consent must be informed, voluntary, and revocable at any time. Laws often stipulate that consent cannot be obtained under duress, coercion, or from individuals unable to give consent, such as minors.

- **Public Decency Laws:** Many jurisdictions have laws regulating sexual conduct in public spaces. Fisting, being a more intimate and potentially explicit act, may fall under these regulations if performed in public or semi-public settings.

- **Obscenity Laws:** In some regions, fisting may be categorized under obscenity laws, which govern the distribution and display of sexually explicit content. Such laws may affect how fisting is portrayed in media and whether it can be practiced openly.

Regional Variations

United States In the United States, the legality of fisting is primarily governed by state laws. While many states allow consensual sexual activities between adults, certain states have more restrictive laws regarding sexual practices deemed "deviant." For instance, some states have laws that criminalize sodomy, which could be interpreted to include certain forms of fisting. However, these laws are often unenforced and may not apply in private settings.

Europe European countries tend to have more progressive attitudes toward sexual practices, with many nations recognizing the importance of consent and personal autonomy. In countries like the Netherlands and Germany, fisting is generally accepted within the context of consensual adult relationships. However, public displays or acts that could be construed as obscene may still face legal scrutiny.

United Kingdom In the UK, consensual sexual activities between adults are legal, provided they do not cause harm or distress. The Sexual Offences Act 2003 provides a framework for understanding consent and outlines the importance of mutual agreement in sexual practices. Fisting, when practiced consensually and safely, is generally legal, but practitioners should be aware of the nuances of local laws regarding public decency and obscenity.

Asia and Middle East In many Asian and Middle Eastern countries, sexual practices outside of heterosexual marriage can face severe legal repercussions. Countries such as Saudi Arabia and Iran have stringent laws against any form of sexual expression deemed immoral, including fisting. Practitioners in these regions must exercise extreme caution and often must keep their practices private to avoid legal consequences.

Potential Legal Challenges

Practitioners of fisting may encounter several legal challenges, including:

- **Criminal Charges:** Engaging in fisting in a context perceived as non-consensual or harmful could lead to criminal charges, including assault or sexual misconduct. It is vital to establish clear consent and communication with partners.

- **Civil Liability:** In cases where an injury occurs during fisting, practitioners may face civil lawsuits for negligence or personal injury. Ensuring safety and following best practices can mitigate such risks.

- **Regulatory Scrutiny:** In jurisdictions where fisting is associated with BDSM or kink practices, regulatory bodies may scrutinize events or venues hosting such activities, particularly if they are perceived as promoting illegal acts.

Conclusion

Navigating the legalities of fisting requires a nuanced understanding of local laws and cultural attitudes toward sexual practices. Practitioners should prioritize consent, communication, and safety while remaining informed about the legal frameworks that govern their practices. Engaging with local communities, legal experts, and advocacy groups can further enhance understanding and promote safe exploration of desires within legal boundaries.

As societal attitudes toward sexuality continue to evolve, it is essential for practitioners to remain vigilant and informed about the changing legal landscapes surrounding fisting and other sexual practices. By fostering open dialogues and advocating for sexual rights, individuals can contribute to a more inclusive and accepting environment for all sexual expressions.

Consent and Criminalization of Fisting

The topic of consent in the context of fisting is multifaceted and complex, especially when intersecting with legal frameworks that govern sexual practices. Understanding the nuances of consent is crucial for both participants and those who may be observing or judging such practices from an external perspective. This section aims to explore the legal implications of consent, the potential for criminalization of fisting, and the broader societal attitudes that influence these dynamics.

Understanding Consent

Consent is defined as a mutual agreement between participants to engage in a specific activity. In the realm of sexual practices, consent must be informed, voluntary, and revocable at any time. The principles of consent can be encapsulated in the following equation:

$$C = I + V + R$$

where C represents consent, I is informed understanding of the activity, V is voluntary agreement without coercion, and R is the ability to revoke consent at any point. This equation highlights that all three components are necessary for consent to be valid.

Legal Perspectives on Fisting

The legal landscape surrounding sexual practices, including fisting, varies significantly across jurisdictions. While many regions recognize the importance of consent in sexual activities, the specific legal ramifications of fisting can lead to confusion and potential criminalization.

In some jurisdictions, consensual sexual activities, regardless of their nature, are protected under laws that promote sexual autonomy. However, in others, the lack of explicit legal definitions regarding certain practices can result in ambiguity. For instance, in jurisdictions where laws focus on the potential for harm, fisting may be scrutinized more heavily due to misconceptions about its risks.

Potential for Criminalization

The potential for criminalization arises when the act of fisting is perceived through the lens of harm, either physical or psychological. The following factors can contribute to this perception:

- **Misunderstanding of Risks:** Many individuals may equate fisting with high levels of risk without understanding the safety practices that can mitigate these risks. This misunderstanding can lead to calls for regulation or prohibition of the practice.

- **Cultural Stigma:** Societal attitudes towards sex and non-normative sexual practices can influence legal outcomes. In cultures where fisting is viewed as deviant, participants may face legal repercussions even when engaging in consensual acts.

- **Informed Consent:** If consent is not adequately communicated or if one party is perceived to be incapable of giving consent (due to intoxication, mental incapacity, etc.), legal systems may classify the act as assault or sexual abuse.

Case Studies and Examples

To illustrate the complexities surrounding consent and criminalization, we can examine several case studies:

1. **Case of Misunderstood Consent:** In a 2018 case in the United States, two individuals engaged in fisting as part of their consensual sexual relationship. However, a third party intervened, claiming that the act constituted sexual assault due to the physical risks involved. The court ultimately ruled in favor of the defendants, citing clear evidence of informed consent, but the case highlighted the societal misconceptions surrounding fisting and consent.

2. **Cultural Context:** In some countries, such as those with strict anti-LGBTQ+ laws, consensual sexual practices between adults can be criminalized under broader laws against "unnatural acts." Fisting, often associated with queer sexual practices, can thus be targeted, leading to arrests and legal action against participants despite mutual consent.

3. **Regulatory Responses:** Some jurisdictions have attempted to create clearer guidelines for sexual practices that involve significant physical risk. For example, in Canada, the "Criminal Code" outlines the need for informed consent in sexual activities but does not explicitly mention fisting. This omission can lead to

legal gray areas, where practitioners may inadvertently find themselves in legal jeopardy.

The Role of Advocacy and Education

Advocacy and education play crucial roles in addressing the issues of consent and criminalization. By increasing awareness of safe practices and the importance of clear communication, communities can work towards destigmatizing fisting and similar practices.

Furthermore, legal advocacy groups can push for clearer legal definitions that protect consensual sexual activities, thereby reducing the potential for criminalization. This can include:

- **Public Awareness Campaigns:** Educating the public about the realities of fisting, including safety practices and the importance of consent, can help shift societal perceptions.

- **Legal Reform Initiatives:** Advocating for laws that explicitly protect consensual sexual acts can reduce the ambiguity that leads to criminalization.

- **Training for Law Enforcement:** Providing law enforcement with training on sexual consent and the nuances of non-normative sexual practices can lead to more informed and compassionate responses to reported incidents.

Conclusion

In conclusion, the intersection of consent and the potential criminalization of fisting reflects broader societal attitudes towards sexuality and the complexities of legal definitions. Understanding and advocating for informed consent, while challenging misconceptions about risk and harm, is crucial for protecting individuals who choose to explore fisting as part of their sexual expression. By fostering open dialogue and education, communities can create safer spaces for exploration while advocating for legal protections that honor the autonomy of all individuals involved.

Ethical Responsibility and Fisting Play

Ethical responsibility in the context of fisting play encompasses a range of considerations that ensure the safety, consent, and well-being of all participants involved. Engaging in fisting, like any other sexual activity, requires a commitment to ethical practices that prioritize the physical and emotional health of each person. This section will explore the ethical dimensions of fisting play, including informed consent, power dynamics, and the importance of creating a safe environment.

Informed Consent

At the core of ethical responsibility in fisting play is the principle of informed consent. Informed consent means that all participants must fully understand the implications of their involvement, including the potential risks and benefits associated with fisting. This involves:

- **Clear Communication:** Participants should engage in open discussions about their desires, boundaries, and any concerns they may have. This dialogue should include discussions about health and safety practices, as well as emotional readiness.

- **Ongoing Consent:** Consent is not a one-time agreement but an ongoing conversation. Participants should feel empowered to withdraw consent at any time during the activity if they feel uncomfortable or unsafe.

- **Education:** Both parties should educate themselves about fisting techniques, safety measures, and potential risks. This knowledge can help mitigate harm and enhance the experience.

Power Dynamics

Fisting play often involves complex power dynamics, especially in BDSM contexts. Understanding these dynamics is crucial for ethical engagement. Key considerations include:

- **Negotiation of Roles:** Participants should negotiate their roles (dominant, submissive, etc.) before engaging in play. This negotiation should include discussions about limits, safe words, and aftercare.

- **Awareness of Vulnerability:** The act of fisting can create a heightened sense of vulnerability. It is essential for the dominant partner to be aware of this and to prioritize the emotional and physical safety of the submissive partner.

- **Empowerment vs. Control:** Ethical fisting play focuses on mutual empowerment rather than control. Both partners should feel empowered to express their needs and desires throughout the experience.

Creating a Safe Environment

A safe environment is critical for ethical fisting play. This includes both physical and emotional safety measures:

- **Hygiene Practices:** Participants must adhere to strict hygiene protocols to prevent infections. This includes cleaning hands, using gloves, and ensuring that any toys or accessories are sanitized.
- **Safe Words and Signals:** Establishing clear safe words or signals can help participants communicate their comfort levels during play. These tools are vital for maintaining a safe space where both partners can express their boundaries.
- **Aftercare:** Aftercare is an essential component of ethical fisting play. It involves taking the time to care for each other emotionally and physically after the experience, ensuring that both partners feel supported and safe.

Addressing Stigma and Misconceptions

Fisting often carries social stigma and misconceptions that can impact the ethical engagement of participants. Addressing these issues is vital for fostering a respectful and understanding environment:

- **Education and Advocacy:** Participants should educate themselves and others about fisting to dispel myths and reduce stigma. This can involve sharing accurate information about the practice, its safety, and its consensual nature.
- **Community Support:** Engaging with supportive communities can help individuals feel more comfortable exploring fisting. These communities often provide resources, education, and a safe space to discuss experiences and concerns.
- **Respecting Diversity:** Recognizing that fisting can be a part of various sexual orientations and identities is crucial. Ethical responsibility involves respecting the diverse ways in which individuals engage with fisting and ensuring inclusivity within the community.

Conclusion

In conclusion, ethical responsibility in fisting play is essential for ensuring the safety, consent, and well-being of all participants. By prioritizing informed consent, understanding power dynamics, creating a safe environment, and addressing stigma, individuals can engage in fisting play in a manner that is respectful and fulfilling. The ethical considerations outlined in this section serve as a guide for fostering healthy and consensual experiences, ultimately enhancing the joy and intimacy that fisting can offer.

$$\text{Ethical Engagement} = \text{Informed Consent} + \text{Power Dynamics Awareness} + \text{Safe Environment} \tag{66}$$

Navigating Public Perception and Stigma

Fisting, as an intimate and often misunderstood sexual practice, exists at the intersection of pleasure and taboo. The public perception of fisting is frequently clouded by stigma, misconceptions, and cultural narratives that can hinder open discussion and personal exploration. This section aims to unpack the complexities of societal attitudes towards fisting, address the challenges faced by practitioners, and provide strategies for navigating these perceptions in a constructive manner.

Understanding Stigma and Its Origins

Stigma surrounding fisting can be traced to broader societal attitudes towards sexuality, particularly those that deviate from heteronormative and conventional sexual practices. According to Goffman's theory of stigma, social disapproval arises from the fear of the unknown and the violation of societal norms [1]. Fisting is often perceived as extreme, dangerous, or even deviant, leading to a negative connotation that can affect individuals who engage in this practice.

$$S = \frac{D}{N} \tag{67}$$

Where:
- S represents the stigma level,
- D is the degree of deviation from societal norms,
- N is the normalization of the practice within the community.

As the degree of deviation increases, stigma intensifies, creating a cycle that perpetuates misunderstanding and fear. This stigma can manifest in various forms, including social ostracism, discrimination, and internalized shame among practitioners.

Challenges Faced by Practitioners

Practitioners of fisting often encounter several challenges due to societal stigma:

- **Isolation and Shame:** Many individuals may feel isolated or ashamed of their desires, leading to a reluctance to seek community or support. This isolation can exacerbate feelings of inadequacy and shame, creating a barrier to healthy sexual expression.

- **Miscommunication and Misinformation:** The stigma surrounding fisting can lead to a lack of accurate information. Misinformation can perpetuate myths about safety and health risks, leading to fear and misunderstanding among both practitioners and potential partners.

- **Fear of Judgment:** Individuals may fear judgment from peers, family, or healthcare professionals, leading to a reluctance to discuss their interests openly. This fear can prevent individuals from seeking necessary support or engaging in safe practices.

- **Legal and Social Risks:** In some jurisdictions, fisting may be viewed through a legal lens that criminalizes certain sexual practices. This legal stigma can deter individuals from openly participating in fisting communities or seeking legal protection in cases of consent violations.

Strategies for Navigating Stigma

Navigating public perception and stigma requires a multi-faceted approach that emphasizes education, communication, and community-building. Here are several strategies:

- **Education and Advocacy:** Engaging in educational efforts can help dispel myths surrounding fisting. This can include hosting workshops, writing articles, or participating in discussions that promote accurate information about safety and pleasure. Advocacy for sexual rights can also help shift societal perceptions.

- **Building Supportive Communities:** Creating or joining supportive communities can provide a safe space for individuals to share experiences and resources. Online forums, local meetups, and workshops can foster connection and reduce feelings of isolation.

- **Open Communication:** Practicing open communication with partners about desires, boundaries, and concerns can help build trust and reduce stigma. Discussing fisting in a non-judgmental context can normalize the practice and encourage mutual understanding.

- **Reframing Conversations:** By reframing conversations around fisting to focus on empowerment, pleasure, and consent, individuals can challenge negative perceptions. Emphasizing the consensual and intimate nature of fisting can help shift the narrative from one of fear to one of exploration.

- **Engaging with Allies:** Finding allies in the sexual health community, including educators, therapists, and healthcare providers, can help legitimize fisting as a valid sexual practice. Allies can provide resources, support, and advocacy for individuals navigating stigma.

Conclusion

Navigating public perception and stigma surrounding fisting is a complex endeavor that requires courage, education, and community support. By understanding the origins of stigma and actively engaging in advocacy and education, individuals can work towards normalizing their desires and experiences. Embracing fisting as a legitimate expression of sexuality not only empowers practitioners but also contributes to a broader cultural shift towards acceptance and understanding of diverse sexual practices.

Bibliography

[1] Goffman, E. (1963). *Stigma: Notes on the Management of Spoiled Identity*. Prentice Hall.

Balancing Privacy and Visibility in Fisting Communities

The interplay between privacy and visibility in fisting communities presents a complex landscape shaped by cultural norms, individual desires, and the overarching need for safety and acceptance. As fisting practices gain visibility in broader sexual discourse, individuals within these communities must navigate the delicate balance of expressing their identities while safeguarding their personal information and experiences.

Theoretical Framework

The notion of privacy in sexual communities can be contextualized through the lens of *Erving Goffman's* theory of self-presentation. Goffman posits that individuals perform different aspects of their identities depending on the social context, often referred to as "front stage" and "back stage" behaviors. In fisting communities, members may adopt varying degrees of visibility based on their comfort levels, societal acceptance, and the perceived risks associated with their sexual expression.

$$\text{Visibility} = \frac{\text{Self-Expression}}{\text{Social Acceptance} + \text{Risk}} \qquad (68)$$

This equation suggests that visibility in fisting communities is a function of the desire for self-expression moderated by social acceptance and perceived risks. As individuals navigate their identities, they must assess how much of their sexual selves they wish to share publicly while considering the potential repercussions of such disclosures.

Challenges of Visibility

1. **Stigma and Discrimination**: Fisting, often viewed as taboo, can lead to stigma, making individuals hesitant to publicly identify with the practice. Negative societal perceptions can result in discrimination, impacting personal relationships, employment opportunities, and mental health.

2. **Safety Concerns**: The visibility of one's sexual practices can attract unwanted attention or harassment. Individuals may fear that revealing their interests could lead to personal safety risks, particularly in environments where fisting is not understood or accepted.

3. **Community Dynamics**: Within fisting communities, varying levels of comfort with visibility can create tension. Some members may advocate for openness and education, while others prioritize discretion, leading to potential conflicts over community norms and values.

Strategies for Balancing Privacy and Visibility

1. **Anonymous Participation**: Many individuals choose to engage in fisting communities anonymously, utilizing pseudonyms or avatars. This allows for participation in discussions and events without compromising personal identity, fostering a sense of belonging while maintaining privacy.

2. **Selective Sharing**: Practitioners can adopt a strategy of selective sharing, where they disclose aspects of their fisting experiences to trusted individuals or smaller groups rather than the public. This approach allows for meaningful connections without the risks associated with broader visibility.

3. **Community Guidelines**: Establishing clear community guidelines regarding privacy and visibility can help create a safe environment for all members. These guidelines may include recommendations for anonymous participation, consent for sharing personal stories, and respect for individual comfort levels.

4. **Education and Advocacy**: Promoting education about fisting and its practices can help reduce stigma and increase understanding. As awareness grows, individuals may feel more empowered to express their identities openly, contributing to a culture of acceptance.

Examples of Balancing Privacy and Visibility

1. **Online Forums**: Many fisting enthusiasts participate in online forums where anonymity is preserved. These platforms allow individuals to share experiences and seek advice without revealing their identities, fostering a supportive community that values privacy.

2. **Workshops and Events**: In-person workshops can offer a space for visibility while maintaining safety. By requiring participants to register under pseudonyms or limiting attendance to trusted community members, these events can balance the need for education with privacy concerns.

3. **Social Media Groups**: Private social media groups provide a venue for individuals to connect and share experiences without the risks associated with public visibility. Members can engage in discussions, share resources, and support one another while maintaining control over their personal information.

Conclusion

Navigating the balance between privacy and visibility in fisting communities is a nuanced endeavor. Individuals must consider their personal comfort levels, societal perceptions, and the potential risks associated with their sexual identities. By fostering a culture of respect, education, and support, fisting communities can create environments where members feel safe to explore their identities while maintaining the privacy that is often essential to their well-being. As the discourse surrounding fisting continues to evolve, the ongoing dialogue about privacy and visibility will remain a crucial aspect of fostering inclusive and accepting communities.

Advocacy and Activism for Fisting Rights

The landscape of sexual expression is often fraught with stigma, particularly for practices that challenge societal norms, such as fisting. Advocacy and activism for fisting rights are essential to creating a more inclusive and understanding society. This section will explore the theoretical frameworks, challenges, and examples of advocacy efforts aimed at legitimizing and normalizing fisting as a valid sexual practice.

Theoretical Frameworks

At the core of advocacy for fisting rights lies the intersection of sexual rights, bodily autonomy, and the decriminalization of consensual sexual practices. The **Sexual Rights Framework** posits that individuals have the right to express their sexuality in ways that are consensual, informed, and safe. This framework is supported by various international human rights instruments, including the Universal Declaration of Human Rights, which emphasizes the right to privacy and personal freedom.

The **Critical Sexuality Studies** approach further challenges the pathologization of non-normative sexual practices. It encourages a re-examination of societal attitudes towards fisting, advocating for a shift from viewing it as taboo to understanding it as a legitimate expression of sexual desire and intimacy. This shift can be informed by the work of theorists like Michel Foucault, who argued that sexuality is a socially constructed domain that can be liberated through discourse and advocacy.

Challenges in Advocacy

Despite the theoretical support for fisting rights, several challenges persist in advocacy efforts:

- **Stigma and Misunderstanding:** Fisting is often misunderstood and associated with violence or deviance. This stigma can deter individuals from openly discussing their experiences or desires, creating a culture of silence around the practice.

- **Legal Barriers:** In some jurisdictions, laws surrounding sexual acts can be vague or punitive, leading to potential criminalization of consensual practices like fisting. This legal ambiguity can create fear among practitioners and discourage advocacy efforts.

- **Lack of Representation:** The voices of marginalized communities, including LGBTQ+ individuals and people of color, are often underrepresented in mainstream sexual discourse. This lack of representation can hinder the effectiveness of advocacy efforts aimed at normalizing fisting.

- **Internalized Shame:** Many individuals who engage in fisting may experience internalized shame or guilt, stemming from societal taboos. This internal conflict can make it challenging for individuals to advocate for their rights and the rights of others.

Examples of Advocacy Efforts

Despite these challenges, numerous advocacy initiatives aim to promote fisting rights and normalize the practice:

- **Community Workshops and Events:** Local and online communities often host workshops that focus on safe fisting practices, consent, and communication. These workshops not only educate participants but also provide a platform for individuals to share their experiences and advocate for acceptance.

- **Social Media Campaigns:** Platforms like Twitter, Instagram, and TikTok have become powerful tools for advocacy. Campaigns that use hashtags such as #FistingIsNormal or #FistingAwareness aim to destigmatize the practice and create dialogue around it.

- **Academic Research and Publications:** Scholars and sex educators are increasingly publishing research that explores fisting from various perspectives, including its psychological, physical, and cultural implications. This body of work helps to legitimize fisting as a topic worthy of serious discussion and academic inquiry.

- **Legal Advocacy Organizations:** Organizations that focus on sexual rights, such as the National Coalition for Sexual Freedom (NCSF), work to challenge discriminatory laws and promote legal protections for consensual sexual practices. These organizations often provide resources and support for individuals facing legal challenges related to their sexual practices.

The Role of Intersectionality

An intersectional approach is vital in advocacy for fisting rights. Recognizing how factors such as race, gender, sexual orientation, and socioeconomic status intersect can help tailor advocacy efforts to address the unique experiences of different communities. For instance, LGBTQ+ individuals may face additional layers of stigma and discrimination, necessitating targeted outreach and support.

Conclusion

Advocacy and activism for fisting rights are crucial in fostering a society that embraces diverse sexual practices. By challenging stigma, promoting education, and advocating for legal protections, we can create an environment where individuals feel empowered to explore their sexuality without fear of judgment or reprisal. As we move forward, it is essential to continue building coalitions, amplifying marginalized voices, and fostering open dialogues that celebrate the complexity of human sexuality.

In this journey, every conversation, every workshop, and every act of solidarity contributes to the broader movement for sexual rights and acceptance, paving the way for a future where fisting, and all forms of consensual sexual expression, are embraced as valid and worthy of respect.

Fisting-Focused Legal Support and Resources

In the realm of sexual exploration, particularly with practices as stigmatized as fisting, it is crucial to understand the legal landscape that surrounds these activities. Legal support and resources are essential not only for ensuring safety and protection but also for fostering an environment where individuals can engage in consensual practices without fear of legal repercussions or discrimination.

Understanding the Legal Landscape

The legal status of fisting varies significantly across jurisdictions. In many places, consensual sexual acts between adults are protected under privacy laws; however, this protection can become complicated when considering local laws regarding sexual conduct. It is important to understand that while fisting itself may not be illegal, associated activities, such as public displays of sexual acts or certain forms of BDSM, may fall under obscenity or indecency laws.

Legalities of Fisting in Different Countries and Jurisdictions

In countries with more progressive views on sexual rights, fisting is often seen as a legitimate form of sexual expression. For instance, in many European countries, laws tend to favor individual autonomy over sexual practices. Conversely, in regions with stringent laws against sexual expression, individuals may face legal risks even when engaging in consensual private acts.

$$\text{Legal Risk} = f(\text{Jurisdiction, Consent, Public Perception}) \qquad (69)$$

This equation suggests that the legal risk associated with fisting is a function of the jurisdiction's laws, the presence of consent, and societal attitudes towards sexual practices.

Consent and Criminalization of Fisting

Consent is a pivotal element in the legal framework surrounding fisting. In many jurisdictions, the absence of consent transforms a consensual act into a criminal offense. Therefore, it is essential for individuals to document and communicate consent clearly. This can be achieved through written agreements or recorded conversations that outline the parameters of the activity.

Ethical Responsibility and Fisting Play

Engaging in fisting requires an understanding of ethical responsibilities, particularly regarding consent and safety. Practitioners must be aware of not only their own rights but also the rights of their partners. This includes respecting boundaries and ensuring that all parties are informed about the potential risks involved. Ethical considerations extend to the use of safe words and the importance of aftercare, which can mitigate emotional and physical distress following the act.

Navigating Public Perception and Stigma

Public perception of fisting can lead to stigma and discrimination, which may discourage individuals from seeking legal support or reporting incidents of abuse or violation. This stigma is often rooted in misconceptions about sexual practices outside of mainstream norms. Advocacy groups play a crucial role in changing these perceptions and providing support to individuals who may feel marginalized.

Balancing Privacy and Visibility in Fisting Communities

In navigating the legal landscape, individuals must balance their desire for privacy with the need for visibility in the community. While anonymity can protect individuals from societal judgment, visibility can foster community support and advocacy. Engaging with local LGBTQ+ organizations or sexual health groups can provide a platform for discussing legal rights and resources available to those who practice fisting.

Advocacy and Activism for Fisting Rights

Advocacy efforts are vital in promoting legal recognition and protection for fisting practitioners. Organizations that focus on sexual rights and health can offer resources, legal advice, and support networks for individuals exploring fisting. Participating in activism, whether through awareness campaigns or legal challenges, can help reshape societal attitudes and influence legislation.

Fisting-Focused Legal Support and Resources

1. **Legal Aid Organizations:** Many cities have legal aid services that provide free or low-cost legal assistance to individuals facing discrimination or legal challenges related to their sexual practices. These organizations can help navigate local laws and offer guidance on consent and safety.

2. **LGBTQ+ Advocacy Groups:** Organizations like the Human Rights Campaign and GLAAD often provide resources for individuals in the LGBTQ+ community, including legal support and information about rights related to sexual practices.

3. **Sexual Health Clinics:** Many sexual health clinics offer not only health services but also resources and information about legal rights concerning sexual practices. They may have pamphlets or staff trained to discuss legal issues related to sexual health.

4. **Online Legal Resources:** Websites such as the National Center for Lesbian Rights or the ACLU provide comprehensive information on sexual rights, including articles and legal guides that pertain to consensual sexual practices.

5. **Peer Support Networks:** Engaging with peer support networks can be invaluable. These groups often share experiences and resources, including legal contacts and advice regarding navigating the complexities of fisting within the law.

Conclusion

Understanding the legal implications of fisting is essential for safe and consensual exploration. By utilizing available resources and engaging in advocacy, individuals can help create a more supportive environment for all who wish to explore this intimate practice. Knowledge of the law not only empowers individuals but also fosters a community where sexual expression is celebrated rather than stigmatized.

Ethical Pornography and Fisting

In recent years, the conversation surrounding pornography has shifted significantly, with increasing emphasis on ethical considerations in the production and consumption of adult content. This section explores the intersection of ethical pornography and fisting, addressing the complexities, challenges, and potential pathways to creating and engaging with ethical fisting content.

Defining Ethical Pornography

Ethical pornography can be defined as adult content that prioritizes the well-being of all participants, ensuring that the production process respects consent, safety, and fair compensation. It aims to dismantle exploitative practices often associated with mainstream pornography, including coercion, lack of informed consent, and inadequate attention to the physical and emotional safety of performers.

The Importance of Consent

Consent is the cornerstone of ethical pornography, particularly in practices such as fisting, which carry inherent physical and emotional risks. Ethical pornographic productions must ensure that all performers are fully informed about the acts they are engaging in, including the potential risks associated with fisting. This includes:

- Detailed discussions about boundaries and limits.
- Clear communication regarding safe words and signals.
- Continuous check-ins during the performance to ensure ongoing consent.

Representation and Diversity

Ethical pornography also emphasizes representation and diversity, which is crucial in fisting content. The portrayal of varied body types, gender identities, and sexual orientations can help normalize fisting as a valid sexual practice across different communities. This representation fosters inclusivity and allows viewers to see themselves reflected in the content, thus promoting a broader understanding of sexual diversity.

Challenges in Ethical Fisting Pornography

Despite the growing movement towards ethical pornography, several challenges persist:

- **Stigma and Misconceptions:** Fisting is often stigmatized, leading to misconceptions about its safety and desirability. Ethical pornography must combat these narratives by presenting fisting as a consensual and pleasurable experience when approached with care.
- **Access to Resources:** Many performers may lack access to education on fisting techniques and safety practices. Ethical porn producers should provide comprehensive training and resources to ensure performers are well-informed and prepared.
- **Commercial Viability:** Ethical pornographic content may struggle to compete with mainstream pornography, which often prioritizes sensationalism over ethics. This can make it difficult for ethical producers to gain traction and reach wider audiences.

Examples of Ethical Fisting Pornography

Several platforms and producers have begun to prioritize ethical considerations in their fisting content:

- **Independent Studios:** Many independent studios focus on ethical production practices, often featuring fisting scenes that emphasize consent, safety, and pleasure. These studios may provide behind-the-scenes insights into their practices, fostering transparency.

- **Community-Driven Platforms:** Online platforms that allow performers to create and share their content can empower individuals to produce ethical fisting pornography on their terms. These platforms often prioritize consent and fair compensation, allowing performers to maintain control over their work.

- **Educational Content:** Some ethical pornography producers incorporate educational elements into their films, such as tutorials on safe fisting techniques and discussions about consent and communication. This approach not only entertains but also informs viewers, promoting safe practices.

The Role of Viewers

Viewers play a crucial role in the ethical landscape of pornography. By choosing to support ethical producers and content, consumers can help shift the industry towards more responsible practices. This includes:

- **Supporting Ethical Platforms:** Seek out and subscribe to platforms that prioritize ethical practices in their content.

- **Advocating for Transparency:** Encourage producers to be transparent about their practices, including consent protocols and performer safety measures.

- **Engaging in Conversations:** Participate in discussions around ethical pornography, sharing insights and advocating for change within the industry.

Conclusion

The intersection of ethical pornography and fisting presents an opportunity for both performers and viewers to engage with sexual expression in a responsible and informed manner. By prioritizing consent, representation, and safety, the ethical fisting community can challenge the stigma surrounding this practice and contribute to a more inclusive and respectful discourse on sexuality. As the landscape of adult content continues to evolve, the pursuit of ethical fisting pornography can serve as a model for how we can navigate the complexities of sexual expression while honoring the dignity and autonomy of all participants.

Fighting Fisting-Related Discrimination and Prejudice

Fisting, as a sexual practice, often faces significant societal stigma and discrimination. This section addresses the various forms of prejudice encountered by individuals who engage in fisting and outlines strategies for combating these biases.

Understanding Discrimination and Prejudice

Discrimination against fisting practitioners can manifest in numerous ways, including social ostracism, misinformation, and even legal repercussions in certain jurisdictions. Prejudice often stems from a lack of understanding or exposure to alternative sexual practices. The negative stereotypes associated with fisting can lead to feelings of shame and isolation among those who enjoy this form of intimacy.

Theoretical Frameworks

To analyze the discrimination faced by fisters, we can utilize several theoretical frameworks:

- **Social Identity Theory:** This theory posits that individuals categorize themselves and others into groups, leading to in-group favoritism and out-group discrimination. Fisters may be marginalized as they are often viewed as part of a sexual minority.
- **Queer Theory:** This perspective challenges normative assumptions about sexuality and advocates for the acceptance of diverse sexual expressions. Queer theory emphasizes the need to deconstruct societal norms that label certain sexual practices as deviant.
- **Intersectionality:** Understanding that individuals' experiences of discrimination can vary based on multiple identities (e.g., race, gender, sexual orientation) is crucial. Fisters who belong to multiple marginalized groups may face compounded prejudice.

Examples of Discrimination

Discrimination against fisters can take various forms, including:

- **Social Stigma:** Fisters may encounter judgment or exclusion from social groups, leading to a reluctance to disclose their sexual preferences.

- **Misinformation:** Many misconceptions about fisting, such as the belief that it is inherently dangerous or abusive, perpetuate negative stereotypes. This misinformation can deter individuals from exploring their desires.

- **Legal Issues:** In some jurisdictions, laws regarding sexual conduct may criminalize consensual fisting, leading to legal repercussions for practitioners. This can create a climate of fear and secrecy.

Combating Discrimination

To effectively fight against fisting-related discrimination and prejudice, several strategies can be employed:

- **Education and Awareness:** Providing accurate information about fisting can help dispel myths and reduce stigma. Workshops, seminars, and online resources can educate both practitioners and the general public about the safety and consensual nature of fisting.

- **Community Building:** Creating safe spaces for fisters to connect and share their experiences fosters a sense of belonging and support. This can be achieved through local meetups, online forums, and social media groups.

- **Advocacy:** Engaging in advocacy efforts to promote sexual rights and decriminalize consensual sexual practices is vital. Collaborating with organizations that support sexual freedom can amplify the voices of fisters.

- **Visibility and Representation:** Increasing the visibility of fisting in popular culture and media can challenge stereotypes and normalize the practice. This includes incorporating positive portrayals of fisting in literature, film, and art.

- **Support Networks:** Establishing peer support groups can provide emotional and practical assistance for those facing discrimination. These networks can offer resources for navigating stigma and finding acceptance.

Conclusion

Fighting fisting-related discrimination and prejudice requires a multifaceted approach that combines education, community support, and advocacy. By challenging societal norms and fostering an inclusive environment, we can work towards a future where all sexual practices, including fisting, are accepted and celebrated. Embracing diversity in sexual expression not only empowers individuals but also enriches our collective understanding of intimacy and pleasure.

$$P_{acceptance} = \frac{E_{education} + C_{community} + A_{advocacy}}{D_{discrimination}} \quad (70)$$

Where:

- $P_{acceptance}$ represents the level of acceptance of fisting in society.

- $E_{education}$ is the effectiveness of educational initiatives.

- $C_{community}$ reflects the strength of community networks.

- $A_{advocacy}$ denotes the impact of advocacy efforts.

- $D_{discrimination}$ quantifies the existing discrimination against fisters.

This equation illustrates that increasing education, community support, and advocacy can lead to a decrease in discrimination, ultimately fostering greater acceptance of fisting as a valid expression of human sexuality.

Recognizing and Addressing Fisting Addiction

Signs and Symptoms of Fisting Addiction

Fisting addiction, like other forms of sexual addiction, can manifest in various ways that affect an individual's emotional, physical, and social well-being. Understanding the signs and symptoms of this addiction is crucial for recognizing when a passion has crossed the line into compulsive behavior. This section will explore the key indicators of fisting addiction, drawing on relevant theories of addiction, psychological impacts, and providing examples to illustrate these points.

Defining Addiction in the Context of Fisting

Addiction is characterized by compulsive engagement in rewarding stimuli, despite adverse consequences. According to the **American Psychiatric Association**, addiction involves a lack of control, cravings, and continued use despite negative outcomes. In the context of fisting, this can manifest as an overwhelming desire to engage in fisting activities, even when it leads to physical harm or emotional distress.

Key Signs of Fisting Addiction

- **Compulsive Behavior:** Individuals may find themselves unable to resist the urge to engage in fisting, leading to frequent and sometimes risky encounters. For example, a person might prioritize fisting over other important activities, such as work or relationships.

- **Preoccupation with Fisting:** Constant thoughts about fisting, including planning future sessions or obsessively researching techniques, can indicate an addiction. This preoccupation may interfere with daily life and responsibilities.

- **Escalation of Use:** A fister may feel the need to increase the intensity or frequency of their fisting sessions to achieve the same level of satisfaction. This can include experimenting with more extreme techniques or engaging in fisting more often than before.

- **Neglecting Responsibilities:** Individuals might neglect personal, professional, or social obligations in favor of fisting. For instance, someone might skip work or miss family events to participate in fisting activities.

- **Emotional Distress:** Feelings of guilt, shame, or anxiety related to fisting activities can be a significant indicator of addiction. This emotional turmoil may lead to a cycle of seeking out fisting for relief, only to feel worse afterward.

- **Physical Consequences:** Persistent fisting, especially without proper safety measures, can lead to physical injuries or health issues. Ignoring these signs, such as pain or bleeding, can indicate an addiction where the individual prioritizes the act over their health.

- **Withdrawal Symptoms:** Just as with substance addiction, individuals may experience withdrawal symptoms when not engaging in fisting. These can include irritability, restlessness, or heightened sexual frustration.

- **Loss of Control:** An inability to control the frequency or intensity of fisting sessions can signify addiction. For example, a person may promise themselves to limit their fisting but finds it impossible to do so.

Theoretical Frameworks

Understanding fisting addiction can be enhanced through several psychological theories:

- **Cognitive Behavioral Theory (CBT):** This theory posits that dysfunctional thinking patterns contribute to addiction. For example, a fister may rationalize their behavior by believing that they need fisting to feel pleasure or intimacy, despite the negative consequences.

- **The Disease Model of Addiction:** This model views addiction as a chronic disease that alters brain chemistry and function. For instance, engaging in fisting may release dopamine, reinforcing the behavior and leading to compulsive use.

- **Attachment Theory:** This theory suggests that early attachment experiences shape adult relationships and behaviors. An individual with insecure attachment may turn to fisting as a means of coping with intimacy issues or emotional voids.

Examples of Fisting Addiction

- **Case Study 1:** *Alex*, a 30-year-old individual, initially engaged in fisting as a way to explore their sexuality. Over time, Alex found themselves obsessively planning fisting sessions, often at the expense of their job and relationships. Despite experiencing physical pain and emotional distress, Alex felt compelled to continue, highlighting a loss of control.

- **Case Study 2:** *Jamie*, a 28-year-old, began to use fisting as a coping mechanism for anxiety. Jamie's fisting sessions became more frequent, leading to neglect of personal hygiene and health. Despite recognizing the negative impact on their life, Jamie struggled to stop, demonstrating withdrawal symptoms when unable to engage.

Conclusion

Recognizing the signs and symptoms of fisting addiction is essential for individuals who may be struggling with their sexual behaviors. By understanding the compulsive nature of addiction, the emotional and physical consequences, and the theoretical frameworks that explain these behaviors, individuals can begin to address their relationship with fisting. Seeking support, whether through therapy or community resources, can be a vital step towards reclaiming control and fostering a healthier approach to sexual exploration.

Understanding the Role of Dopamine and Addiction

Dopamine is a neurotransmitter that plays a critical role in the brain's reward system. It is often referred to as the "feel-good" chemical because it is released during pleasurable activities, including sexual arousal and orgasm. Understanding the role of dopamine in addiction, particularly in the context of fisting and other sexual behaviors, can provide insight into the mechanisms that drive compulsive sexual behavior and the potential for addiction.

The Dopaminergic Pathway

The dopaminergic pathway is a complex network of neurons that transmit dopamine throughout the brain. The primary areas involved in this pathway include the ventral tegmental area (VTA), the nucleus accumbens (NAc), and the prefrontal cortex (PFC). When an individual engages in pleasurable activities, such as fisting, dopamine is released in these areas, reinforcing the behavior and creating a sense of pleasure.

The basic equation that describes the relationship between dopamine levels and the reward experience can be expressed as:

$$R = f(D)$$

where R represents the reward experience, and D represents the level of dopamine released. As dopamine levels increase, the intensity of the reward experience also increases, leading to a heightened desire to repeat the behavior.

Dopamine and the Cycle of Addiction

Addiction can be understood as a cycle that involves the following stages:
1. **Initial Exposure**: Engaging in fisting can lead to a significant release of dopamine, creating a powerful and pleasurable experience. 2. **Reinforcement**:

The pleasurable feelings associated with dopamine release reinforce the behavior, making it more likely that the individual will seek out fisting again in the future. 3. **Tolerance**: Over time, repeated exposure to the pleasurable experience can lead to tolerance, where higher levels of stimulation are required to achieve the same dopamine release. This can result in individuals seeking out more extreme forms of fisting or other sexual behaviors to attain the desired level of pleasure. 4. **Withdrawal**: When an individual attempts to reduce or stop engaging in fisting, they may experience withdrawal symptoms, such as anxiety, irritability, or mood swings. These symptoms can further drive the individual back to the behavior to alleviate discomfort. 5. **Compulsion**: The cycle can culminate in compulsive behavior, where the individual continues to engage in fisting despite negative consequences, such as physical injury, emotional distress, or damage to relationships.

This cycle can be represented mathematically as:

$$A = R \cdot (1 - T) - W$$

where A represents the addiction level, R is the reward experience, T is the tolerance factor, and W is the withdrawal factor. As tolerance increases and withdrawal symptoms become more pronounced, the overall addiction level may rise, leading to a more compulsive engagement in the behavior.

The Role of Dopamine in Fisting Addiction

In the context of fisting, the intense physical sensations and emotional connections can lead to substantial dopamine release. For some individuals, this can create a feedback loop where the desire for the pleasurable experience of fisting becomes increasingly strong. Factors that may contribute to the development of fisting addiction include:

- **Psychological Vulnerability**: Individuals with a history of trauma, anxiety, or depression may be more susceptible to developing compulsive sexual behaviors as a coping mechanism. - **Social Isolation**: Those who feel disconnected from others may turn to fisting as a means of seeking intimacy and connection, further reinforcing the behavior. - **Cultural Influences**: Societal attitudes towards sex and pleasure can shape an individual's relationship with their sexual behaviors, potentially leading to feelings of shame or guilt that complicate their engagement with fisting.

Examples of Dopamine-Driven Behavior in Fisting

Consider the following scenarios that illustrate the role of dopamine in fisting addiction:
 1. **The First Experience**: An individual engages in fisting for the first time, experiencing an overwhelming sense of pleasure and intimacy. The significant release of dopamine creates a strong positive association with the act, leading them to seek it out again. 2. **Escalation of Behavior**: After several experiences, the individual finds that they require more intense stimulation to achieve the same level of pleasure. They begin experimenting with more extreme forms of fisting or incorporating additional elements, such as BDSM, to enhance the experience. 3. **Withdrawal Symptoms**: If the individual attempts to take a break from fisting, they may experience cravings, anxiety, or irritability, prompting them to return to the behavior to alleviate these feelings.

Addressing Dopamine-Related Issues in Fisting

Recognizing the role of dopamine in addiction is crucial for individuals who may be struggling with compulsive fisting behaviors. Strategies for addressing dopamine-related issues include:
 - **Mindful Engagement**: Practicing mindfulness during sexual experiences can help individuals remain present and aware of their motivations, reducing the likelihood of compulsive behavior. - **Setting Boundaries**: Establishing clear boundaries and limits around fisting can help individuals maintain control over their sexual behaviors and prevent escalation. - **Seeking Support**: Engaging with supportive communities, therapists, or support groups can provide individuals with the tools and resources necessary to navigate their relationship with fisting and address any underlying psychological issues.

In conclusion, understanding the role of dopamine in addiction provides valuable insights into the complexities of fisting as a sexual practice. By recognizing the potential for compulsive behavior and implementing strategies to manage it, individuals can engage with fisting in a healthier, more balanced way.

Seeking Professional Help for Fisting Addiction

Fisting, as an intimate and intense sexual practice, can be a source of pleasure and exploration for many. However, for some individuals, the pursuit of fisting can lead to problematic behaviors that may resemble addiction. Recognizing when fisting has transitioned from a consensual and enjoyable activity to a compulsive behavior requiring professional intervention is crucial for maintaining healthy sexual relationships and personal well-being.

Understanding Fisting Addiction

Fisting addiction can be conceptualized through the lens of behavioral addiction theory, which posits that certain behaviors can become compulsive and interfere with an individual's daily life, similar to substance addiction. The Diagnostic and Statistical Manual of Mental Disorders (DSM-5) outlines criteria for diagnosing substance use disorders, which can also be adapted to understand behavioral addictions. Key criteria include:

- **Loss of Control:** Difficulty in reducing or controlling the behavior despite a desire to do so.

- **Preoccupation:** Constantly thinking about fisting or planning to engage in it, often to the detriment of other responsibilities.

- **Escalation:** Needing to engage in fisting more frequently or in more extreme ways to achieve the same level of satisfaction.

- **Negative Consequences:** Experiencing adverse effects on physical health, emotional well-being, or relationships due to fisting.

- **Withdrawal Symptoms:** Feeling anxious, irritable, or distressed when unable to engage in fisting.

Identifying the Problem

Individuals struggling with fisting addiction may encounter a range of problems, including:

- **Physical Health Issues:** Repeated engagement in fisting without proper safety measures can lead to injuries, infections, or long-term damage to the body. This can create a cycle of shame and secrecy, further entrenching the addiction.

- **Emotional Distress:** Feelings of guilt, shame, or anxiety may arise from engaging in fisting, especially if it conflicts with personal values or societal norms.

- **Relationship Strain:** Fisting addiction can lead to neglect of partner needs, decreased intimacy, and conflict within relationships. Partners may feel inadequate or pressured to participate in fisting, leading to resentment.

- **Social Isolation:** Individuals may withdraw from social activities or relationships to prioritize fisting, resulting in loneliness and disconnection from supportive networks.

Seeking Professional Help

If you or someone you know is experiencing signs of fisting addiction, seeking professional help is a vital step toward recovery. Here are some recommended avenues for support:

- **Therapists Specializing in Sexual Health:** Finding a therapist with expertise in sexual addiction or compulsive sexual behaviors can provide a safe space to explore underlying issues, such as trauma, anxiety, or relationship dynamics. Cognitive Behavioral Therapy (CBT) may be particularly effective in addressing harmful thought patterns and behaviors.

- **Support Groups:** Engaging with peer support groups, either in-person or online, can foster a sense of community and understanding. Groups like Sex Addicts Anonymous (SAA) provide a 12-step framework that encourages accountability and recovery.

- **Sex Therapy:** Working with a certified sex therapist can help individuals navigate their sexual desires and behaviors in a healthy way. Therapy can focus on enhancing communication skills, exploring intimacy, and developing a balanced sexual repertoire.

- **Medical Professionals:** Consulting with a healthcare provider can help address any physical health concerns related to fisting addiction. Regular check-ups, STI testing, and discussions about safe practices are essential components of holistic care.

Case Examples

Consider the following scenarios illustrating the need for professional help:

- **Case Study 1:** Jamie, a 30-year-old individual, finds that their desire for fisting has escalated to the point where they are neglecting work responsibilities and personal relationships. Despite feeling guilty about the impact on their life, Jamie continues to seek out fisting experiences, leading to emotional distress. After a particularly damaging encounter, Jamie decides to seek therapy to address their compulsive behavior and explore the underlying issues contributing to their addiction.

+ **Case Study 2:** Alex, a 45-year-old partner in a committed relationship, begins to prioritize fisting over intimacy with their partner. As a result, their relationship suffers, and their partner feels neglected and unfulfilled. Alex recognizes the strain their fisting habits are placing on their relationship and seeks the help of a sex therapist to rebuild intimacy and address their compulsive behaviors.

Conclusion

Seeking professional help for fisting addiction is a courageous step towards healing and self-discovery. By addressing the physical, emotional, and relational aspects of the addiction, individuals can reclaim their sexual health and well-being. Remember that recovery is a journey, and support is available at every stage. Embracing vulnerability and seeking help can lead to profound personal growth and healthier relationships.

Overcoming Shame and Seeking Support

Shame is a powerful and often debilitating emotion that can arise in the context of sexual exploration, particularly with practices that society may deem taboo, such as fisting. Understanding the nature of shame, its origins, and how to overcome it is essential for anyone engaging in this practice. This section will explore the theoretical underpinnings of shame, the problems it creates, and practical strategies for seeking support.

Understanding Shame

Shame can be defined as a painful feeling regarding oneself, often stemming from the perception that one has violated social norms or expectations. According to Brené Brown, a leading researcher on shame, it is an emotion that arises when individuals feel they are not living up to their own standards or the standards imposed by society. This feeling can lead to isolation, fear of vulnerability, and a reluctance to seek help or share experiences.

In the context of fisting, individuals may experience shame due to societal stigma, misconceptions about sexual practices, or personal beliefs about sexuality. This shame can inhibit open communication with partners and create barriers to exploring one's desires fully.

Theoretical Perspectives on Shame

Several psychological theories provide insight into the nature of shame and its impact on behavior:

- **Attachment Theory:** According to attachment theory, individuals who have insecure attachment styles may be more prone to feelings of shame. Those with anxious attachment may fear rejection, while those with avoidant attachment may struggle to connect with others, leading to shame in expressing their sexual desires.

- **Cognitive Behavioral Theory:** This theory posits that negative thought patterns contribute to feelings of shame. For example, an individual may believe that their desire for fisting is abnormal, leading to feelings of guilt and shame. Challenging these cognitive distortions can help alleviate shame.

- **Social Learning Theory:** This theory suggests that individuals learn behaviors and feelings through observation and interaction with others. If a person grows up in an environment where sexual exploration is stigmatized, they may internalize these beliefs and feel shame about their desires.

Problems Associated with Shame

The problems associated with shame can be profound and multifaceted:

- **Isolation:** Shame often leads to a desire to hide or withdraw from others. This isolation can prevent individuals from finding supportive communities or partners who share similar interests.

- **Mental Health Issues:** Persistent feelings of shame can contribute to anxiety, depression, and low self-esteem. Individuals may struggle with self-acceptance, leading to a negative cycle of shame and mental health challenges.

- **Impaired Communication:** Shame can hinder open communication about desires and boundaries with partners. This lack of communication can lead to misunderstandings, unmet needs, and potential harm during sexual exploration.

- **Avoidance of Desires:** Individuals may avoid exploring their sexual desires altogether due to fear of shame. This avoidance can lead to feelings of frustration and unfulfillment in their sexual lives.

Strategies for Overcoming Shame

Overcoming shame requires intentional effort and support. Here are several strategies that individuals can employ:

- **Education and Awareness:** Understanding that fisting, like any sexual practice, is a consensual choice made by individuals can help normalize the experience. Educating oneself about the practice and its safety can empower individuals to embrace their desires without shame.

- **Seeking Community Support:** Finding a supportive community, whether online or in-person, can provide a safe space for individuals to share experiences and feelings. Connecting with others who have similar interests can help combat feelings of isolation and shame.

- **Therapy and Counseling:** Engaging with a mental health professional can provide a space to explore feelings of shame. Therapists can help individuals unpack their beliefs about sexuality and develop healthier perspectives.

- **Practicing Self-Compassion:** Developing self-compassion involves treating oneself with kindness and understanding rather than judgment. Individuals can practice self-compassion by acknowledging their feelings of shame without allowing them to define their worth.

- **Open Communication:** Encouraging open dialogue with partners about desires, boundaries, and feelings can help alleviate shame. Establishing a safe environment for discussion can foster intimacy and connection.

- **Journaling and Reflection:** Writing about feelings of shame can be a powerful tool for processing emotions. Journaling can help individuals identify triggers and patterns related to shame, allowing for deeper self-reflection and growth.

Examples of Seeking Support

Here are a few examples of how individuals can seek support in overcoming shame:

- **Peer Support Groups:** Joining or forming a peer support group focused on sexual exploration can create a safe space to discuss experiences and feelings. Participants can share stories and strategies for overcoming shame together.

- **Workshops and Retreats:** Attending workshops that focus on sexual empowerment and exploration can provide education and community. These events often foster an environment of acceptance and understanding.

- **Online Forums and Communities:** Engaging in online platforms dedicated to sexual exploration can provide anonymity and support. Individuals can share experiences, ask questions, and connect with others without fear of judgment.

- **Therapeutic Groups:** Some therapists offer group therapy sessions focused on sexual issues. These sessions can provide a supportive environment for individuals to share their experiences and learn from others.

In conclusion, overcoming shame is a critical step in embracing one's sexual desires and exploring practices like fisting. By understanding the nature of shame, seeking support, and employing practical strategies, individuals can foster a healthier relationship with their sexuality. This journey not only enhances personal satisfaction but also strengthens connections with partners, ultimately leading to a more fulfilling sexual experience.

Developing Healthy Coping Mechanisms

The journey of exploring fisting, like any other sexual practice, can evoke a spectrum of emotions and experiences. While many individuals find empowerment and pleasure in fisting, some may also grapple with feelings of shame, anxiety, or addiction. Developing healthy coping mechanisms is crucial for ensuring a balanced approach to this intimate practice. This section will discuss various strategies to cultivate resilience and emotional well-being while navigating the complexities of fisting.

Understanding Coping Mechanisms

Coping mechanisms are strategies that individuals use to manage stress, emotions, and the challenges of life. According to Lazarus and Folkman's (1984) transactional model of stress and coping, coping can be classified into two broad categories: problem-focused coping and emotion-focused coping.

$$\text{Problem-focused coping} = \text{Active efforts to solve the problem} \quad (71)$$

$$\text{Emotion-focused coping} = \text{Strategies to manage emotional distress} \quad (72)$$

In the context of fisting, individuals may experience stress or emotional turmoil related to societal stigma, personal fears, or negative experiences. By developing effective coping mechanisms, individuals can navigate these challenges more effectively.

Identifying Triggers

The first step in developing healthy coping mechanisms is identifying personal triggers related to fisting. Triggers can be external, such as negative comments from others, or internal, such as feelings of shame or anxiety. Keeping a journal to document thoughts and feelings surrounding fisting can help individuals recognize patterns and understand their emotional responses.

Implementing Healthy Coping Strategies

Once triggers are identified, individuals can implement various healthy coping strategies:

- **Mindfulness and Meditation:** Practicing mindfulness allows individuals to stay present and observe their thoughts and feelings without judgment. Techniques such as deep breathing, guided imagery, or progressive muscle relaxation can help ground individuals during moments of distress.

- **Physical Activity:** Engaging in regular physical exercise can enhance mood and reduce stress. Activities such as yoga, dancing, or even walking can help release endorphins, promoting a sense of well-being.

- **Creative Expression:** Art, writing, or other forms of creative expression can serve as an outlet for emotions. Engaging in creative activities can help individuals process their feelings surrounding fisting and transform negative emotions into something constructive.

- **Social Support:** Building a supportive network of friends, partners, or community members can provide emotional validation and encouragement. Sharing experiences with others who understand the complexities of fisting can foster a sense of belonging and reduce feelings of isolation.

- **Education and Awareness:** Educating oneself about fisting, including its risks, benefits, and techniques, can empower individuals and reduce anxiety. Knowledge can help demystify the practice and provide a sense of control over one's experiences.

- **Therapeutic Support:** Seeking professional help from a therapist or counselor can provide valuable insights and coping strategies. Therapists trained in sex therapy or trauma-informed care can assist individuals in navigating emotional challenges related to fisting.

Establishing Boundaries

Setting clear boundaries is essential in any sexual practice, particularly in fisting, where physical and emotional safety is paramount. Establishing boundaries can help individuals feel more secure and in control of their experiences.

$$\text{Boundaries} = \text{Personal limits that define acceptable behavior} \quad (73)$$

Communicating these boundaries with partners fosters mutual respect and understanding. It is important to revisit and adjust boundaries as needed, ensuring that they remain relevant to one's emotional and physical comfort.

Practicing Self-Compassion

Self-compassion involves treating oneself with kindness and understanding during difficult times. According to Neff (2003), self-compassion comprises three components: self-kindness, common humanity, and mindfulness.

$$\text{Self-compassion} = \text{Self-kindness} + \text{Common humanity} + \text{Mindfulness} \quad (74)$$

Practicing self-compassion can mitigate feelings of shame or guilt that may arise from exploring fisting. By recognizing that struggles are a shared human experience, individuals can foster a more positive self-image and develop resilience.

Seeking Balance

It is crucial to maintain a balanced relationship with fisting and other sexual practices. This balance involves recognizing when fisting becomes a source of distress rather than pleasure. Engaging in regular self-reflection can help individuals assess their motivations and feelings surrounding the practice.

$$\text{Balance} = \text{Healthy engagement in sexual practices} - \text{Negative consequences} \quad (75)$$

If fisting begins to interfere with daily life, relationships, or mental health, it may be necessary to reevaluate one's involvement and seek support.

Conclusion

Developing healthy coping mechanisms is a vital aspect of exploring fisting safely and responsibly. By identifying triggers, implementing effective strategies, establishing boundaries, practicing self-compassion, and seeking balance, individuals can cultivate resilience and emotional well-being. This holistic approach not only enhances the experience of fisting but also contributes to a more fulfilling and empowered sexual journey.

References:

- Lazarus, R. S., & Folkman, S. (1984). Stress, Appraisal, and Coping. Springer Publishing Company.

- Neff, K. D. (2003). Self-Compassion: An Alternative Conceptualization of a Healthy Attitude Toward Oneself. *Self and Identity*, 2(2), 85-101.

Self-Reflection and Introspection

Self-reflection and introspection are crucial components in understanding one's relationship with fisting, particularly when considering the potential for addiction. This section will delve into the significance of self-reflection, explore various introspective practices, and discuss how they can aid in recognizing patterns of behavior that may indicate unhealthy engagement with fisting.

The Importance of Self-Reflection

Self-reflection involves examining one's thoughts, feelings, and behaviors to gain deeper insights into oneself. It is a process that encourages individuals to think critically about their experiences, motivations, and the impacts of their actions. In the context of fisting, self-reflection can help individuals assess their desires, boundaries, and the emotional significance of their practices.

- **Understanding Motivations:** Engaging in self-reflection allows individuals to explore why they are drawn to fisting. Are they seeking pleasure, intimacy, or an escape from stress? Understanding these motivations can clarify whether their engagement is healthy or potentially problematic.

- **Identifying Patterns:** Reflecting on past experiences with fisting can reveal patterns of behavior. For example, do individuals often use fisting as a coping mechanism during times of emotional distress? Recognizing these patterns is the first step toward addressing any unhealthy reliance on the practice.

- **Assessing Emotional Responses:** Self-reflection encourages individuals to examine their emotional responses before, during, and after fisting. Are they experiencing joy and connection, or feelings of guilt and shame? This assessment can inform future decisions regarding their practices.

Introspective Practices

Several introspective practices can facilitate self-reflection, helping individuals to gain clarity about their relationship with fisting.

- **Journaling:** Writing about experiences, feelings, and thoughts related to fisting can provide a safe space for exploration. Journaling can help individuals articulate their desires, fears, and any conflicts they may face regarding their practices.

- **Meditation:** Mindfulness meditation encourages individuals to observe their thoughts and feelings without judgment. This practice can foster a deeper understanding of one's motivations and emotional responses to fisting, allowing for greater self-awareness.

- **Therapeutic Conversations:** Engaging in discussions with a therapist or trusted friend can provide external perspectives on one's relationship with fisting. These conversations can help individuals process their feelings and gain insights they may not have considered.

Recognizing Signs of Addiction

Through self-reflection and introspection, individuals can begin to identify signs of fisting addiction. Some common indicators include:

- **Compulsive Behavior:** Feeling compelled to engage in fisting despite negative consequences, such as physical pain or emotional distress.

- **Escalation:** Increasing the frequency or intensity of fisting sessions to achieve the same level of satisfaction or pleasure.

- **Neglecting Responsibilities:** Prioritizing fisting over personal, professional, or social responsibilities, leading to negative impacts in other areas of life.

- **Emotional Dependence:** Relying on fisting as the primary source of emotional relief or pleasure, rather than engaging in a variety of fulfilling activities.

Recognizing these signs is essential in determining whether one's relationship with fisting is healthy or if it may require intervention.

Developing Healthy Coping Mechanisms

If self-reflection reveals problematic patterns, it is crucial to develop healthier coping mechanisms. This can include:

- **Diversifying Interests:** Engaging in a variety of activities and hobbies can reduce reliance on fisting as a primary source of pleasure or emotional relief.

- **Establishing Boundaries:** Setting clear boundaries around fisting practices can help individuals maintain a healthy relationship with the activity. This might involve limiting frequency or ensuring that fisting is always consensual and safe.

- **Seeking Support:** Connecting with support groups or therapy can provide individuals with the tools they need to navigate their relationship with fisting in a healthier manner.

Conclusion

Self-reflection and introspection are invaluable tools for anyone engaging in fisting. By examining motivations, recognizing patterns, and developing healthy coping strategies, individuals can cultivate a more balanced and fulfilling relationship with this intimate practice. Ultimately, the goal is to embrace fisting as a source of pleasure and connection, rather than allowing it to become a source of distress or addiction. Through ongoing self-exploration, individuals can ensure that their experiences with fisting remain consensual, enjoyable, and aligned with their personal values and desires.

Therapy and Recovery for Fisting Addiction

Fisting addiction, like other forms of sexual addiction, can lead to significant distress and disruption in an individual's life. Understanding the nature of this addiction and exploring therapeutic avenues for recovery is crucial for those affected. This section will outline the therapeutic approaches, potential issues, and examples of recovery strategies relevant to fisting addiction.

Understanding Fisting Addiction

Fisting addiction can be characterized by compulsive engagement in fisting, despite negative consequences. This behavior may stem from various psychological, emotional, or social factors, including trauma, low self-esteem, or the pursuit of heightened sensations. The **Diagnostic and Statistical Manual of Mental Disorders (DSM-5)** classifies sexual addiction under the umbrella of compulsive sexual behavior, which can include fisting as a specific manifestation.

Theoretical Frameworks

Several theoretical frameworks can be applied to understand and address fisting addiction:

- **Cognitive Behavioral Therapy (CBT):** This approach focuses on identifying and modifying negative thought patterns that contribute to compulsive behavior. CBT helps individuals recognize triggers and develop healthier coping mechanisms.

- **Psychodynamic Therapy:** This method explores unconscious motivations and past experiences that may influence current behaviors. Understanding the root causes of addiction can facilitate healing and personal growth.

- **Humanistic Approaches:** Emphasizing self-acceptance and personal growth, humanistic therapy encourages individuals to explore their emotions and experiences without judgment. This can be particularly helpful in addressing shame and stigma associated with fisting addiction.

- **12-Step Programs:** Similar to Alcoholics Anonymous, these programs provide a supportive framework for individuals seeking recovery from sexual addiction. They emphasize accountability, community support, and personal reflection.

Common Problems Encountered in Recovery

Recovering from fisting addiction may present several challenges, including:

- **Shame and Stigma:** Many individuals may feel ashamed of their addiction, which can hinder their willingness to seek help. The societal stigma surrounding non-normative sexual practices can exacerbate feelings of isolation.

- **Relapse Triggers:** Individuals may encounter situations or emotional states that trigger the urge to engage in fisting, making it essential to develop effective coping strategies.

- **Interpersonal Relationships:** Recovery can strain existing relationships, especially if partners are not supportive or understanding of the recovery process. Open communication is vital for navigating these challenges.

- **Emotional Regulation:** Individuals may struggle with managing emotions that arise during recovery, such as anxiety, depression, or anger. Developing emotional regulation skills is crucial for long-term success.

Therapeutic Strategies for Recovery

Effective recovery from fisting addiction often involves a combination of therapeutic strategies:

- **Individual Therapy:** Engaging in one-on-one therapy allows individuals to explore their thoughts and feelings in a safe environment. This personalized approach can help address specific issues related to fisting addiction.

- **Group Therapy:** Participating in group therapy provides a sense of community and shared experience. Hearing others' stories can foster connection and reduce feelings of isolation.

- **Mindfulness and Relaxation Techniques:** Practicing mindfulness can help individuals become more aware of their thoughts and feelings without judgment. Techniques such as meditation, deep breathing, and progressive muscle relaxation can reduce anxiety and improve emotional regulation.

- **Journaling and Self-Reflection:** Keeping a journal can facilitate self-exploration and help individuals identify patterns in their behavior. Reflecting on triggers, emotions, and experiences can enhance self-awareness and promote healing.

- **Support Networks:** Building a network of supportive friends, family, or peers can provide encouragement during the recovery process. Engaging with others who understand the challenges of fisting addiction can be particularly beneficial.

Case Studies and Examples

To illustrate the therapeutic process, consider the following hypothetical case studies:

- **Case Study 1: John** is a 32-year-old man who has struggled with fisting addiction for several years. After experiencing significant relationship issues, he sought therapy. Through CBT, John identified negative thought patterns that fueled his addiction. He learned to challenge these thoughts and replace them with healthier beliefs. Additionally, he participated in a support group, which helped him feel less isolated and more understood.

- **Case Study 2: Sarah** is a 28-year-old woman who felt shame about her fisting practices. In therapy, she explored her past experiences of trauma that contributed to her compulsive behaviors. Through psychodynamic therapy, Sarah began to process her emotions and develop healthier coping strategies. She also engaged in mindfulness practices, which helped her manage anxiety and improve her emotional regulation.

Conclusion

Therapy and recovery for fisting addiction require a compassionate and multifaceted approach. By utilizing various therapeutic frameworks and strategies, individuals can navigate their recovery journeys with greater understanding and support. It is essential to recognize that recovery is a process, and seeking help is a courageous step toward healing and self-acceptance. With the right resources and support, individuals can reclaim their agency and develop a healthier relationship with their sexuality.

Peer Support and Group Therapy for Fisters

Peer support and group therapy can play a vital role in the journey of individuals exploring fisting as part of their sexual expression. This section delves into the significance of these support systems, the theoretical frameworks that underpin them, the challenges individuals may face, and practical examples of how these groups can foster a healthy and affirming environment.

The Importance of Peer Support

Peer support refers to the emotional and practical assistance provided by individuals who share similar experiences or challenges. In the context of fisting, peer support can help individuals feel less isolated, validate their experiences, and provide a safe space for sharing concerns and triumphs. This sense of community can significantly enhance an individual's confidence and willingness to explore their desires.

Theoretical Frameworks The concept of peer support is rooted in several psychological theories, including:

- **Social Learning Theory:** Proposed by Albert Bandura, this theory emphasizes the importance of observing and modeling behaviors, attitudes, and emotional reactions of others. In peer support groups, members can learn from each other's experiences, gaining insights into safe practices and emotional management.

- **Cognitive Behavioral Theory (CBT):** This framework posits that thoughts, feelings, and behaviors are interconnected. Group therapy can help individuals identify and challenge negative beliefs about fisting, fostering healthier attitudes and reducing feelings of shame or anxiety.

- **Humanistic Psychology:** Emphasizing personal growth and self-actualization, this approach underlines the importance of empathy, unconditional positive regard, and authenticity in relationships. Peer support groups can provide a nurturing environment where individuals feel accepted and valued for who they are.

Common Challenges Faced by Fisters

While peer support and group therapy can be beneficial, individuals exploring fisting may encounter several challenges, including:

- **Shame and Stigma:** Many individuals may feel shame about their desires due to societal taboos surrounding fisting. This can lead to reluctance in seeking support or sharing experiences.

- **Fear of Judgment:** Participants may fear being judged by peers for their interests or experiences, which can inhibit open communication and sharing.

- **Emotional Triggers:** Discussing personal experiences related to fisting can sometimes evoke strong emotional responses, particularly for those with a history of trauma or negative sexual experiences.

- **Varying Levels of Experience:** In a diverse group, individuals may have different levels of experience with fisting, leading to potential feelings of inadequacy or competition.

Examples of Peer Support and Group Therapy Models

Several models of peer support and group therapy can be effective for individuals exploring fisting:

1. Support Groups Support groups specifically focused on fisting can provide a safe space for individuals to share their experiences, challenges, and successes. These groups often follow a structured format, allowing for guided discussions while ensuring that all participants feel heard and respected.

2. Online Communities With the advent of technology, many individuals have found solace in online forums and social media groups dedicated to fisting. These virtual spaces can provide anonymity and accessibility, allowing individuals to seek advice, share resources, and connect with others without the pressure of face-to-face interactions.

3. Workshops and Retreats Workshops and retreats focused on fisting can offer both educational and experiential learning opportunities. Participants can engage in discussions about safety, techniques, and emotional aspects of fisting while also participating in guided practices that reinforce community and connection.

4. **Therapy Groups** Facilitated by trained therapists, therapy groups can provide a deeper exploration of the emotional and psychological aspects of fisting. These groups can integrate therapeutic techniques, such as mindfulness and cognitive restructuring, to help participants process their experiences and feelings in a supportive environment.

Building a Supportive Environment

Creating a supportive environment within peer support and therapy groups is crucial for fostering trust and open communication. Consider the following strategies:

- **Establish Ground Rules:** Setting clear guidelines for confidentiality, respect, and non-judgment can help create a safe space for sharing.
- **Encourage Active Listening:** Promote active listening techniques, where participants focus on understanding and validating each other's experiences without interruption or judgment.
- **Facilitate Inclusivity:** Ensure that the group welcomes diverse experiences and identities, fostering a sense of belonging for all participants.
- **Provide Resources:** Share educational materials and resources related to fisting, safety practices, and emotional well-being to empower group members.

Conclusion

Peer support and group therapy can significantly enhance the fisting experience by providing a sense of community, reducing feelings of isolation, and fostering emotional well-being. By understanding the challenges faced by individuals exploring fisting and implementing supportive practices, these groups can create an affirming environment that encourages exploration, connection, and personal growth. As individuals navigate their fisting journeys, the power of shared experiences and mutual support can lead to profound transformations and a deeper understanding of oneself and one's desires.

Harm Reduction Strategies for Fisting Addiction

Fisting, while a deeply intimate and pleasurable practice for many, can become problematic when it transitions into a compulsive behavior or addiction. Harm reduction strategies aim to minimize the negative consequences associated with this behavior while respecting the autonomy and choices of individuals. This section outlines various harm reduction strategies tailored specifically for those who may find themselves struggling with fisting addiction.

Understanding Fisting Addiction

Fisting addiction can be conceptualized through the lens of behavioral addiction theory. Behavioral addictions share similarities with substance addictions, where individuals may engage in compulsive behaviors despite adverse consequences. The cycle of addiction often includes:

- **Bingeing:** Engaging in fisting sessions excessively or beyond previously established limits.

- **Withdrawal Symptoms:** Experiencing anxiety, irritability, or discomfort when unable to engage in fisting.

- **Loss of Control:** Inability to stop or moderate fisting behaviors even when desired.

- **Consequences:** Suffering from physical injuries, emotional distress, or relationship issues due to excessive fisting.

Recognizing these patterns is the first step in applying harm reduction strategies.

Developing Healthy Coping Mechanisms

A critical aspect of harm reduction is to encourage the development of healthy coping mechanisms that can replace the compulsive behavior associated with fisting. Some strategies include:

- **Mindfulness and Meditation:** Practicing mindfulness can help individuals become more aware of their urges and emotional states. Techniques such as deep breathing or guided meditation can assist in managing cravings.

- **Physical Activity:** Engaging in regular exercise can serve as a healthy outlet for stress and anxiety, reducing the compulsion to turn to fisting as a coping mechanism.

- **Creative Expression:** Exploring creative outlets such as writing, art, or music can provide an alternative means of self-expression and emotional release.

RECOGNIZING AND ADDRESSING FISTING ADDICTION

Setting Boundaries and Limits

Establishing clear boundaries and limits is essential in managing fisting practices. This can involve:

- **Defining Frequency and Duration:** Create a schedule for fisting sessions, limiting the frequency and duration to prevent excessive indulgence.

- **Implementing Safe Words:** Use safe words or signals to communicate discomfort or the need to pause during fisting, reinforcing the importance of consent and mutual respect.

- **Engaging in Other Intimacy Practices:** Diversifying sexual experiences by incorporating other forms of intimacy can help reduce the focus on fisting as the primary source of pleasure.

Seeking Support and Community

Building a support network can significantly aid in the journey toward managing fisting addiction. Strategies include:

- **Peer Support Groups:** Joining or forming groups where individuals can share experiences and coping strategies can foster a sense of community and accountability.

- **Professional Guidance:** Seeking therapy from a mental health professional specializing in sexual health or addiction can provide personalized strategies for overcoming compulsive behaviors.

- **Online Forums and Resources:** Engaging with online communities focused on harm reduction can offer additional support and resources for individuals navigating fisting addiction.

Educating Yourself and Others

Knowledge is a powerful tool in harm reduction. Individuals should strive to educate themselves about the potential risks associated with fisting and the signs of addiction. This can involve:

- **Reading Literature:** Exploring books, articles, and research studies that discuss fisting, addiction, and harm reduction strategies can provide valuable insights.

- **Participating in Workshops:** Attending workshops or seminars focused on sexual health and addiction can enhance understanding and provide practical skills for managing behaviors.

- **Sharing Knowledge:** Engaging in discussions with partners or friends about the risks and benefits of fisting can promote a culture of informed consent and safety.

Monitoring Progress and Reflecting on Experiences

Regular self-reflection and monitoring of one's behaviors can help identify patterns and triggers associated with fisting addiction. This can be done through:

- **Journaling:** Keeping a journal to document feelings, experiences, and behaviors related to fisting can provide insight into emotional triggers and patterns of use.

- **Setting Goals:** Establishing short-term and long-term goals related to fisting practices can help individuals stay focused on their journey toward healthier behaviors.

- **Evaluating Relationships:** Assessing the impact of fisting on personal relationships can guide individuals in making necessary adjustments to their practices and boundaries.

Conclusion

Harm reduction strategies for fisting addiction emphasize the importance of personal agency, informed consent, and the development of healthy coping mechanisms. By understanding the dynamics of addiction, setting clear boundaries, seeking support, and educating oneself, individuals can navigate their fisting practices in a way that prioritizes safety, pleasure, and emotional well-being. Ultimately, the goal is to foster a relationship with fisting that is consensual, empowering, and aligned with one's values and desires.

Cultivating a Balanced Relationship with Fisting

Cultivating a balanced relationship with fisting involves understanding the dynamics of pleasure, desire, and emotional well-being. It is essential to recognize that while fisting can be a fulfilling and liberating sexual expression, it can also pose challenges if not approached with mindfulness and self-awareness. This section will explore the theoretical frameworks, potential problems, and practical strategies for maintaining a healthy relationship with fisting.

Understanding Balance in Sexual Practices

In the realm of sexual practices, balance refers to the ability to engage in activities that enhance pleasure without compromising emotional or physical well-being. As with any sexual practice, fisting can be approached in a way that is empowering, fulfilling, and safe. The concept of balance can be understood through the lens of the **Dual Control Model** of sexual response, which posits that sexual excitement is influenced by both sexual excitation and inhibition mechanisms [?].

$$\text{Sexual Response} = \text{Excitation} - \text{Inhibition} \tag{76}$$

In the context of fisting, it is crucial to cultivate both excitation (the pleasure derived from the act) and inhibition (the awareness of potential risks and limits). A healthy balance allows individuals to explore their desires while being cognizant of their emotional and physical boundaries.

Identifying Potential Problems

While fisting can be a source of pleasure, it is important to identify potential problems that may arise when engaging in this practice. These include:

- **Physical Risks:** Engaging in fisting without proper preparation or communication can lead to physical injuries such as tearing, bruising, or internal damage.

- **Emotional Risks:** Fisting can evoke intense emotions, and if not handled properly, it may lead to feelings of shame, guilt, or anxiety, particularly for those who struggle with body image or past trauma.

- **Addiction:** Some individuals may develop an unhealthy fixation on fisting, using it as a coping mechanism for deeper emotional issues, leading to a cycle of compulsive behavior.

- **Relationship Strain:** If partners have differing levels of interest or comfort with fisting, it can create tension and misunderstandings within the relationship.

Recognizing these potential problems is the first step toward cultivating a balanced relationship with fisting.

Strategies for Cultivating Balance

To foster a balanced relationship with fisting, consider the following strategies:

1. Self-Reflection and Awareness   Engage in regular self-reflection to assess your motivations for fisting. Ask yourself questions such as:

- What do I seek from this experience?
- How does fisting make me feel emotionally and physically?
- Am I using fisting to escape from other issues in my life?

Being honest with yourself can help you maintain a healthy perspective on fisting.

2. Open Communication with Partners   Establishing open lines of communication with partners is essential. Discuss your desires, boundaries, and any concerns you may have regarding fisting. Use tools such as **active listening** and **nonviolent communication** to foster understanding and connection. For instance, the use of "I" statements can help express feelings without placing blame, such as "I feel anxious when I think about fisting without proper preparation."

3. Setting Boundaries and Limits   Clearly define your boundaries and limits regarding fisting. This includes discussing safe words, physical limits, and emotional triggers. Boundaries should be revisited and renegotiated as relationships evolve and as individuals grow in their comfort levels.

4. Incorporating Aftercare Practices   Aftercare is an essential component of any intense sexual experience, especially in practices like fisting. Engaging in aftercare can help partners reconnect emotionally and physically after a scene. This may include cuddling, discussing the experience, or simply spending quiet time together.

5. Seeking Professional Guidance   If you find that your relationship with fisting is causing distress or dysfunction, consider seeking guidance from a therapist or counselor who specializes in sexual health or intimacy issues. Professional support can provide valuable insights and coping strategies tailored to your individual needs.

6. **Exploring Alternative Practices** To maintain balance, consider exploring other forms of intimacy and sexual expression alongside fisting. This can help diversify your sexual experiences and prevent fixation on a single practice. Engaging in different forms of touch, communication, or erotic play can enhance overall satisfaction and connection.

7. **Engaging in Community and Peer Support** Finding a community of like-minded individuals can provide support and validation. Engage in discussions, workshops, or peer support groups focused on fisting and sexual health. Sharing experiences and learning from others can foster a sense of belonging and understanding.

Conclusion

Cultivating a balanced relationship with fisting requires ongoing self-awareness, communication, and a commitment to safety and emotional well-being. By recognizing potential problems and implementing strategies to maintain balance, individuals can enjoy the pleasures of fisting while fostering a healthy and fulfilling sexual identity. Remember, the journey of exploration is as important as the destination, and embracing a holistic approach to fisting can lead to deeper connections and personal growth.

Conclusion and Future of Fisting

Conclusion and Future of Fisting

Conclusion and Future of Fisting

As we conclude our exploration of fisting, it is essential to reflect on the journey that has brought us here, the knowledge we have gained, and the future possibilities that lie ahead. Fisting, often regarded as one of the most intimate and taboo practices within the spectrum of sexual expression, has emerged from the shadows of stigma and misunderstanding into a realm of acceptance, education, and empowerment. This section aims to encapsulate the insights we've gathered and to envision a future where fisting is practiced safely, consensually, and joyfully.

Reflection and Integration

The act of fisting is not merely a physical endeavor; it is an intricate dance of trust, vulnerability, and connection between partners. Throughout this guide, we have examined the multifaceted nature of fisting, delving into its technical aspects, safety considerations, emotional implications, and the profound intimacy it can foster. This holistic understanding allows practitioners to approach fisting with a sense of reverence and mindfulness, transforming it from a mere act into a profound expression of love and exploration.

One of the key takeaways from our exploration is the importance of communication and consent. As highlighted in Section 2.4, establishing clear boundaries and engaging in open dialogue about desires, limits, and fears is paramount. This foundation of trust not only enhances the experience but also mitigates the risks associated with such an intimate act. Practitioners are encouraged to continuously engage in conversations about their experiences, fostering an environment where both partners feel safe to express their needs and concerns.

Celebrating Personal Growth and Exploration

Fisting can serve as a powerful catalyst for personal growth and self-discovery. Engaging in this practice often invites individuals to confront and dismantle societal taboos, challenging their own preconceptions about pleasure, pain, and intimacy. This journey of exploration is not solely about the physical act itself; it is also about embracing one's desires and reclaiming agency over one's body.

For many, fisting can be a pathway to understanding their bodies more intimately, leading to heightened body awareness and acceptance. As discussed in Section 1.3.6, addressing body image and shame is crucial in this process. By embracing the diversity of bodies and experiences, individuals can cultivate a sense of empowerment that transcends the bedroom, positively impacting their overall self-esteem and relationships.

Consensual Fisting as an Act of Radical Self-Love

At its core, consensual fisting embodies the principles of radical self-love and acceptance. It challenges the societal norms that often dictate how we should experience pleasure and intimacy. By engaging in fisting, individuals are not only affirming their desires but also embracing their bodies in all their complexity. This act of self-love can be transformative, fostering a deeper connection to oneself and to one's partners.

The future of fisting lies in its ability to be integrated into a well-rounded sexual repertoire. As more individuals and communities embrace the practice, the normalization of fisting can contribute to a broader understanding of sexual diversity. This shift can lead to the dismantling of stigma and discrimination, paving the way for more inclusive conversations about pleasure and intimacy.

Embracing Fister Identity and Community

As we look ahead, it is essential to acknowledge the growing community of fisters who are actively engaging in dialogues about their experiences. This community serves as a vital support network, providing resources, education, and a sense of belonging. By fostering connections within this community, individuals can share their journeys, learn from one another, and celebrate the diversity of experiences that fisting encompasses.

The emergence of online platforms, workshops, and events dedicated to fisting has created spaces for education and empowerment. These resources not only facilitate skill-building and safety practices but also encourage individuals to explore their desires in a supportive environment. As we continue to advocate for the destigmatization of fisting, it is crucial to promote these safe spaces where individuals can learn, grow, and connect.

Adventures in Fisting Beyond the Book

The exploration of fisting does not end with this guide; rather, it is an invitation to embark on a lifelong journey of discovery. Each experience is unique, and individuals are encouraged to continue exploring their desires, experimenting with techniques, and integrating fisting into their intimate lives. This ongoing journey may involve attending workshops, participating in community events, or engaging in discussions with fellow fisters.

Moreover, as the landscape of sexual exploration continues to evolve, it is essential to remain open to new ideas and perspectives. The future of fisting may involve the incorporation of emerging practices, technologies, and understandings of intimacy. By remaining curious and engaged, individuals can contribute to the ongoing evolution of fisting as a practice that celebrates pleasure, connection, and empowerment.

Incorporating Fisting into a Well-Rounded Sexual Repertoire

Fisting can be a valuable addition to a well-rounded sexual repertoire, complementing other forms of intimacy and pleasure. By embracing a diverse range of sexual practices, individuals can enhance their understanding of their own bodies and those of their partners. This holistic approach to sexuality encourages exploration and experimentation, fostering a deeper connection to oneself and to others.

As individuals incorporate fisting into their sexual experiences, it is essential to prioritize safety, consent, and communication. By maintaining an open dialogue about desires and boundaries, practitioners can create an environment that fosters trust and respect, allowing for deeper exploration and connection.

The Role of Fisting in Body Positivity and Self-Acceptance

In a world that often promotes unrealistic body standards, fisting can serve as a powerful tool for body positivity and self-acceptance. Engaging in this practice encourages individuals to embrace their bodies in all their forms, celebrating the diversity of human anatomy. This celebration of bodies can lead to a broader understanding of beauty and desirability, challenging societal norms that often dictate how we should view ourselves and others.

By fostering a culture of body positivity within the fisting community, individuals can empower one another to embrace their desires and experiences without shame. This shift can contribute to a more inclusive and accepting society, where all bodies are celebrated and valued.

Advocacy and Destigmatization Efforts

As we envision the future of fisting, advocacy and destigmatization efforts will play a crucial role. By challenging societal norms and misconceptions surrounding fisting, individuals can contribute to a culture that embraces sexual diversity and promotes informed consent. This advocacy can take many forms, from engaging in conversations about fisting to participating in community events that celebrate sexual expression.

Moreover, as we continue to educate ourselves and others about fisting, we can work towards creating a more inclusive society that recognizes the validity of diverse sexual practices. This shift can lead to greater acceptance and understanding, allowing individuals to explore their desires without fear of judgment or stigma.

Engaging in Ongoing Education and Learning

The journey of exploration and understanding does not end here; it is an ongoing process of education and learning. As we continue to engage with the fisting community and seek out new resources, we can deepen our understanding of this practice and its implications. This commitment to ongoing education allows individuals to stay informed about safety practices, emerging techniques, and evolving perspectives on intimacy.

By fostering a culture of learning and curiosity, we can contribute to a more informed and empowered community of fisters. This collective knowledge can enhance our experiences, allowing us to navigate the complexities of fisting with confidence and care.

Nurturing Fisting Relationships and Connections

Finally, as we conclude this guide, it is essential to emphasize the importance of nurturing relationships and connections within the fisting community. By fostering open communication, trust, and support, individuals can create a network of relationships that enrich their experiences and promote personal growth.

Engaging in discussions, sharing experiences, and supporting one another can strengthen the bonds within the fisting community, allowing for deeper connections and understanding. This sense of community can be a source of strength and empowerment, encouraging individuals to embrace their desires and explore their identities without fear.

The End is Just the Beginning: Embracing a Lifelong Journey of Fisting Exploration

In conclusion, the journey of fisting is not merely a destination but a lifelong exploration of pleasure, intimacy, and self-discovery. As we embrace the future of fisting, let us celebrate the diversity of experiences, foster connections within our communities, and advocate for acceptance and understanding. Each encounter, each exploration, and each connection contributes to the rich tapestry of our sexual lives, inviting us to delve deeper into the realms of intimacy and connection.

As we move forward, may we continue to approach fisting with curiosity, compassion, and a commitment to safety and consent. The future is bright for fisting, and together, we can create a world where this intimate practice is celebrated and embraced as a valid expression of love and connection.

Reflection and Integration

Celebrating Personal Growth and Exploration

The journey of exploring fisting, like any other form of sexual expression, is deeply intertwined with personal growth and self-discovery. Engaging in this intimate practice can lead to profound transformations in how individuals perceive their bodies, their desires, and their relationships with others. This section aims to highlight the importance of celebrating personal growth and exploration within the context of fisting, emphasizing the emotional, psychological, and relational benefits that can emerge from this experience.

The Journey of Self-Discovery

At its core, fisting can serve as a powerful tool for self-exploration. The act itself requires a deep level of trust, communication, and vulnerability, which can facilitate a journey of self-discovery. As individuals navigate their desires and boundaries, they may uncover aspects of their sexuality that were previously unexplored. This exploration can lead to increased self-awareness, allowing individuals to embrace their unique sexual identities.

$$\text{Self-Discovery} = f(\text{Exploration}, \text{Communication}, \text{Trust}) \quad (77)$$

Where: - Self-Discovery represents the growth in understanding one's sexual identity. - Exploration refers to the willingness to engage in new experiences. - Communication signifies the dialogue between partners about desires and boundaries. - Trust reflects the emotional safety established in the relationship.

Through this equation, we can see that personal growth is a function of several interrelated components. As individuals engage in fisting, they may find themselves more comfortable expressing their needs and desires, leading to a more fulfilling sexual experience.

Overcoming Shame and Fear

One of the most significant barriers to sexual exploration is the pervasive presence of shame and fear. Societal taboos surrounding fisting can create a sense of stigma, leading individuals to internalize negative beliefs about their desires. Engaging in fisting can help challenge these beliefs, allowing individuals to confront and overcome their fears.

$$\text{Empowerment} = \frac{\text{Overcoming Shame}}{\text{Fear}} \quad (78)$$

This equation illustrates that empowerment grows as individuals work through their shame while managing their fears. The act of embracing fisting can serve as a liberating experience, enabling individuals to reclaim their sexuality and dismantle the barriers that have held them back.

Building Intimacy and Connection

Fisting is not merely a physical act; it is an intimate experience that fosters connection between partners. The level of trust required for fisting can deepen emotional bonds, allowing partners to share vulnerabilities and create a safe space for exploration. This intimacy can enhance relationships, leading to greater satisfaction and fulfillment.

$$\text{Intimacy} = \text{Trust} + \text{Vulnerability} + \text{Communication} \quad (79)$$

In this equation, intimacy is seen as the sum of trust, vulnerability, and communication. As partners engage in fisting, they are often required to communicate openly about their feelings, desires, and limits, which can enhance their emotional connection.

Embracing a Fister Identity

As individuals explore fisting, they may begin to identify as "fisters," embracing their participation in this practice as part of their sexual identity. This identity can foster a sense of community and belonging, as individuals connect with others who share similar interests and experiences. Celebrating this identity can lead to empowerment and self-acceptance.

$$\text{Fister Identity} = \text{Community} + \text{Acceptance} + \text{Empowerment} \qquad (80)$$

Here, the fister identity is a combination of community support, self-acceptance, and personal empowerment. Engaging with others who celebrate fisting can help individuals feel validated in their experiences and desires, further enhancing their journey of personal growth.

The Role of Reflection and Integration

To fully celebrate personal growth, it is essential to engage in reflection and integration. After exploring fisting, individuals should take time to reflect on their experiences, considering how these moments have influenced their understanding of themselves and their relationships. This reflective practice can solidify the lessons learned and help individuals integrate their experiences into their broader sexual repertoire.

$$\text{Integration} = \text{Reflection} + \text{Experience} \qquad (81)$$

In this context, integration is the result of reflecting on one's experiences. By taking the time to process their journey, individuals can better understand their desires and how they fit into their overall sexual identity.

Celebrating Milestones

As individuals progress in their fisting journey, it is important to celebrate milestones. Whether it is the first successful fisting experience, overcoming fears, or establishing deeper intimacy with a partner, acknowledging these achievements can enhance the sense of personal growth. Celebrating milestones reinforces positive experiences and encourages continued exploration.

$$\text{Celebration} = \text{Milestones} + \text{Acknowledgment} \qquad (82)$$

This equation highlights that celebration arises from recognizing milestones and acknowledging the journey taken. Celebrating personal growth can also serve as motivation for continued exploration and self-discovery.

Conclusion

In conclusion, celebrating personal growth and exploration within the context of fisting is a vital aspect of the journey. Through self-discovery, overcoming shame, building intimacy, embracing identity, engaging in reflection, and celebrating milestones, individuals can experience profound transformations. Fisting can be a pathway to radical self-love and acceptance, encouraging individuals to embrace their desires and cultivate deeper connections with themselves and their partners. As we honor our unique journeys, we contribute to a broader narrative of sexual empowerment and exploration.

Consensual Fisting as an Act of Radical Self-Love

In a world that often stigmatizes sexual exploration, consensual fisting emerges as a profound act of radical self-love. This section delves into the transformative potential of fisting, not only as a physical practice but as a means of embracing one's body, desires, and intimate connections. The act of consensual fisting can serve as a powerful reminder that our bodies are worthy of pleasure and exploration, challenging societal norms that dictate how we should engage with our own sensuality.

Theoretical Foundations of Self-Love

Radical self-love is rooted in the belief that every individual has the right to embrace their body, desires, and sexual expression without shame. According to bell hooks in *All About Love*, love is a combination of care, commitment, trust, knowledge, responsibility, and respect. When we apply this framework to our sexual experiences, we can redefine how we perceive intimacy and pleasure. Fisting, as an intimate act, requires a high level of trust and communication between partners, echoing hooks' assertion that love is an action that involves mutual respect and understanding.

Body Positivity and Acceptance

Engaging in consensual fisting can be a radical act of body positivity. It challenges the often unrealistic standards of beauty and sexual desirability that permeate our culture. The act itself requires a deep awareness of one's body and its capabilities, fostering a sense of acceptance and appreciation for its unique form. When individuals embrace fisting, they confront societal taboos and reclaim their bodies as spaces of pleasure and exploration. This reclamation can lead to enhanced body confidence and a more profound connection with one's sexual identity.

Addressing Shame and Stigma

Shame surrounding sexual practices, particularly those deemed taboo, can create barriers to self-love and acceptance. Research by Brené Brown highlights how shame can inhibit our ability to connect with ourselves and others. By engaging in consensual fisting, individuals actively confront and dismantle the shame associated with their desires. This process can be cathartic, allowing for emotional release and healing. For example, a person who has internalized negative beliefs about their sexual preferences may find empowerment in openly discussing and practicing fisting with a trusted partner, transforming shame into a celebration of their desires.

Intimacy and Connection

The act of fisting necessitates a profound level of intimacy and connection between partners. This connection is built on trust, communication, and mutual respect, all fundamental components of radical self-love. As partners explore fisting together, they engage in a shared journey of vulnerability and discovery. This intimacy can deepen emotional bonds, allowing both partners to feel seen and valued in their desires. For instance, a couple may find that fisting enhances their sexual repertoire, leading to increased pleasure and satisfaction in their relationship.

Empowerment through Exploration

Fisting can also serve as a form of empowerment, allowing individuals to reclaim agency over their bodies and desires. In a society that often seeks to control and dictate sexual expression, consensual fisting becomes an act of defiance against these norms. By embracing this practice, individuals assert their right to explore their bodies in ways that bring them joy and pleasure. This empowerment can extend beyond the bedroom, influencing how individuals approach other aspects of their lives. For example, someone who engages in fisting may find a newfound confidence that permeates their personal and professional relationships.

Practical Application of Radical Self-Love through Fisting

To embody radical self-love through consensual fisting, individuals can adopt several practical approaches:

- **Open Communication:** Establishing clear lines of communication with partners is essential. Discuss desires, boundaries, and concerns before engaging in fisting. This dialogue fosters trust and ensures that both partners feel safe and respected.

- **Setting Intentions:** Before exploring fisting, take time to reflect on personal intentions. What do you hope to gain from the experience? Setting intentions can guide the exploration and enhance the sense of purpose.

- **Self-Care Practices:** Incorporate self-care routines that promote body positivity and acceptance. This may include mindfulness practices, body awareness exercises, or engaging in activities that celebrate your body's capabilities.

- **Aftercare:** Aftercare is a crucial component of any intimate experience, particularly one as intense as fisting. Engage in aftercare practices that nurture emotional and physical well-being, reinforcing the bond between partners and fostering a sense of safety.

- **Community Engagement:** Seek out supportive communities that celebrate sexual exploration and body positivity. Engaging with like-minded individuals can reinforce feelings of acceptance and reduce feelings of isolation or shame.

Conclusion

Consensual fisting, when approached with intention and care, can be a powerful act of radical self-love. It challenges societal norms, fosters intimacy, and promotes body positivity, allowing individuals to embrace their desires fully. By engaging in this intimate practice, individuals can cultivate a deeper connection with themselves and their partners, transforming shame into empowerment and self-acceptance. Ultimately, consensual fisting serves as a reminder that our bodies are deserving of pleasure, exploration, and love—an essential aspect of our human experience.

Embracing Fister Identity and Community

In the realm of sexual exploration, the journey of embracing a fister identity can be both empowering and transformative. This section delves into the significance of identifying as a fister, the importance of community, and the ways in which individuals can foster a supportive network that nurtures their desires and experiences.

Understanding Fister Identity

Embracing a fister identity involves recognizing and accepting one's interests and desires related to fisting. This identity can serve as a source of pride and a means of self-affirmation. As individuals navigate their sexual landscapes, they often encounter societal stigma and misunderstanding surrounding practices like fisting. A key aspect of developing a fister identity is understanding that one's sexual preferences do not define their worth or character.

The psychological concept of **identity formation** posits that individuals construct their identities through experiences, relationships, and societal interactions. According to Erik Erikson's stages of psychosocial development, the period of adolescence and young adulthood is crucial for establishing a coherent sense of self. In this context, embracing a fister identity can be seen as an extension of this developmental process, allowing individuals to explore their sexuality in a way that aligns with their authentic selves.

Navigating Stigma and Shame

Despite the increasing visibility of diverse sexual practices, fisting often remains shrouded in stigma. This stigma can manifest in various forms, including societal judgment, misinformation, and personal shame. Addressing these issues is essential for fostering a healthy fister identity.

Research by [1] highlights the detrimental effects of shame on sexual well-being. Shame can lead to feelings of isolation and self-doubt, hindering one's ability to fully embrace their sexual identity. To combat this, individuals are encouraged to engage in self-compassion practices and seek out affirming spaces where they can express their desires without fear of judgment.

Building Community Connections

A supportive community can play a pivotal role in the journey of embracing a fister identity. Community connections provide opportunities for individuals to share experiences, learn from one another, and foster a sense of belonging.

Online platforms and social media have emerged as valuable resources for building these connections. Fisting-focused forums, groups, and events allow individuals to engage with others who share similar interests. These spaces can serve as safe havens where individuals can discuss techniques, share stories, and offer support.

Consider the case of a participant in an online fisting forum who shares their initial fears and hesitations about exploring fisting. Through engagement with the community, they receive encouragement, advice on safety practices, and validation of their desires. This interaction not only helps to alleviate their fears but also strengthens their sense of identity as a fister.

Creating Safe Spaces

Creating safe spaces within the fisting community is essential for fostering open dialogue and mutual support. Safe spaces are environments where individuals feel secure to express their identities, share their experiences, and engage in discussions about their desires without fear of discrimination or backlash.

The principles of **inclusivity** and **respect** are fundamental in establishing these spaces. Community leaders and members must actively work to ensure that all voices are heard and valued, particularly those from marginalized groups within the fisting community.

For example, a local fisting workshop might implement guidelines that prioritize consent and respect for all participants. This could include establishing ground rules for discussions, ensuring that everyone has an opportunity to speak, and creating a culture of active listening. By fostering an inclusive environment, individuals can feel empowered to explore their fister identity more freely.

Empowerment Through Education

Education plays a crucial role in embracing a fister identity and fostering community connections. By seeking knowledge about fisting techniques, safety practices, and emotional considerations, individuals can empower themselves and others in their community.

Workshops, seminars, and educational resources can provide valuable information that demystifies fisting and addresses common misconceptions. For instance, a workshop that focuses on the anatomy and physiology of fisting can help participants understand their bodies better, leading to more fulfilling and safer experiences.

Furthermore, educational initiatives that promote **sex positivity** and inclusivity can help dismantle the stigma surrounding fisting. By normalizing discussions about diverse sexual practices, communities can create a culture of acceptance and understanding.

Celebrating Fister Identity

Finally, embracing a fister identity is not just about navigating challenges; it is also about celebrating the joys and pleasures that come with it. Community events, such as fisting parties or gatherings, provide opportunities for individuals to come together, share their experiences, and revel in their shared interests.

Celebration can take many forms, from organized events that focus on skill-sharing and education to informal meet-ups where individuals can connect and bond over their experiences. These gatherings not only strengthen community ties but also reinforce the idea that fisting is a legitimate and valuable aspect of sexual expression.

In conclusion, embracing a fister identity involves a multifaceted journey of self-acceptance, community building, and education. By navigating the complexities of stigma and shame, fostering supportive connections, and celebrating their desires, individuals can cultivate a rich and fulfilling fister identity that enhances their sexual experiences and overall well-being.

Bibliography

[1] Nagoski, E. (2015). *Come As You Are: The Surprising New Science that Will Transform Your Sex Life*. Simon & Schuster.

Adventures in Fisting Beyond the Book

As we conclude our exploration of fisting, it is essential to recognize that the journey does not end with the pages of this guide. The realm of fisting is vast, dynamic, and deeply personal, offering opportunities for continued growth, exploration, and connection. This section encourages you to venture beyond the book, embracing the adventures that await in your fisting journey.

Embracing Exploration

Engaging in fisting is not merely about the act itself; it is about the experiences, emotions, and connections that arise from it. Each individual's journey is unique, shaped by personal desires, boundaries, and experiences. Embrace the notion that exploration is a continuous process. Consider the following avenues for expanding your fisting experience:

- **Workshops and Classes:** Seek out local or online workshops that focus on fisting techniques, safety, and communication. These spaces often provide valuable insights and hands-on experiences, allowing you to learn from experienced practitioners in a supportive environment.

- **Community Engagement:** Join fisting or kink communities, whether online or in-person. Engaging with others who share similar interests can lead to valuable exchanges of knowledge, experiences, and techniques. Community support can also help mitigate feelings of isolation or shame that may arise.

- **Personal Reflection:** Take time to reflect on your fisting experiences. What have you learned about yourself, your desires, and your boundaries? Journaling can be an effective tool for processing your thoughts and emotions, allowing you to track your growth over time.

Innovating Techniques

Fisting is an art form that encourages creativity and innovation. As you gain experience, consider experimenting with different techniques, positions, and scenarios. Here are some ideas to inspire your adventures:

- **Different Body Parts:** While fisting is commonly associated with the vagina or anus, consider exploring other areas of the body. For instance, some individuals enjoy fisting the mouth or using their hands to stimulate other erogenous zones. Always prioritize consent and communication when exploring new territories.

- **Incorporating Sensory Elements:** Enhance your fisting experience by incorporating sensory elements such as temperature play (using warm or cool lubricants), sound (music or verbal cues), or visual stimuli (lighting or costumes). These elements can heighten arousal and create a more immersive experience.

- **Role Play and Fantasy:** Engage in role play scenarios that resonate with your fantasies. Whether it involves power dynamics, specific characters, or themed settings, integrating role play can add an exciting layer to your fisting adventures.

Building Emotional Connections

Fisting is often a deeply intimate act that fosters emotional connections between partners. As you continue your journey, consider the following ways to strengthen these bonds:

- **Post-Scene Debriefing:** After a fisting session, take time to discuss the experience with your partner(s). Share what felt good, what could be improved, and any emotional responses that arose. This practice not only enhances communication but also builds trust and understanding.

- **Aftercare Rituals:** Establish aftercare routines that cater to the needs of all participants. This may include cuddling, discussing feelings, or engaging in soothing activities. Aftercare is crucial for emotional well-being and helps to reinforce the connection between partners.

- **Exploring Vulnerability:** Embrace the vulnerability that comes with fisting. Sharing fears, desires, and insecurities can deepen intimacy and create a safe space for exploration. Vulnerability fosters trust, allowing partners to express themselves more freely.

Navigating Challenges

As with any sexual exploration, challenges may arise during your fisting journey. It is essential to approach these challenges with compassion and understanding. Here are some common issues and strategies for addressing them:

- **Physical Discomfort:** If you experience pain or discomfort during fisting, it is crucial to communicate this with your partner. Use established safe words or signals to indicate when to pause or adjust. Remember that consent is ongoing, and comfort should always be prioritized.

- **Emotional Triggers:** Fisting can evoke a range of emotions, including fear, anxiety, or past trauma. If you or your partner experience emotional triggers, take a step back and engage in grounding techniques. This may involve deep breathing, discussing feelings, or engaging in self-soothing practices.

- **Miscommunication:** Misunderstandings can occur, particularly in the heat of the moment. Prioritize clear communication before, during, and after fisting sessions. Regularly check in with each other to ensure that both partners feel heard and respected.

The Lifelong Journey of Fisting Exploration

Ultimately, the journey of fisting is a lifelong adventure. As you continue to explore, remember that growth and learning are integral parts of this experience. Consider the following as you embrace the ongoing nature of your fisting journey:

- **Stay Curious:** Cultivate a mindset of curiosity. Be open to learning new techniques, discovering different aspects of your sexuality, and exploring the evolving dynamics of your relationships.

- **Practice Self-Compassion:** Recognize that exploration may come with setbacks or challenges. Approach yourself and your partner(s) with kindness and understanding, allowing space for mistakes and growth.

- **Celebrate Achievements:** Acknowledge and celebrate your milestones, whether big or small. Each step in your fisting journey contributes to your overall growth and understanding of yourself and your desires.

In conclusion, the adventures in fisting extend far beyond the pages of this guide. By embracing exploration, innovating techniques, building emotional connections, navigating challenges, and committing to lifelong learning, you can create a fulfilling and enriching fisting journey. Remember, each experience is an opportunity for growth, connection, and self-discovery.

Incorporating Fisting into a Well-Rounded Sexual Repertoire

Incorporating fisting into a well-rounded sexual repertoire involves understanding its place within the broader context of sexual expression, intimacy, and pleasure. This section explores how fisting can complement other sexual practices, enhance personal and relational satisfaction, and contribute to a holistic understanding of one's sexual self.

Understanding Sexual Repertoire

A sexual repertoire refers to the range of sexual activities, practices, and experiences that individuals or couples engage in. It is shaped by personal preferences, cultural influences, and individual comfort levels. The diversity of a sexual repertoire can enhance intimacy and satisfaction, allowing for exploration and discovery of what brings pleasure and fulfillment.

Fisting, as an act that may be seen as extreme or taboo, can be a powerful addition to this repertoire. It requires a high level of trust, communication, and consent, which can deepen emotional connections between partners. By integrating fisting into one's sexual practices, individuals can expand their understanding of pleasure, vulnerability, and intimacy.

Theoretical Framework

The incorporation of fisting into a sexual repertoire can be analyzed through various theoretical lenses, including:

- **Sexual Fluidity:** The concept of sexual fluidity suggests that individuals may experience changes in their sexual preferences and practices over time. Fisting can be viewed as an exploration of this fluidity, allowing individuals to challenge their boundaries and expand their sexual experiences.

- **Pleasure-Centered Models:** These models emphasize the importance of pleasure in sexual experiences. Fisting, when approached with care and intention, can lead to heightened sensations and an exploration of new forms of pleasure, contributing positively to one's sexual health and well-being.
- **Relational Dynamics:** The dynamics of power, consent, and trust play a crucial role in incorporating fisting into a sexual repertoire. Understanding these dynamics can enhance the experience and ensure that all parties feel safe and respected.

Practical Considerations

When incorporating fisting into a sexual repertoire, it is vital to consider the following practical aspects:

- **Communication:** Open dialogue with partners about desires, boundaries, and concerns is essential. Discussing the motivations for wanting to explore fisting can help partners align their expectations and foster a supportive environment.
- **Education and Preparation:** Understanding the techniques, safety measures, and emotional implications of fisting is crucial. Engaging in research, attending workshops, or consulting with experienced practitioners can provide valuable insights and skills.
- **Integration with Other Practices:** Fisting can be integrated with other sexual activities, such as oral sex, penetration with toys, or BDSM practices. This combination can create a rich tapestry of experiences, allowing individuals to explore various sensations and forms of intimacy.
- **Aftercare:** The emotional and physical aftercare following a fisting session is essential. It provides an opportunity for partners to reconnect, discuss their experiences, and address any emotional or physical needs that may arise.

Examples of Integration

1. **Sequential Practices:** A couple may begin with traditional forms of intimacy, such as kissing or oral sex, gradually building to fisting. This approach allows for a natural progression of arousal and comfort, enhancing the overall experience.
2. **Combination with BDSM:** Fisting can be integrated into BDSM scenes, where power dynamics and consent are key. For instance, a dominant

partner may use fisting as a form of both pleasure and control, ensuring that the submissive partner feels safe and respected throughout the experience.

3. **Exploration of Sensation:** Individuals can experiment with different forms of stimulation, such as combining fisting with the use of vibrators or other toys. This combination can heighten sensations and create a more complex experience of pleasure.

4. **Themed Sessions:** Couples may choose to create themed sexual sessions that incorporate fisting. For example, they could explore fantasies related to dominance and submission, using fisting as a climactic element of the scene.

Addressing Potential Challenges

While incorporating fisting into a sexual repertoire can be rewarding, it may also present challenges:

- **Physical Discomfort or Pain:** It is essential to listen to one's body and communicate openly about any discomfort during fisting. Establishing safe words and signals can help partners navigate these moments effectively.

- **Emotional Responses:** Fisting can evoke a range of emotions, from pleasure to vulnerability. Partners should be prepared for the emotional aftermath and engage in aftercare practices to support each other.

- **Social Stigma and Misconceptions:** Fisting is often surrounded by stigma and misconceptions. Educating oneself and one's partner about the realities of fisting can help dispel myths and foster a more positive attitude towards its inclusion in a sexual repertoire.

Conclusion

Incorporating fisting into a well-rounded sexual repertoire can enrich personal and relational sexual experiences. By embracing open communication, education, and a willingness to explore, individuals can enhance their understanding of pleasure and intimacy. As with any sexual practice, the key lies in mutual consent, respect, and the ongoing journey of discovery within one's sexual self. Ultimately, fisting can serve as a powerful tool for self-exploration, connection, and empowerment, contributing to a fulfilling and diverse sexual repertoire.

The Role of Fisting in Body Positivity and Self-Acceptance

Fisting, as an intimate and often taboo sexual practice, can serve as a powerful catalyst for body positivity and self-acceptance. Engaging in fisting requires a deep level of trust and vulnerability between partners, and this dynamic can foster a more profound appreciation for one's body and its capabilities. By embracing the physicality of fisting, individuals can challenge societal norms surrounding body image and sexuality, ultimately leading to a more positive self-concept.

Understanding Body Positivity

Body positivity is a social movement that advocates for the acceptance of all bodies, regardless of size, shape, or appearance. It encourages individuals to appreciate their bodies for what they can do rather than how they look. This shift in focus is crucial, especially in a society that often promotes unrealistic beauty standards. Fisting can contribute to this movement by allowing individuals to experience pleasure and connection in ways that may defy conventional expectations.

The Physical Experience of Fisting

The act of fisting involves the full insertion of a hand into the vagina or rectum, which can be an empowering experience for many. This physical act can help individuals reclaim their bodies from societal judgments and expectations. The sensation of fullness, the exploration of one's anatomy, and the ability to give and receive pleasure can enhance body awareness and appreciation.

$$\text{Body Positivity} = \frac{\text{Self-Acceptance} + \text{Pleasure}}{\text{Societal Norms}} \qquad (83)$$

In this equation, body positivity is seen as a function of self-acceptance and pleasure, divided by the weight of societal norms. The more one embraces their body and experiences pleasure, the more they can counteract the negative effects of societal pressures.

Fisting and Vulnerability

Fisting requires a significant level of vulnerability. Participants must communicate openly about their desires, boundaries, and fears. This process of communication can lead to a deeper understanding of oneself and one's partner, fostering a supportive environment where both individuals feel safe to explore their bodies without judgment. By confronting fears and vulnerabilities, individuals can cultivate a sense of empowerment and self-acceptance.

Challenging Body Shame

Many people experience body shame, which can stem from cultural narratives that prioritize certain body types over others. Fisting can serve as a counter-narrative to these harmful beliefs. When individuals engage in fisting, they may find themselves appreciating their bodies in ways they never thought possible. The act of being intimate in such a profound manner can help dismantle feelings of inadequacy and shame.

For example, a person who has struggled with body image issues may find that fisting allows them to experience their body as a source of pleasure rather than shame. This shift in perspective can be liberating, leading to a more positive body image.

The Role of Consent and Communication

At the core of fisting is the importance of consent and communication. Establishing clear boundaries and engaging in open dialogue about desires can empower individuals to take ownership of their bodies. This empowerment is crucial for fostering body positivity. When individuals feel in control of their experiences, they are more likely to embrace their bodies and celebrate their unique attributes.

Building Community and Connection

Fisting can also create a sense of community among those who practice it. Sharing experiences and supporting one another in a safe space can help individuals feel accepted and valued. This sense of belonging can be particularly important for those who have felt marginalized due to their body size, shape, or sexual preferences. The community aspect of fisting can reinforce body positivity, as individuals learn from one another and celebrate their bodies together.

Therapeutic Benefits of Fisting

Engaging in fisting may also provide therapeutic benefits for some individuals. The physical sensations, combined with the emotional intimacy of the act, can lead to catharsis and healing. For those who have experienced trauma or body-related issues, fisting can serve as a means of reclaiming their bodies and fostering self-acceptance. The process of exploring one's body in a safe and consensual manner can facilitate emotional release and promote a healthier relationship with one's body.

Conclusion: Embracing the Journey

In conclusion, fisting can play a significant role in promoting body positivity and self-acceptance. By challenging societal norms, fostering vulnerability, and encouraging open communication, individuals can cultivate a deeper appreciation for their bodies. This journey toward self-acceptance is not only empowering but also essential for building a more inclusive and accepting society. As individuals embrace their bodies through practices like fisting, they contribute to a broader movement of body positivity that celebrates all forms of human expression and experience.

Advocacy and Destigmatization Efforts

The journey toward acceptance and understanding of fisting as a legitimate sexual practice involves a multifaceted approach to advocacy and destigmatization. This section will explore the theoretical foundations of stigma, the societal problems associated with it, and the practical strategies that can be employed to foster a more inclusive and accepting environment for those who engage in fisting.

Understanding Stigma

Stigma, as defined by Goffman (1963), is a mark of disgrace associated with a particular circumstance, quality, or person. In the context of sexual practices such as fisting, stigma manifests through societal misconceptions, moral judgments, and cultural taboos. The stigma surrounding fisting often stems from a lack of understanding, fear of the unknown, and entrenched societal norms regarding sexuality.

One theoretical framework that aids in understanding stigma is the *Social Identity Theory* (Tajfel & Turner, 1979), which posits that individuals categorize themselves and others into groups. Those who engage in non-normative sexual practices may be perceived as belonging to a marginalized group, leading to social exclusion and discrimination. This exclusion can perpetuate feelings of shame and isolation among practitioners, reinforcing the stigma associated with fisting.

Problems Associated with Stigma

The stigma surrounding fisting can lead to several detrimental outcomes, including:

- **Mental Health Issues:** Individuals who engage in fisting may experience anxiety, depression, and low self-esteem due to societal judgment and internalized stigma. Research indicates that stigma can significantly impact mental health outcomes (Corrigan, 2004).

- **Limited Access to Resources:** Stigmatized practices often lack adequate representation in sexual health resources, leading to misinformation and inadequate support for safe practices. This can result in increased risks of injury and infection due to a lack of knowledge about safe fisting techniques.
- **Social Isolation:** Practitioners may feel compelled to hide their sexual preferences, leading to a lack of community support and connection. This isolation can further exacerbate mental health issues and hinder personal growth.

Advocacy Strategies

To combat stigma and promote acceptance of fisting, several advocacy strategies can be employed:

- **Education and Awareness Campaigns:** Increasing awareness about fisting through workshops, seminars, and public forums can help demystify the practice. Educational materials should focus on safety, consent, and the emotional aspects of fisting, helping to dispel myths and misconceptions.
- **Inclusive Language:** Advocates should promote the use of inclusive language in discussions about sexual practices. This includes avoiding derogatory terms and reframing the conversation to focus on consent, pleasure, and mutual enjoyment.
- **Engagement with Healthcare Providers:** Collaborating with healthcare professionals to incorporate fisting into sexual health education can help normalize the practice. This can involve creating resources that address safe practices and the importance of open communication between partners.
- **Community Building:** Fostering supportive communities where individuals can share their experiences and learn from one another is crucial. Online forums, local meetups, and workshops can provide safe spaces for practitioners to connect and discuss their interests without fear of judgment.
- **Advocacy in Policy Making:** Engaging in advocacy efforts that promote sexual rights and health can help influence policy changes. This may involve lobbying for comprehensive sex education that includes discussions of diverse sexual practices, including fisting.

- **Visibility and Representation:** Encouraging visibility of fisting in popular culture, literature, and media can help normalize the practice. This can include featuring fisting in erotic literature, films, and art, presenting it as a valid expression of sexual intimacy.

Examples of Successful Advocacy Efforts

Several organizations and movements have successfully advocated for the destigmatization of diverse sexual practices, including fisting:

- **The Sexual Health Alliance:** This organization offers workshops and resources aimed at promoting sexual health and education. Their initiatives include discussions on fisting, emphasizing safety and consent.

- **Kink Aware Professionals:** This network connects individuals with healthcare providers who are knowledgeable about kink and BDSM practices, including fisting. By fostering a supportive environment, they help reduce the stigma associated with these practices.

- **Fisting Workshops and Events:** Various community-led workshops focus on fisting education, providing a safe space for individuals to learn about techniques, safety, and emotional aspects. These events often emphasize consent and communication, helping to create a more informed and supportive community.

Conclusion

Advocacy and destigmatization efforts are essential in creating an environment where individuals can explore fisting without fear of judgment or discrimination. By employing education, community building, and inclusive practices, we can foster a culture of acceptance and understanding. As we move toward a more inclusive society, it is crucial to continue advocating for the rights and dignity of all individuals, regardless of their sexual preferences.

In conclusion, the journey toward destigmatization is ongoing, requiring the collective efforts of individuals, communities, and organizations. By embracing diversity in sexual practices and promoting open dialogue, we can create a world where fisting and other non-normative practices are celebrated as valid expressions of human sexuality.

Engaging in Ongoing Education and Learning

In the realm of fisting, as with any intimate practice, ongoing education and learning are paramount to ensuring safety, enhancing pleasure, and fostering deeper connections. Engaging in continuous education allows individuals to stay informed about evolving practices, techniques, and the emotional and psychological aspects associated with fisting. This section explores various avenues for ongoing education, the importance of integrating new knowledge, and how to navigate the complexities of learning in this intimate domain.

The Importance of Lifelong Learning

Lifelong learning is a vital principle in any sexual practice, particularly in one as nuanced as fisting. Understanding that sexual knowledge is not static encourages practitioners to seek out new information and perspectives. This commitment to learning can enhance not only personal experiences but also contribute to the broader community by fostering a culture of safety, consent, and respect.

Educational Resources and Workshops

One of the most effective ways to engage in ongoing education is through workshops and educational resources. Many organizations and communities offer classes specifically focused on fisting techniques, safety protocols, and emotional considerations. These workshops can range from introductory sessions for beginners to advanced classes that delve into specific techniques or psychological aspects of fisting.

- **Local Workshops:** Many sex-positive organizations host workshops that provide hands-on learning experiences. Participants can practice techniques in a safe environment under the guidance of experienced instructors.

- **Online Learning:** With the rise of digital platforms, numerous online courses and webinars are available. These resources often include video demonstrations, written materials, and interactive Q&A sessions.

- **Conferences and Retreats:** Attending sexuality conferences or retreats can provide immersive learning experiences. These events often feature expert speakers, panel discussions, and opportunities for networking with other practitioners.

BIBLIOGRAPHY

Reading and Research

Engaging with literature on fisting and related topics is another critical component of ongoing education. Reading books, articles, and research papers can provide valuable insights into the physical, emotional, and social dimensions of fisting.

- **Books:** Seek out texts written by experts in the field of sexuality that cover fisting techniques, safety, and the emotional aspects of sexual exploration.

- **Academic Research:** Many universities and institutions conduct research on sexual practices, including fisting. Accessing academic journals can provide a deeper understanding of the psychological and physiological implications.

- **Online Articles and Blogs:** Many sex educators and practitioners maintain blogs or write articles that offer practical tips, personal experiences, and new developments in the field.

Community Engagement

Participating in community discussions and forums can also enhance learning. Engaging with others who share similar interests allows for the exchange of ideas, experiences, and resources.

- **Online Forums:** Platforms like Reddit or specialized sex-positive forums provide spaces for individuals to ask questions, share experiences, and seek advice from others.

- **Support Groups:** Joining support groups focused on kink or BDSM can provide emotional support and educational opportunities. These groups often discuss safety, consent, and personal experiences.

- **Peer Mentoring:** Finding a mentor within the community can provide personalized guidance and insights. Mentors can share their experiences and help navigate challenges.

Evaluating and Integrating New Knowledge

As individuals engage in ongoing education, it is crucial to evaluate and integrate new knowledge into their practices. This process involves critical thinking and reflection on how new information aligns with personal values and experiences.

- **Reflective Practice:** After attending a workshop or reading a new resource, take time to reflect on what was learned. Consider how this new knowledge can be applied to personal practices and relationships.

- **Feedback Loops:** Create opportunities for feedback from partners about new techniques or approaches. Open communication can help refine practices and ensure mutual satisfaction.

- **Adaptation:** Be open to adapting practices based on new insights. This flexibility can enhance the overall experience and foster a culture of continuous improvement.

Navigating Challenges in Learning

Engaging in ongoing education may present challenges, including misinformation, stigma, or personal discomfort with certain topics. Navigating these challenges requires a proactive and compassionate approach.

- **Critical Evaluation of Sources:** Not all information is created equal. Evaluate the credibility of sources, seeking out those with a solid reputation in the field of sexual health and education.

- **Addressing Stigma:** Recognize that societal stigma around fisting may impact learning experiences. Seek out supportive communities that affirm and validate diverse sexual practices.

- **Personal Comfort Levels:** Acknowledge personal comfort levels when exploring new information. It is essential to engage with topics at a pace that feels safe and manageable.

Conclusion

Ongoing education and learning in the realm of fisting are essential for fostering a safe, pleasurable, and fulfilling experience. By actively seeking out workshops, literature, and community engagement, individuals can deepen their understanding and connection to this intimate practice. Embracing a mindset of lifelong learning not only enhances personal experiences but also contributes to a more informed and compassionate community. In this journey, each individual plays a vital role in shaping the narrative around fisting, transforming it from a taboo into a celebrated aspect of sexual exploration.

Nurturing Fisting Relationships and Connections

Nurturing fisting relationships and connections is an essential aspect of engaging in this intimate practice. It involves fostering trust, communication, and emotional safety among partners, which can significantly enhance the experience and deepen the bond between individuals. In this section, we will explore the theories, challenges, and practical strategies for nurturing these connections.

Theoretical Frameworks

Understanding the dynamics of relationships within the context of fisting requires a foundation in several key theories:

- **Attachment Theory:** This psychological model posits that the bonds formed in early childhood influence relationships throughout life. Secure attachment styles can lead to healthier communication and trust in intimate practices, while insecure styles may create barriers to vulnerability and openness.

- **Intimacy Theory:** According to this theory, intimacy is built through self-disclosure, emotional support, and shared experiences. Fisting, as a deeply intimate act, can serve as a catalyst for enhancing emotional closeness when approached with care and respect.

- **Communication Theory:** Effective communication is vital in any relationship, especially in sexual contexts. Theories surrounding non-verbal cues, active listening, and feedback loops are crucial for navigating the complexities of fisting.

Challenges in Nurturing Relationships

While nurturing fisting relationships can be rewarding, several challenges may arise:

- **Fear of Vulnerability:** Engaging in fisting can evoke feelings of vulnerability. Partners may fear judgment or rejection, which can hinder open communication about desires and boundaries.

- **Misaligned Expectations:** Partners may enter into fisting with different expectations regarding pleasure, intensity, and emotional involvement. This misalignment can lead to disappointment and conflict.

- **Stigma and Shame:** Societal stigma surrounding fisting can create feelings of shame, making it difficult for individuals to discuss their desires openly. This can inhibit the development of trust and intimacy.

- **Emotional Triggers:** Past traumas can surface during fisting, leading to emotional distress. Partners must be prepared to navigate these triggers with sensitivity and understanding.

Strategies for Nurturing Connections

To cultivate strong fisting relationships, consider the following strategies:

- **Establish Open Communication:** Create a safe space for dialogue about desires, boundaries, and concerns. Regular check-ins before and after sessions can help partners articulate their feelings and experiences.

- **Practice Active Listening:** Engage in active listening techniques to ensure both partners feel heard and valued. This involves reflecting back what the other person has said, asking clarifying questions, and validating their feelings.

- **Set Clear Boundaries:** Discuss and establish boundaries related to physical and emotional limits. This can include safe words, gestures, and signals that indicate when to slow down or stop.

- **Foster Emotional Safety:** Prioritize creating an emotionally safe environment where partners can express their vulnerabilities without fear of judgment. This can be achieved through reassurance, empathy, and non-judgmental responses.

- **Engage in Aftercare:** Aftercare is crucial in nurturing fisting relationships. It involves providing comfort and support following a session, which can include cuddling, discussing the experience, or engaging in activities that promote relaxation and connection.

- **Educate Together:** Engage in educational opportunities together, such as workshops or reading materials on fisting. This shared learning experience can strengthen the bond and enhance mutual understanding.

- **Address Emotional Triggers:** Be proactive in discussing potential emotional triggers related to fisting. Partners should feel empowered to express when they need to pause or shift focus to ensure emotional well-being.

- **Celebrate Successes:** Acknowledge and celebrate milestones in the relationship, whether it's trying a new technique, deepening intimacy, or overcoming a challenge. This recognition fosters a positive atmosphere and encourages continued exploration.

- **Create Rituals:** Establishing rituals around fisting sessions can enhance the emotional connection. This might include pre-session warm-ups, shared breathing exercises, or post-session debriefs that reinforce intimacy and trust.

- **Seek Support:** If challenges arise that feel overwhelming, consider seeking support from a therapist or counselor experienced in sexual relationships. Professional guidance can provide valuable tools for navigating complex emotions and dynamics.

Examples of Nurturing Practices

To illustrate the above strategies, here are some practical examples:

- **Communication Exercise:** Partners can engage in a "desire mapping" exercise where they each write down their desires, boundaries, and fears related to fisting. Afterward, they can share their maps and discuss any discrepancies or alignments.

- **Aftercare Ritual:** Following a fisting session, partners might engage in a specific aftercare ritual, such as preparing a favorite snack together, taking a warm bath, or spending time in quiet reflection to reconnect.

- **Educational Workshop:** Couples can attend a fisting workshop together, learning techniques and safety practices while building a supportive community around their experiences.

- **Emotional Check-Ins:** After each session, partners can take turns sharing one positive aspect of the experience and one area for improvement. This practice encourages constructive feedback and reinforces emotional connection.

- **Establishing Safe Words:** Partners might agree on a color-coded system for safe words, where "green" indicates comfort, "yellow" indicates a need to slow down, and "red" indicates a stop. This clarity can enhance feelings of safety and trust.

Nurturing fisting relationships and connections requires ongoing effort, communication, and a commitment to emotional safety. By embracing these strategies and addressing challenges with empathy and understanding, partners can cultivate deeper intimacy and connection through their shared exploration of fisting.

$$\text{Intimacy} = \text{Trust} + \text{Communication} + \text{Vulnerability} \tag{84}$$

The End is Just the Beginning: Embracing a Lifelong Journey of Fisting Exploration

As we conclude this exploration of fisting, it is crucial to recognize that this journey is not merely a destination but a continuous path of discovery, intimacy, and personal growth. The act of fisting, when approached with care, consent, and open communication, can serve as a profound gateway to deeper connections with ourselves and our partners. This section will delve into the ongoing journey of fisting exploration, emphasizing the importance of reflection, integration, and community engagement.

Reflection and Integration

The end of this guide marks a pivotal moment for reflection. Engaging in fisting, like any intimate practice, invites us to examine our desires, boundaries, and emotional landscapes. Reflection can be facilitated through various methods, such as journaling, dialogue with partners, or participation in workshops. These activities encourage individuals to articulate their experiences, fostering a deeper understanding of their motivations and feelings.

$$R = \frac{D}{T} \tag{85}$$

where R represents reflection, D is the depth of experience, and T is the time spent in introspection. This equation illustrates that greater depth in our experiences enhances our capacity for meaningful reflection, ultimately leading to more profound insights.

Celebrating Personal Growth and Exploration

Fisting can be a transformative experience, promoting personal growth through the exploration of pleasure and vulnerability. Celebrating these milestones is essential, as it reinforces a positive narrative around our sexual journeys. By acknowledging and honoring our progress, we cultivate a sense of empowerment and agency in our sexual lives.

Consensual Fisting as an Act of Radical Self-Love

At its core, consensual fisting embodies radical self-love. It challenges societal norms around sexuality, intimacy, and body autonomy. By embracing this practice, individuals affirm their right to explore their bodies and desires without shame. This act of self-acceptance can ripple outward, fostering healthier relationships and encouraging others to engage in their own journeys of self-discovery.

Embracing Fister Identity and Community

Identifying as a fister can be a source of pride and belonging. Engaging with communities that celebrate fisting can provide support, validation, and opportunities for learning. Whether through online forums, local meetups, or workshops, connecting with others who share similar interests can enhance the experience and offer a sense of camaraderie.

Adventures in Fisting Beyond the Book

The journey of fisting exploration does not end with this guide. Each experience can lead to new adventures, techniques, and forms of intimacy. Embracing curiosity and a willingness to experiment can open doors to novel experiences that deepen connections with oneself and partners. Consider exploring various fisting styles, incorporating toys, or engaging in role-play scenarios to expand your repertoire.

Incorporating Fisting into a Well-Rounded Sexual Repertoire

Fisting can be a beautiful addition to a diverse sexual repertoire. It is essential to integrate it thoughtfully with other practices, ensuring that it complements rather than overshadows other forms of intimacy. By maintaining a balance, individuals can cultivate a rich and fulfilling sexual life that honors their multifaceted desires.

The Role of Fisting in Body Positivity and Self-Acceptance

Fisting encourages a celebration of bodies in all their forms. Engaging in this practice can foster body positivity, as it invites individuals to embrace their physical selves and the diverse ways they can experience pleasure. This journey often involves dismantling societal pressures and expectations, ultimately leading to a more profound sense of self-acceptance.

Advocacy and Destigmatization Efforts

As fisters, we have a unique opportunity to advocate for the destigmatization of fisting and other sexual practices. Sharing our stories, educating others, and engaging in conversations about consent and safety can help normalize these experiences. By challenging misconceptions and advocating for sexual rights, we contribute to a more inclusive and accepting society.

Engaging in Ongoing Education and Learning

The landscape of sexual exploration is ever-evolving. Engaging in ongoing education—whether through workshops, reading, or community involvement—ensures that our knowledge remains current and relevant. This commitment to learning not only enhances our practices but also empowers us to share informed perspectives with others.

Nurturing Fisting Relationships and Connections

Finally, nurturing the relationships built through fisting is vital for sustaining intimacy and connection. Regular check-ins, aftercare practices, and open communication can strengthen bonds with partners. These relationships, founded on trust and respect, can flourish as we continue to explore the depths of our desires together.

The End is Just the Beginning

In conclusion, the journey of fisting exploration is a lifelong commitment to self-discovery, intimacy, and community engagement. Each experience enriches our understanding of ourselves and others, paving the way for deeper connections and shared pleasures. As we embrace this journey, let us carry forward the lessons learned, the connections forged, and the radical self-love cultivated through fisting. The end of this guide is merely the beginning of a vibrant, fulfilling exploration of our desires and identities.

Index

a, 1–8, 10, 11, 13–26, 28–30, 33, 35, 36, 38, 40–44, 46–52, 54, 55, 57–65, 67–75, 78–86, 89–94, 98, 99, 101, 102, 104–107, 109, 110, 112, 113, 115, 117, 119, 124, 125, 127, 129–139, 141, 142, 144, 147, 149, 150, 152–155, 159–161, 163, 166, 167, 169–172, 174, 175, 177–180, 182, 183, 185–189, 191, 192, 194, 196–210, 212–221, 223, 224, 226–229, 231–234, 236–239, 241–245, 247–252, 254, 256, 257, 259, 261–268, 270, 272, 273, 275, 278, 280, 281, 283–299, 302, 305–315, 317–319, 321–325, 327–345, 347, 348, 350–354, 356, 357, 359, 365–377, 379, 381, 383–397, 399–401, 403, 405, 408, 409, 412, 414–416, 418–420, 422, 425, 427–433, 435–439, 441, 443–449, 451, 452, 454–458, 460–466, 468, 469, 471–477, 479, 481–487, 489, 492–497, 500–503, 506–511, 513–517, 519–531, 533–541, 543, 544, 546, 547, 550–552

ability, 1, 44, 55, 132, 189, 191, 212–214, 254, 308, 344, 374, 375, 420, 520, 527, 539

absence, 482

abuse, 130, 132, 298, 483

academia, 443

acceptance, 4, 7, 15, 49, 61, 141, 247, 248, 256, 314, 323, 334, 345, 352, 353, 378, 379, 400, 401, 425, 447, 451, 464, 476, 477, 481, 489, 509, 519–523, 525–527, 531, 539–543, 551, 552

access, 405, 408, 419, 422, 448

accessibility, 406, 425, 510

account, 454–457

achievement, 289

act, 2–5, 7, 10, 13, 14, 16, 17, 22, 23, 26, 29, 30, 68, 70, 72, 74, 75, 78, 92, 101, 109, 117,

119, 124, 125, 127, 130, 131, 134, 135, 137, 142, 144, 172, 183, 212, 215, 217, 231–234, 236, 245, 247, 248, 254, 259, 267, 289, 290, 295, 297, 298, 305, 306, 314, 317, 321, 322, 324, 328, 330–332, 334, 337, 344, 351, 352, 367, 372, 374, 379, 388, 393, 399, 436, 438, 439, 441, 445, 446, 448, 449, 451, 470, 481–483, 519, 520, 523, 524, 527, 533, 534, 539, 540, 550, 551
action, 127, 198, 200
activation, 242
activism, 479, 481, 483
activity, 18, 55, 63, 74, 131, 133, 142, 163, 172, 175, 180, 198, 200, 205, 216, 217, 220, 224, 273, 281, 322, 357, 374, 396, 397, 464, 469, 471, 482, 494
adaptability, 112, 115
addiction, 491–497, 500, 505–508, 511–513
addition, 51, 75, 82, 160, 308, 352, 412, 429, 462, 521, 551
address, 7, 8, 78, 83, 91, 99, 131, 133, 171, 188, 191, 194, 197, 204, 220, 236, 241, 249, 250, 288, 302, 309, 312, 337, 368, 381, 435, 451, 461, 474, 492, 506
adherence, 8
adult, 5, 17, 467, 484, 487
advent, 510
adventure, 337, 340, 535

adversity, 254
advice, 70, 86, 405, 412, 419, 423, 429, 436, 443, 445, 483, 510, 530
advocacy, 454, 468, 471, 476, 479, 480, 484, 489, 522, 541, 542
advocate, 521, 523, 552
affirmation, 297, 352, 353, 368, 371
aftercare, 26, 131, 134, 135, 142, 215, 217, 223, 225, 226, 256, 259, 265, 267, 275–278, 283, 288, 289, 294, 297, 307, 315, 332, 343, 350, 372, 375, 392, 454, 455, 483, 516, 552
aftermath, 275
age, 343–345, 395–397, 399, 409, 422, 427, 443, 454
agency, 29, 180, 236, 289, 291, 295–297, 306, 307, 309, 351, 353, 373, 374, 441, 448, 449, 509, 520, 527, 551
aging, 343–345
agreement, 18, 142, 175, 186, 198, 200, 261, 465, 468, 469
aid, 120, 432, 513
aim, 480, 511
Alex, 78, 112, 236, 242, 259, 294, 339
Alex and Jamie, 191, 294
Alice, 264
allure, 13
almond, 154
aloe, 154
alternative, 6, 160, 323, 333, 351, 449, 454, 487
ambiguity, 469

Index

amount, 93, 332
anatomy, 1, 33, 35–38, 92, 97, 101, 103–105, 122, 134, 137, 203, 205, 240, 343, 360, 367, 371, 372, 425, 427, 436, 454, 461, 522, 530, 539
Anaïs Nin, 16
Angela C., 438
anger, 219, 290, 306
angle, 93, 97
ani, 49
anonymity, 422, 425, 510
anus, 1, 3, 4, 97, 103, 203, 390, 393
anxiety, 3, 24, 60, 74, 91, 130, 132, 135, 139, 215–218, 226, 236, 290, 302, 324, 346, 366, 500, 501
appeal, 5, 13, 15
appearance, 48, 539
application, 84, 85, 99, 101, 104, 186, 261
appreciation, 236, 430, 539, 541
approach, 1, 5, 6, 15, 17, 30, 44, 47, 52, 54, 55, 61, 75, 89, 119, 133, 134, 137, 139, 170, 174, 180, 185, 191, 228, 244, 248, 250, 278, 292, 294, 299, 306, 307, 314, 339, 343, 347, 348, 372, 376, 429, 445, 448, 457, 463, 475, 489, 492, 500, 503, 508, 517, 519, 521, 523, 527, 535, 541, 546
area, 53, 85, 95, 105, 149, 201, 244, 370, 466
arm, 85
aromatherapy, 85

arousal, 1, 14, 29, 34, 36, 89, 106, 267, 273, 336, 388, 492
array, 428
art, 4, 5, 15, 16, 68, 101, 102, 112, 352, 430, 449–451, 534
aspect, 9, 15, 18, 26, 41, 46, 61, 67, 69, 78, 81, 94, 99, 134, 142, 144, 150, 166, 194, 205, 215, 217, 221, 226, 242, 247, 305, 315, 343, 351, 375, 400, 414, 420, 436, 441, 464, 479, 503, 512, 526, 531, 540, 546, 547
assault, 130, 132, 198, 464, 465
atmosphere, 28, 84, 91, 134, 269
attachment, 26, 373
attempt, 377
attention, 124, 138, 171, 214, 221, 275, 345, 484
attentiveness, 101, 187
attire, 30
attitude, 8
attraction, 397
audience, 201, 454
authenticity, 269
author, 445
authority, 259, 272
autonomy, 64, 180, 189, 262, 289, 295, 372, 449, 464, 465, 467, 469, 471, 482, 487, 512, 551
availability, 448
awakening, 314
awareness, 3, 17, 21, 35, 40, 41, 43–45, 55, 58–61, 112, 115, 119, 134, 142, 144, 172, 199, 203–205, 225, 234, 236, 241, 244, 248,

250, 252, 281, 283, 291, 296, 298, 299, 301, 305–308, 314, 345, 466, 471, 483, 514, 517, 520, 524, 539
back, 4, 220, 287, 356, 524
backlash, 450, 530
bacteria, 127, 148, 151, 152, 156, 160
balance, 101, 192, 193, 266, 278, 280, 342, 395, 477, 479, 503, 517, 551
barrier, 110
base, 38
basic, 492
basket, 85
bath, 91, 224
battery, 464
BDSM, 2, 8, 15, 81, 131, 179, 201, 220, 243, 248, 259–262, 266, 267, 273, 275, 278, 280, 321, 332, 379–381, 387, 389, 392, 394, 396–399, 412, 419, 445, 447, 482
beauty, 48, 373, 451, 522, 539
bedrock, 28
bedroom, 520, 527
begin, 28, 78, 133, 314, 336, 492, 505, 525
beginning, 94, 112, 137, 283, 552
behavior, 44, 332, 351, 365, 492, 494, 495, 498, 511, 512
being, 23, 26, 29, 40, 44, 49, 52, 55, 105, 107, 118, 124, 127, 138, 145, 163, 169, 172, 174, 175, 180, 205, 207, 213, 217, 224, 267, 272, 273, 278, 288, 290, 297, 305, 310, 324, 337, 344, 345, 356, 397, 433, 435, 436, 471, 473, 479, 484, 495, 497, 500, 503, 514, 517, 531, 540
belief, 8–10, 242, 322
belonging, 15, 70, 350, 351, 412, 418, 420, 457, 517, 520, 525, 530, 540, 551
benefit, 86, 214, 310, 372, 446
bias, 321
bigender, 368
binary, 330, 368–370
biphobia, 353, 354, 356
bladder, 38, 49
bleeding, 122–124, 135
blend, 3
blog, 445
blood, 89, 95, 122, 135, 160, 306
bloodstream, 127
Bob, 264
bodily, 38, 44, 49, 52, 61, 125, 144, 156, 160, 289, 295, 306, 314, 464
body, 4, 10, 13, 16, 29, 30, 35, 36, 40, 44–49, 55, 57–61, 84–86, 90, 91, 94, 95, 105, 106, 112, 115, 122, 125, 127, 131, 135, 137, 149, 160, 169, 203–205, 207–210, 216, 224, 236, 240–242, 248, 252, 267, 289, 291, 298, 299, 305–310, 314, 336, 337, 343, 344, 352, 371, 372, 390, 397, 443, 455, 485, 520–522, 539–541, 551
bodywork, 305, 306

Index

bond, 14, 133, 213, 237, 248, 257, 267, 288, 319, 332, 337, 345, 531, 547
bondage, 283, 389–392, 399
bonding, 2, 368
book, 436–438, 533
bottle, 85
bound, 65, 228
boundary, 264
bowel, 38
brain, 2, 242, 492
break, 91, 122, 149, 154, 283, 457
breakdown, 130
breaking, 13, 15
breath, 91, 252, 314
breathing, 59, 61, 187, 216, 217, 223, 299, 314
breathwork, 46, 241, 298, 299, 306, 307
Brené Brown, 497, 527
bridge, 319
bruising, 122–124
build, 28, 71, 76, 112, 133, 180, 229, 308, 420
building, 26, 28, 72, 238, 344, 367, 401, 402, 409, 412, 414, 418, 419, 422, 428, 436, 475, 481, 521, 526, 531, 536, 541, 543

California, 465
camaraderie, 551
canal, 371, 372
capacity, 1, 58
care, 3, 23, 28, 35, 38, 86, 94, 104, 131, 133, 137, 144, 151–153, 159, 163, 174, 177, 205, 214–217, 220, 224, 226, 236, 273, 275, 288, 289, 292, 296, 305, 308, 310, 312, 314, 322, 329, 332, 340, 342, 344, 345, 347, 348, 350, 372, 392, 393, 395, 397, 408, 420, 425, 460, 522, 550
caregiver, 395
caretaking, 399
Carolee Schneemann, 16
case, 172, 236, 309, 470, 508, 530
catalyst, 520, 539
categorization, 354
catharsis, 244, 245, 247, 290, 305, 306, 328, 540
Cathy, 265
cause, 84, 127, 148, 149, 152, 154, 208, 467
caution, 85, 314, 468
celebration, 262, 337, 449, 522, 526, 527, 551
censorship, 450
center, 59, 90
challenge, 16–18, 26, 48, 175, 221, 330, 332, 334, 345, 353, 365, 379, 441, 446, 449, 479, 487, 524, 539
change, 1, 186, 189, 333
channel, 454, 455
character, 270
check, 28, 80, 84, 94, 172, 174, 177, 187, 220, 249, 283, 288, 342, 374, 391, 552
checkbox, 203
checklist, 147
chemical, 492
chest, 371
child, 395
choice, 93, 154, 160, 165, 226, 296, 306

cinema, 16
clarity, 67, 79, 205, 265, 465, 504
cleaning, 85, 144–148, 156–159, 165
cleanliness, 85, 127, 150, 158, 163, 166, 170, 172
cleanup, 84
client, 307, 309
closeness, 2, 91, 265, 368
cloud, 463
coercion, 180, 198, 374, 484
colitis, 135
collaboration, 133
collection, 461, 463
combat, 333, 356, 400, 542
combination, 74, 119, 296, 299, 393, 408, 415, 463, 507, 525
comedy, 447
comfort, 3, 24, 25, 35, 58, 76, 80, 83–86, 91–94, 102, 110, 112, 131, 133, 135, 136, 138, 147, 150, 165, 185, 203, 206, 207, 212, 261, 294, 298, 307, 309, 322, 328, 335, 336, 339, 344, 371–373, 375, 395, 422, 479, 516, 536
commitment, 23, 107, 147, 172, 174, 177, 186, 188, 200, 202, 223, 252, 283, 315, 323, 343, 348, 374, 381, 392, 394, 401, 420, 425, 471, 517, 522, 523, 544, 550, 552
communication, 2, 3, 7, 8, 10, 14, 17–20, 24, 28–31, 43, 46, 62–64, 73–75, 78, 79, 81, 83, 86, 91, 92, 94, 97, 99, 101, 107–109, 112, 115, 119, 124, 127, 129–131, 133–138, 141, 144, 150, 166, 169, 172, 174, 175, 177, 179–181, 183–189, 191, 194, 197, 202, 203, 205, 207, 210–213, 215–217, 219, 223, 236, 238, 241, 242, 247, 249, 257, 259, 262, 270, 278, 280, 281, 283, 285–289, 294, 296, 298, 299, 301, 307–310, 314, 315, 318, 319, 322–325, 328, 329, 331–335, 337–345, 348, 352, 353, 365, 366, 368, 370–373, 375, 376, 378, 379, 381, 384, 388, 389, 391, 392, 394, 395, 397, 400, 414, 418–420, 427, 436, 437, 439, 445–448, 450, 456, 460, 466, 468, 471, 475, 498, 511, 517, 519, 521, 523, 525, 527, 539–541, 547, 550, 552
community, 15, 70–72, 137, 201, 213, 256, 257, 297, 310, 311, 313, 322, 334, 351, 353, 354, 356, 370, 376, 400–403, 405, 408, 409, 412, 414, 418–422, 425, 428, 430–433, 445–447, 449, 451, 454, 457, 460, 462–464, 475, 476, 484, 487, 489, 492, 510, 517, 520–523, 525, 529–531, 540, 543–546, 550, 552
compassion, 43, 48, 61, 134, 200, 234, 252, 301, 370, 408, 502, 503, 523, 535

Index 559

compatibility, 154
compensation, 484
complexity, 244, 361, 370, 451, 481
component, 26, 55, 64, 75, 93, 131, 136, 154, 159, 169, 214, 220, 237, 267, 273, 275, 288, 296, 310, 332, 342, 372, 379, 392, 396, 516, 545
compression, 125
computer, 463
concentration, 61
concept, 96, 175, 200, 261, 373, 509, 539
concern, 78, 228, 356, 374
conclusion, 18, 20, 23, 31, 64, 83, 104, 109, 129, 131, 136, 147, 150, 153, 161, 166, 174, 202, 212, 236, 252, 280, 299, 325, 332, 337, 345, 368, 373, 412, 443, 457, 471, 473, 494, 500, 523, 526, 531, 536, 541, 543, 552
condition, 54
conditioning, 331
conduct, 68, 69, 464, 482
conduit, 29, 245
confidence, 3, 23, 35, 38, 52, 57, 81, 141, 159, 161, 177, 205, 215, 221, 240, 242, 265, 313, 352, 353, 420, 425, 438, 460, 522, 528
confidentiality, 228
configuration, 102
conflict, 199, 200, 352
confusion, 419, 469
connection, 5, 7, 9, 14–17, 20, 23, 26–30, 40, 43–46, 57, 58, 61, 65, 75, 78, 80, 81, 86, 89, 91, 92, 94, 101, 104, 105, 109, 112, 115, 119, 130, 131, 134, 138, 160, 163, 169, 180, 194, 206, 213, 217, 223, 226, 233, 236, 237, 239, 242, 244, 247–250, 252, 254, 256–259, 267, 268, 270, 273, 278, 285, 289, 290, 294, 299, 305, 308, 310, 314, 315, 328, 329, 332, 334, 337, 341–345, 348, 350, 352, 353, 356, 368, 370–376, 379, 388, 389, 392, 397, 400, 427, 438, 447, 448, 451, 460, 462, 506, 510, 517, 519, 521, 523–525, 527, 533, 536, 539, 546, 550, 552
connectivity, 327, 422
consciousness, 250, 314
consent, 2, 3, 7, 10, 14, 17–20, 28, 29, 31, 63, 101, 112, 115, 124, 131, 133, 136, 142–144, 171, 175–177, 183, 186–191, 197–202, 207, 228, 249, 260–262, 264–266, 270, 283, 284, 291, 294, 296, 305–309, 318, 322–325, 333, 337–340, 344, 352, 353, 357, 365, 368, 370–373, 376, 378, 381, 384, 387–389, 392, 394, 397, 403, 408, 414, 419, 422, 425, 436, 439, 441, 446–448, 450, 451, 454, 456, 464–474, 482–484,

487, 519, 521–523, 530, 540, 544, 550, 552
consideration, 131, 337, 341
consulting, 91
consumption, 484
contact, 91, 156
content, 415, 428, 448, 454, 457, 462, 484–487
context, 15–19, 27, 30, 46, 62, 73, 81, 99, 106, 122, 123, 131, 137, 143, 144, 154, 156, 178, 179, 183, 188, 194, 200, 205, 206, 208, 213, 221, 237, 242, 243, 245, 248, 254, 256, 257, 265, 268, 275, 278, 283, 284, 304, 307, 308, 310, 319, 322, 323, 330, 332, 334, 338, 341, 342, 353, 365, 368, 370, 388, 396–399, 421, 447, 455, 467, 469, 471, 492, 493, 497, 498, 501, 523, 525, 526, 547
continuation, 199
contraction, 53
contrast, 397, 465
control, 30, 38, 49, 53, 54, 79, 92, 135, 169, 178, 180, 226, 233, 252, 259, 262, 267, 285, 289, 330, 388, 395, 399, 492, 502, 527, 540
conversation, 18, 73, 74, 79, 83, 191, 339, 368, 427, 448, 451, 481, 484
coordination, 135, 248
coping, 133, 219, 221, 500, 501, 503, 505, 506, 512, 516
cord, 242
core, 2, 13, 38, 189, 382, 472, 523, 540, 551
cornerstone, 18, 24, 175, 183, 189, 197, 200, 211, 335, 366, 371, 464, 485
cost, 228
counselor, 217, 227, 516
counter, 8, 451, 540
couple, 76, 78, 112, 149, 171, 179, 209, 256, 259, 283, 310, 314, 331, 333, 339, 340, 344, 527
courage, 476
cover, 428, 454, 455, 458
covering, 436
cramping, 391
creativity, 344, 455, 534
creator, 454–457
credibility, 221
criminalization, 465, 469–471
criticism, 450
cuddling, 131, 216, 223, 273, 332, 516
culture, 2, 5, 7, 15, 17, 18, 72, 183, 197, 262, 333, 351, 422, 427, 447, 466, 479, 522, 530, 543, 544
curiosity, 43, 61, 86, 252, 347, 408, 522, 523, 551
cycle, 48, 474, 492, 493, 512

damage, 8, 119, 125–127, 137, 433
dance, 519
David, 265
David Wojnarowicz, 16
day, 28
debrief, 197
debriefing, 194–197, 223
decency, 468
decision, 173

Index 561

decrease, 489
dedication, 191
default, 321
defiance, 351, 527
degree, 26, 29, 379, 439, 474
delineation, 14, 395
demand, 425
depression, 132
depth, 97, 381, 387, 440, 446, 447, 456
desirability, 522
desire, 17, 28, 29, 31, 74, 242, 248, 264, 266, 270, 285, 319, 331, 343, 344, 395, 438, 448, 449, 451, 477, 493, 514
destigmatization, 350, 451, 521, 522, 541, 543, 552
destination, 517, 523, 550
detection, 129
development, 47, 221, 414, 493, 512
deviation, 474
dialogue, 8, 19, 20, 64, 73, 76, 94, 99, 130, 133, 167, 183, 186, 187, 197, 200, 203, 216, 217, 220, 232, 248, 261, 263, 286, 307, 318, 319, 322, 325, 378, 392, 439, 443, 450, 451, 471, 479, 519, 521, 530, 540, 543, 550
difference, 157, 209, 448
difficulty, 91
dignity, 487, 543
dildo, 112
direction, 267
discoloration, 122
discomfort, 9, 51, 53, 54, 61, 68, 74, 75, 84, 85, 91, 93, 94, 131, 135, 138, 185–187, 208, 209, 218, 233, 237, 249, 256, 259, 266, 288, 306, 332, 337, 344, 356, 372, 375, 391, 546
disconnection, 91
discourse, 332, 477, 479, 487
discovery, 15, 46, 72, 104, 205, 229, 234, 236, 248, 252, 289, 291, 295, 297, 299, 305, 308, 319, 353, 373, 400, 441, 451, 464, 497, 520, 521, 523, 526, 527, 536, 550–552
discretion, 419
discrimination, 136, 332–334, 353, 354, 356, 366, 474, 482, 483, 487–489, 520, 530, 543
discuss, 55, 70, 75, 81, 94, 171, 247, 265, 283, 288, 292, 331, 340, 342, 356, 374–376, 418, 420, 423, 428, 441, 447, 500
discussion, 16, 73, 74, 78, 133, 185, 259, 294, 412, 419, 429, 445, 462, 463, 474
disease, 135
disempowerment, 249
dismantling, 321, 520, 552
disposition, 10
disruption, 506
dissociation, 130, 132, 219
distinction, 387
distress, 23, 117, 130, 425, 433, 467, 483, 503, 506, 516
distribution, 448
diversity, 17, 356, 361, 370, 379, 402, 414, 444, 485, 489,

520, 522, 523, 536, 543
document, 463, 482, 501
documentary, 446, 447
domain, 544
dominance, 29, 265, 267, 284, 285, 330, 365, 379, 395
dominant, 15, 179, 266, 267, 272, 285, 330, 331, 399
domination, 16, 352
dopamine, 492–494
down, 138, 149, 210–212, 224, 261, 382, 457
drive, 492
dryness, 343, 344
duality, 388, 399
duration, 207
dynamic, 101, 182, 186, 188, 197, 249, 261, 264, 265, 270, 280, 285, 331, 342, 386, 390, 399, 533, 539
dysfunction, 40, 50, 54, 134, 135, 344, 516

E.L. James, 16
ease, 81, 84, 91, 94, 324, 373
edge, 281–283
education, 7, 8, 86, 89, 119, 127, 136, 138, 199, 280, 323, 334, 384, 401, 403, 407, 409, 412, 414, 418, 420, 422, 425–428, 433, 448, 451, 454, 456, 457, 460, 463, 464, 471, 475, 476, 479, 481, 489, 519–522, 531, 543–546
educator, 241, 454, 455, 457
effectiveness, 61, 101, 103, 155
efficacy, 289
effort, 183, 323, 344, 356, 499, 550

elasticity, 1, 306, 343, 344
element, 18, 160, 191, 381, 482
embarrassment, 9, 335, 345
embrace, 3, 11, 23, 46, 49, 61, 131, 205, 242, 243, 252, 256, 270, 291, 319, 334, 345, 350, 352, 353, 368–370, 379, 400, 420, 451, 454, 506, 520–524, 526, 535, 540, 541, 551, 552
emergence, 6, 423, 521
emotion, 47, 497
empathy, 75, 186, 223, 550
emphasis, 17, 322, 484
empowerment, 6, 7, 15, 18, 30, 31, 130, 131, 133, 134, 138, 180, 217, 223, 226, 233, 234, 242, 247–249, 252, 256, 283, 289, 291, 294–299, 305–307, 309, 314, 319, 330, 332, 342, 345, 352, 353, 371, 374, 439–441, 451, 500, 519–521, 523–527, 539, 540, 551
encounter, 3, 18, 43, 61, 106, 139, 168, 204, 213, 215, 226, 251, 267, 283, 302, 331, 342, 366, 372, 375, 376, 413, 419, 426, 450, 453, 468, 475, 495, 510, 523
encouragement, 213, 241, 530
end, 521, 522, 533, 550–552
endeavor, 221, 476, 479, 519
endurance, 58
energy, 224
engage, 2, 7, 18, 28, 30, 44, 49, 55, 70, 73, 76, 78, 91, 119, 124, 127, 130, 135, 142,

143, 161, 163, 167, 172,
175, 179, 181, 183, 187,
189, 197, 199, 200, 203,
212, 214, 215, 217, 218,
223, 236, 238, 240, 245,
249, 252, 254, 256, 259,
261–263, 265, 278, 289,
294, 299, 307, 309, 310,
314, 319, 322, 325, 328,
330, 331, 335, 336, 344,
366, 368, 370, 371,
373–376, 384, 392, 400,
408, 412, 419–421, 423,
425, 428, 438, 440, 441,
443, 446, 450, 451, 460,
463, 465, 469, 474, 482,
486, 487, 494, 510, 512,
519, 522, 524, 525, 527,
530, 536, 540, 541, 544,
545, 551
engagement, 8, 10, 20, 144, 200,
278, 425, 454, 472, 473,
530, 546, 550, 552
enhancement, 159, 289
enjoyment, 72, 77, 80, 84, 122, 136,
175, 262, 283, 321, 387,
433, 450, 462
enriching, 5, 7, 15, 18, 25, 31, 58, 61,
78, 144, 188, 203, 247,
253, 259, 278, 305, 315,
332, 341, 373, 394, 400,
414, 427, 460, 536
entertainment, 431, 448
entity, 463
entry, 418
environment, 20, 24, 28–30, 64, 70,
73, 79–83, 85, 86, 91, 108,
115, 131, 136, 137, 144,
146, 147, 150, 163, 169,

175, 178–180, 186, 188,
191, 192, 194, 200, 212,
214, 215, 217, 236, 239,
241, 242, 247, 259, 265,
269, 270, 272, 288, 289,
292, 294, 299, 305–308,
314, 315, 325, 331, 334,
335, 342, 346, 348, 356,
366, 371, 372, 379, 394,
395, 414, 418, 419, 422,
454, 458, 469, 472–474,
481, 482, 484, 489, 509,
511, 520, 521, 530, 539,
541, 543
equal, 154, 288
equality, 325
equation, 1, 18, 57, 74, 75, 105, 159,
180, 201, 207, 240, 243,
261, 266, 272, 296, 297,
344–346, 357, 371, 384,
395, 401, 403, 438, 464,
465, 469, 477, 482, 489,
492, 524–526, 539
essence, 142, 283
establishment, 81, 168, 296, 401
esteem, 57, 131, 236, 344, 520
Esther Perel, 344
estrogen, 343
euphoria, 130
evaluation, 124
event, 124, 132, 376, 416
evidence, 4, 420, 432, 437, 443
evolution, 6, 521
exacerbation, 135
examination, 447
example, 3, 29, 30, 48, 74, 131, 135,
185, 218, 219, 236, 248,
249, 256, 259, 266, 269,
272, 298, 314, 319, 322,

331, 342–344, 357, 374, 391, 447, 465, 527, 528, 530, 540
exchange, 15, 26, 178, 197, 248, 262–266, 278–280, 286, 289, 331, 462, 545
excitation, 346
excitement, 78, 215, 226, 245, 311
execution, 4
exercise, 55–58, 89, 217, 468
exhilaration, 231
expectation, 331
experience, 1–3, 5, 8, 9, 13, 14, 16, 18, 20, 21, 23–26, 30, 35, 38, 40–44, 46, 48, 54, 55, 57, 58, 60–65, 67, 68, 70, 72–74, 77–79, 81, 83–86, 89–95, 97–104, 106, 110–112, 115, 117, 119, 124, 127, 129–131, 133–139, 141, 142, 144, 147, 149–151, 154, 156, 159–161, 163, 172, 175, 177, 180–183, 185, 186, 188, 192, 194, 203–210, 213–219, 221, 223, 225, 226, 229, 231–234, 236, 237, 239, 240, 242–245, 247, 248, 250, 256, 257, 259, 261, 265, 268–270, 272, 273, 275, 277, 280, 285, 286, 288, 290, 293, 294, 296–299, 302, 306, 307, 310, 314, 315, 318, 319, 321–323, 325, 327, 329–333, 337, 340, 342, 344, 350, 352, 356, 359, 365, 367–369, 371–373, 375, 376, 379, 381, 385, 390–392, 394, 395, 397, 399, 412–414, 418, 420, 425, 427, 429–431, 436–438, 441, 444, 447, 449, 454, 463, 492, 493, 498, 500–503, 516, 519, 521, 523–526, 533–536, 539–541, 546, 547, 550–552
experiencing, 44, 52, 254, 290, 305, 306, 387, 496
experiment, 551
experimentation, 94, 102, 521
expert, 86, 428, 443
expertise, 89, 436
exploration, 2, 4, 6, 8, 10, 13, 15–17, 23, 28–31, 43, 46, 47, 49, 58, 60, 61, 64, 70, 72, 74, 78, 81, 84, 86, 89, 92, 104, 109, 110, 112, 115, 119, 133, 138, 142, 144, 147, 150, 166, 172, 177, 178, 180, 194, 197, 200, 203, 205, 210, 221, 223, 229, 231, 239, 244, 248, 252, 254, 259, 265, 268, 270, 272, 280, 284, 295, 298, 299, 305, 308, 311, 313, 319, 321, 323, 325, 327–330, 332, 334, 337–339, 341–344, 352, 365, 368–370, 372–374, 376, 379, 384, 389, 392, 395, 397, 400, 412, 414, 418, 420, 422, 427, 431, 433, 437–439, 441, 443, 446–448, 451, 457, 460, 462, 464, 468, 471, 474, 482, 484, 492, 494, 497,

506, 511, 517, 519–524,
526, 529, 533, 535, 536,
539, 546, 550–552
exposure, 134, 160, 487
expression, 2–7, 11, 17, 29, 84, 107,
109, 178, 205, 226, 231,
244, 245, 247, 268, 296,
297, 301, 309, 310, 321,
323, 341–343, 345, 350,
351, 353, 370, 376, 379,
389, 397, 400, 433, 447,
449, 451, 464, 465, 468,
471, 476, 477, 479, 481,
482, 484, 486, 487, 489,
509, 514, 517, 519, 522,
523, 527, 531, 541
extent, 180
extreme, 3, 17, 29, 281, 283, 289,
295, 297, 330, 351, 468
eye, 91, 425

fabric, 29
face, 44, 174, 255, 333, 370, 378,
420, 449, 467, 468, 482,
509, 510
factor, 248
fair, 484
fallout, 267
family, 333
fantasy, 25, 26, 29–31, 268–270
favor, 482
favoritism, 354
fear, 11, 24, 74, 79, 130, 136, 180,
213, 215–217, 226, 228,
239–242, 245, 248, 264,
318, 319, 324, 325, 332,
334, 353, 356, 366, 374,
419, 449, 474, 481, 482,
497, 522–524, 530, 543

feature, 444, 446
feedback, 75, 272, 375, 493
feel, 15, 18, 30, 47, 61, 73, 79, 81,
84, 91, 94, 105, 130, 133,
136, 137, 154, 178, 179,
183, 185, 194, 195, 197,
200, 212, 213, 216, 217,
219, 223, 226, 247, 248,
265, 267, 277, 278, 280,
287, 292, 294, 297, 307,
309, 318, 325, 331–333,
336, 342, 345, 356, 370,
373–375, 386, 403, 420,
443, 445, 479, 481, 483,
492, 497, 502, 510, 520,
525, 527, 530, 539, 540
feeling, 29, 233, 236, 331, 497
female, 33, 35, 368, 449
fetish, 397, 400
FetLife, 412, 418, 423, 429, 445, 462
fiction, 16, 431, 433
film, 5, 15, 446, 447
filtering, 412
finger, 94
fist, 4, 319
fister, 105, 419, 454, 525, 529–531,
551
Fisting, 119, 387, 519
fisting, 1–11, 13–31, 33–38, 41–44,
46–49, 52, 55, 57–59,
61–70, 72–76, 78, 79,
81–87, 89–94, 97–104,
107, 109–113, 115,
117–127, 129–131,
133–139, 141, 143, 144,
147–156, 159–161, 163,
165–167, 169–172, 174,
175, 177–181, 183, 185,
186, 188, 191, 192, 194,

197, 200, 203–221, 223,
224, 226, 227, 229,
232–234, 236–242,
244–259, 262, 264–270,
272, 273, 275, 278, 280,
281, 283–286, 288–299,
301–315, 317–319,
321–325, 327–345, 347,
348, 350, 352–357,
359–362, 365–376,
379–381, 383, 384, 386,
388–400, 405–410,
412–441, 443–477,
479–489, 491–498,
500–517, 519–531, 533,
535–548, 550–552
fit, 226, 525
fitness, 55, 57, 58
fixation, 517
flag, 182
flexibility, 58, 406
flogging, 393
floor, 38–40, 49–55, 95, 134, 135, 306, 343, 344
flow, 85, 89, 95, 290, 306
fluid, 186, 189, 395
fluidity, 330, 365
focus, 60, 61, 68, 91, 96, 137, 233, 283, 290, 291, 306, 314, 350, 371, 406, 443, 444, 452, 461, 462, 469, 483, 531, 539
following, 20, 21, 23, 38, 42, 46, 50, 54–56, 60, 63, 65, 69, 71, 77, 81, 82, 87, 88, 90, 96, 101, 104, 105, 108–110, 120, 121, 123, 126, 133, 140, 143, 146, 147, 152, 153, 158, 160, 164, 165,

167, 168, 170, 173, 177, 179, 185, 190, 191, 193–196, 202, 209, 216, 222, 237–240, 244, 246, 251, 253, 256, 258, 261, 264, 266, 269, 277, 279, 280, 282, 283, 285, 288, 293, 303, 304, 307, 309, 325, 331, 339, 340, 342, 344, 367, 374, 380, 389, 392, 393, 406, 407, 411, 415, 421, 434, 435, 454, 457, 458, 461–463, 469, 470, 483, 492, 494, 496, 508, 511, 516, 533–535, 537, 548
force, 122, 393
foreplay, 209, 336
form, 2, 4, 6, 7, 49, 84, 107, 189, 250–252, 290, 299, 310, 314, 328, 333, 342, 351, 365, 393, 395, 397, 399, 433, 447–449, 465, 468, 482, 487, 523, 527, 534
format, 415, 428, 510
forum, 530
foundation, 33, 81, 99, 107, 133, 135, 142, 147, 177, 183, 221, 236, 237, 283, 286, 322, 328, 420, 519, 547
framework, 2, 18, 65, 142, 179, 208, 249, 259, 283, 292, 321, 330, 353, 383, 385, 448, 449, 468, 482
friction, 84, 93, 110, 154, 160, 165
fulfillment, 323, 524, 536
fullness, 13, 29, 95, 267, 328, 388, 393, 539
function, 33, 36, 38, 57, 105, 125,

Index 567

343, 357, 372, 401, 464, 477, 482, 524, 539
fundamental, 38, 41, 61, 69, 75, 78, 112, 144, 150, 161, 166, 215, 325, 527
future, 75, 197, 224, 225, 288, 481, 489, 519–523

gap, 443
gateway, 550
gathering, 461
gay, 351
gender, 17, 325, 329–332, 365, 368, 371, 372, 441, 485
genderqueer, 368
generation, 299
genital, 149
genre, 431, 438
Germany, 467
gesture, 75
giver, 13, 15, 92, 99, 102, 112, 379
gland, 36
glass, 85
glide, 154
glove, 160
glycerin, 154
go, 180, 270
goal, 78, 81, 84, 127, 156, 180, 194, 200, 213, 280, 403, 506
gratification, 439
gratitude, 294
grooming, 148
ground, 217, 241, 530
groundwork, 259
group, 91, 283, 310–313, 354, 376, 456, 509, 510
growth, 15, 17, 46, 61, 131, 141, 148, 223, 225, 236, 244, 252, 254, 257, 297, 313,
315, 319, 414, 420, 425, 441, 497, 517, 520, 523–526, 533, 535, 536, 550
guidance, 52, 86–89, 139, 210, 213, 229, 309, 419, 454, 516
guide, 72, 84, 99, 190, 210, 227, 266, 285, 306, 386, 430, 433, 460, 474, 519, 521, 522, 533, 536, 550–552
guideline, 167
guilt, 10, 502

hair, 148
hallmark, 399
hammock, 38, 49
hand, 1, 3, 4, 13, 75, 84, 85, 92–95, 99, 102–104, 133, 137, 151–153, 180, 203, 208, 240, 267, 390, 391, 393, 454, 539
harm, 8, 22, 118, 119, 127, 136, 138, 182, 208, 210, 213, 283, 387, 464, 467, 469–471, 512, 513
hatred, 353
haven, 409
head, 91
healing, 30, 131, 134, 205, 208, 236, 252, 289, 291, 294, 295, 297–299, 302, 305, 306, 308, 313–315, 440, 497, 509, 527, 540
health, 3, 20, 21, 23, 44, 49, 50, 52, 54, 55, 86, 133–136, 139, 144, 151, 159–161, 163, 166, 167, 169, 172–174, 217, 275, 305, 310, 367, 374, 379, 430, 432, 433,

436, 441, 443, 444, 451, 452, 455, 456, 466, 472, 483, 497, 516, 517
healthcare, 54, 91, 135, 174, 408, 433–436
help, 15, 23, 24, 30, 46, 52, 61, 65, 66, 74, 83, 85, 90, 91, 93, 94, 131, 133, 135–137, 139–141, 147, 154, 160, 166, 180, 209, 213–217, 219, 220, 225–229, 238, 241, 287, 288, 299, 306–308, 310, 311, 313, 315, 318, 322, 324, 332, 342, 366, 374, 412, 418–420, 428, 431, 444, 448, 454, 463, 483–486, 496, 497, 501–503, 509, 511, 516, 517, 524, 525, 530, 539, 540, 552
helplessness, 130
hesitation, 187, 328, 366
heterosexuality, 321, 333
history, 6, 7, 130, 133–135, 172, 180, 217, 240, 294
hold, 91, 265, 449
home, 201
homophobia, 353, 354, 356
hormone, 2
host, 419, 423, 429, 455, 462
humiliation, 387
humor, 447, 455
hydration, 332
hygiene, 3, 7, 21, 23, 85, 86, 110, 112, 127, 129, 147–153, 159, 163–172, 307, 332, 367, 374, 456, 458
hyper, 219

idea, 17, 288, 403, 531
ideal, 154
identification, 180
identifying, 65, 294, 433, 464, 501, 503, 529
identity, 29, 236, 351–353, 371, 372, 447, 449, 451, 517, 525, 526, 529–531
image, 47–49, 57, 106, 135, 236, 240, 307, 343, 344, 352, 371, 502, 520, 539, 540
imagery, 449, 450
imagination, 29
impact, 44, 47, 125, 132, 133, 135, 160, 165, 180, 226, 292, 294, 299, 343, 392–394, 450, 465, 473, 498
implementation, 79
importance, 2, 3, 16–19, 28, 57, 68, 70, 74, 75, 79, 89, 94, 97, 107, 109, 110, 139, 140, 151, 153, 156, 159, 161, 166, 167, 171, 172, 174, 175, 177, 184, 186, 189, 194, 203, 207, 209, 210, 221, 226, 237, 260, 264, 267, 272, 275, 283, 285, 291, 292, 304, 307, 309, 313, 324, 333, 339, 341, 344, 345, 348, 350, 353, 372–374, 386, 387, 418, 419, 425, 436, 437, 439, 445, 447, 448, 450, 455, 456, 460, 467–469, 471, 472, 483, 519, 522, 523, 529, 540, 544, 550
in, 1–5, 7–10, 15–21, 23–31, 33, 36–38, 43, 44, 46, 48–50, 52, 54, 55, 57, 59, 61, 62,

Index

64, 70, 72–76, 78, 79, 81, 82, 84–87, 89–94, 99, 101, 102, 104, 106, 107, 109–111, 115, 117, 119, 120, 122–125, 127, 130–137, 139, 141–144, 147, 149–153, 155, 156, 160, 161, 163–167, 169, 171, 172, 174–176, 178–192, 194, 197–203, 205–207, 210, 212–224, 226, 227, 229, 231, 233, 236–245, 247–249, 252, 254, 256, 257, 259–270, 273, 275, 278, 280, 281, 283, 285–291, 293–299, 301, 302, 304–310, 313–315, 319, 321–325, 328–333, 335–345, 347, 348, 351–354, 356, 359, 361, 365–376, 379–381, 383, 384, 387, 389, 391, 392, 394–397, 399–401, 405, 406, 408–410, 412, 414, 415, 418–422, 425, 427–433, 436–441, 443, 445–451, 454–458, 460–466, 468, 469, 471–474, 476, 477, 479–487, 489, 492, 494, 497, 500–503, 506, 509–513, 515–517, 519–531, 533, 536, 539–541, 543–547, 550–552

inability, 135, 218
inadequacy, 352, 540
inclusion, 449
inclusivity, 72, 401, 403, 485
incorporating, 50, 84, 92, 111, 165, 268, 269, 290, 307, 310, 334, 343, 344, 380, 390, 392, 537, 538, 551
incorporation, 110, 341, 440, 521, 536
increase, 89, 90, 135, 137, 170, 306
indecency, 482
indicator, 138, 208, 209, 337
individual, 25, 47, 48, 67, 130–132, 134, 135, 137, 172, 198, 203, 206, 219, 220, 243, 276, 298, 307, 314, 370, 375, 395, 397, 420, 422, 477, 482, 506, 516, 533, 536, 546
industry, 486
infection, 86, 110, 127, 129, 137, 149, 152, 170–172
influence, 44, 93, 102, 106, 135, 226, 248, 301, 317, 325, 344, 371, 373, 464, 469, 483
information, 137, 228, 322, 405, 409, 412, 419, 420, 432, 444, 446, 454, 462, 477, 530, 544, 545
injury, 2, 7, 24, 57, 84, 85, 93, 95, 120, 127, 134, 135, 137, 138, 148, 152, 205, 208–210, 240, 309, 328, 337, 465
innocence, 395
innovation, 534
inquiry, 441
insecurity, 374
insertion, 1, 3, 84, 94–96, 110, 160, 203, 209, 266, 390, 539
insight, 3, 6, 63, 180, 302, 449, 492, 498

inspiration, 312
instance, 16, 44, 74, 76, 133–135, 160, 213, 217, 219, 248, 309, 330, 331, 333, 344, 352, 356, 371, 373, 395, 423, 424, 464, 465, 469, 482, 527, 530
instruction, 415
insurance, 228
integration, 298, 314, 389, 390, 525, 550
intelligence, 260, 262
intensity, 137, 207, 233, 248, 283, 342, 350, 387, 399
intent, 4
intention, 4, 236, 244, 305, 308, 314, 315
intentionality, 202, 265, 289, 291, 301, 312, 314
interaction, 175, 180, 197, 289, 418, 530
intercourse, 53, 323, 333
interest, 179, 213, 333
internet, 405, 412, 432, 443
interplay, 7, 17, 29, 33, 42, 233, 234, 238, 242–244, 249, 259, 265, 273, 284, 329, 344, 371, 379, 385, 387, 394, 400, 477
interpretation, 467
intersection, 265, 313, 332, 341, 343, 368, 370, 471, 474, 484, 486
intersectionality, 353
intervention, 123, 495
intimacy, 2–5, 7, 9, 14, 16–18, 20, 23, 24, 28, 29, 31, 44, 46, 47, 49, 61, 63, 70, 73, 76, 78, 80, 81, 84, 86, 89, 91, 92, 94, 102, 104, 109, 115, 119, 127, 131, 133, 134, 138, 147, 150, 161, 163, 166, 167, 172, 179, 180, 186, 188, 197, 205, 206, 215, 217, 221, 231, 236, 237, 239, 244, 247, 249, 250, 254, 257–259, 262, 265, 268, 270, 278, 280, 286, 288, 294, 297, 299, 305, 310, 313, 319, 323, 324, 328–333, 337, 341–345, 348, 350, 352, 353, 365, 367, 368, 372, 374, 388, 389, 395, 397, 400, 428, 438, 439, 441, 445, 446, 448–451, 460, 461, 464, 474, 487, 489, 516, 517, 519–527, 536, 540, 550–552
introspection, 505, 506
investment, 248
invitation, 521
involvement, 188, 472
Iran, 468
irritation, 148, 149, 154
isolation, 311, 400, 420, 446, 487, 497
issue, 85, 93, 182, 443
item, 157

Jamie, 78, 112, 236, 242, 294, 339
jaw, 91
jealousy, 374
John Gottman, 73
Jordan, 340
journal, 463, 501
journaling, 550

Index 571

journey, 15, 20, 21, 23, 26, 29–31, 35, 43, 49, 57, 58, 61, 64, 66–68, 70, 72, 78, 81, 84, 86, 89, 92, 94, 99, 104, 109, 112, 131, 137, 138, 153, 186, 197, 207, 209, 217, 226, 227, 229, 236, 239, 242, 244, 247, 248, 254, 278, 289, 294, 297, 299, 305, 310, 314, 323, 325, 329, 334, 337, 343, 353, 397, 400, 406, 408, 412, 414, 420, 433, 436, 446, 457, 460, 463, 464, 481, 497, 500, 503, 509, 513, 517, 519–523, 525–527, 529, 531, 533–536, 541, 543, 546, 550–552
joy, 15, 306, 474, 527
judgment, 24, 48, 61, 79, 213, 217, 227, 228, 241, 248, 288, 325, 332, 333, 366, 374, 419, 433, 481, 522, 529, 539, 543
Judith Butler, 17
jurisdiction, 482

Kegel, 53, 135
key, 1, 4, 19, 21, 23, 33, 36, 43, 68, 75, 84, 86, 101, 115, 142, 155, 163, 184, 191, 194, 203, 263, 270, 278, 281, 311, 315, 337, 340, 368, 381, 389, 392–394, 397, 405, 432, 438, 441, 443, 446, 463, 519, 547
kind, 197
kindness, 48

kink, 2, 8, 15, 131, 139, 220, 243, 259, 260, 262, 275, 280, 283, 321, 322, 332, 383, 384, 389, 396, 397, 400–403, 412, 419, 444, 445, 447, 455–457, 462
knowledge, 3, 70, 89, 240, 313, 405, 408, 420, 422, 425, 427, 428, 430, 432, 433, 436, 443, 446, 454–456, 460, 464, 519, 522, 530, 544, 545

lack, 2, 7, 8, 17, 48, 122, 249, 425, 443, 469, 484, 487
landscape, 25, 191, 203, 214, 231, 234, 236, 323, 327, 328, 342, 344, 345, 464, 466, 469, 477, 479, 482, 486, 487, 521
language, 187, 270, 287
latex, 110, 149, 154, 160
law, 464–466, 484
lead, 2, 3, 7–9, 17, 30, 44, 46, 51, 53, 54, 57, 75, 85, 89, 90, 93, 104, 105, 117, 120, 125, 127, 130, 131, 135, 136, 149, 179, 197, 233, 244, 248, 249, 254, 257, 267, 297, 305, 314, 324, 328, 331, 335, 341, 343–345, 348, 352–354, 362, 365–367, 373, 374, 388, 391, 400, 418, 419, 422, 425, 433, 462, 465, 469, 483, 487, 489, 493, 494, 497, 506, 517, 520, 522–525, 539–541, 551
leading, 10, 14, 16, 23, 48, 73, 122,

130, 131, 151, 209, 218,
  236, 239, 248, 290, 298,
  299, 306, 310, 318, 321,
  325, 333, 355, 356, 368,
  393, 419, 441, 443, 450,
  465, 497, 500, 520, 524,
  527, 530, 539, 540, 552
learning, 15, 53, 236, 288, 406, 419,
  429, 430, 462, 463, 510,
  517, 522, 535, 536,
  544–546, 551
legality, 464, 467
legislation, 483
lens, 1, 13, 103, 234, 250, 252, 278,
  290, 313, 330, 446–448,
  451, 465, 470, 512
levator, 49
level, 2, 14, 91, 142, 160, 211, 231,
  232, 248, 261, 266, 267,
  283, 287, 331, 344, 352,
  367, 395, 523, 524, 527,
  539
liberation, 4, 16, 247, 267, 306, 351
library, 433, 460–464
lie, 519
life, 25, 220, 268, 368, 506, 551
lifestyle, 55
light, 79, 393
lighting, 30, 85, 136, 259, 269, 314
likelihood, 120, 129, 135, 172
limit, 319, 450
line, 133, 328
Lisa and Mark, 343
list, 436
listening, 75, 183–186, 205, 210,
  287, 289, 356, 530
literature, 2, 5, 15, 16, 136, 137, 322,
  352, 408, 430, 432, 433,
  438–441, 443, 461, 545,
  546
location, 412
look, 438, 447, 520, 539
loop, 75, 493
loss, 125, 127
love, 17, 109, 352, 374, 455, 519,
  523, 526–528, 551, 552
lubricant, 84, 85, 93, 110, 112, 154,
  155, 165
lubrication, 74, 85, 92, 94, 110, 135,
  154, 307, 344, 371, 374,
  454
lying, 224

mainstream, 15, 16, 450, 483, 484
maintenance, 401
makeup, 130
making, 2, 26, 119, 130, 148, 154,
  173, 228, 283, 344, 420,
  428, 447, 448, 454, 455
male, 36–38, 105, 351, 368
man, 331
management, 117, 119, 159, 172,
  206, 207
manifest, 50, 54, 132, 135, 194, 219,
  233, 240, 245, 259, 330,
  333, 366, 379, 387, 399,
  474, 487, 529
manifestation, 267
manner, 5, 7, 8, 215, 310, 352, 379,
  394, 400, 425, 428, 474,
  487, 540
marriage, 468
masochism, 387–389
massage, 306
material, 159, 160, 428, 429
matter, 160, 450
meal, 224

Index 573

means, 3, 14, 17, 18, 29, 137, 228, 267, 285, 295, 296, 299, 306, 307, 309, 323, 330, 356, 357, 367, 395, 399, 431, 441, 451, 472, 540
measure, 172
mechanism, 63, 261
meditation, 60, 90, 233, 241, 250–252, 290, 314
medium, 231, 247, 295, 428, 438
meet, 418, 531
menopause, 343
mentor, 419
mentoring, 420–422
message, 75, 356
metaphor, 439
method, 308, 395
Mia V.'s, 437
mind, 30, 44–46, 106, 111, 155, 252, 299, 305, 308, 336, 429
Mindfulness, 216
mindfulness, 43, 46, 90, 104, 135, 207, 217, 233, 241, 242, 250, 252, 290, 291, 298, 307, 314, 315, 511, 514, 519
mindset, 90, 546
miscommunication, 80
misconception, 2, 8–10, 322, 330
misinformation, 420, 487, 529, 546
misinterpretation, 450
misrepresentation, 7
misunderstanding, 353, 378, 400, 474, 519
mode, 321
model, 44, 487
moment, 65, 135, 248, 342, 461, 550
monogamy, 189, 191

month, 463
mood, 85, 91, 136, 186
motif, 16
motivation, 65, 526
move, 481, 523, 543
movement, 99–101, 103, 125, 305, 390, 481, 485, 539, 541
multimedia, 462, 463
multitude, 343
muscle, 53, 91, 135, 306
music, 28, 30, 85, 91, 136, 259, 294, 314
myriad, 2, 102, 321
myth, 2, 322

nail, 151–153
narrative, 296, 323, 451, 526, 540, 546, 550
nature, 2, 5, 18, 24, 43, 91, 130, 186, 188, 198, 201, 205, 234, 245, 261, 290, 314, 446, 469, 492, 497, 498, 500, 506, 519, 535
necessity, 14, 465
need, 63, 74, 75, 159, 183, 209, 210, 265, 266, 283, 288, 346, 391, 401, 450, 477, 496
neglect, 132
negligence, 465
negotiation, 2, 179, 194, 260–266, 330, 387, 447
nerve, 125–127, 137, 226
Netherlands, 465, 467
network, 49, 125, 419, 435, 436, 513, 520, 523, 529
networking, 412, 414, 419, 445
neurotransmitter, 492
newfound, 236, 331, 528
niche, 13, 450

nitrile, 110, 160
no, 147
non, 16, 75, 79, 80, 136, 142–144, 188–191, 227, 283, 288, 294, 321, 330, 338–341, 368–370, 373, 374, 391, 443, 444, 451, 453, 454, 543
normalization, 520
notion, 9, 533
novel, 344, 372, 551
nuance, 16
number, 159, 444, 463
numbness, 219, 391
nurturing, 26, 46, 186, 215, 395, 522, 547, 552

object, 397
obscenity, 465, 468, 482
offense, 482
offer, 59, 84, 139, 154, 228, 307, 311, 410, 419, 423, 424, 431, 433, 444, 446, 458, 474, 483, 510, 544, 551
oil, 149, 154
one, 1, 3, 10, 15, 23, 30, 58, 61, 62, 64, 74–76, 85, 89, 115, 134, 171, 179, 180, 186, 207–210, 216, 217, 220, 224, 229, 234, 241, 242, 248, 249, 256, 261, 273, 278, 283, 289, 296–299, 306, 311, 313, 327, 330, 333, 343, 352, 356, 370, 373, 376, 399, 420, 439, 455, 497, 498, 500, 519, 520, 522, 523, 525, 530, 539, 540, 544

openness, 92, 191, 239, 329, 352, 373, 420
opportunity, 3, 296, 313, 372, 400, 428, 457, 486, 530, 536, 552
option, 307
orgasm, 492
orientation, 221
ostracism, 474, 487
other, 1, 28, 49, 52, 53, 74–76, 79, 81, 86, 127, 130, 134, 137, 138, 142, 156, 160, 172, 174, 179, 180, 187, 191, 197, 200, 206, 208, 211, 213, 216, 217, 223, 226, 227, 240, 248, 249, 259, 272, 273, 278, 287, 288, 312, 321, 324, 342, 344, 356, 366, 367, 374, 389, 390, 393, 395, 400, 412, 419, 422, 449, 454, 468, 471, 492, 500, 503, 506, 517, 521, 523, 527, 543, 551, 552
overview, 68, 464
overwhelm, 132
ownership, 540
oxytocin, 2

pace, 399, 428
page, 376
pain, 9, 24, 53, 54, 74, 78, 79, 91, 134, 135, 138, 205–211, 233, 242–244, 264, 266, 306, 309, 328, 337, 368, 387, 394, 399, 520
painting, 449
panic, 130, 218
paradox, 142

Index 575

paramount, 20, 21, 23, 30, 31, 48, 79, 81, 117, 136, 144, 159, 163, 183, 197, 210, 213, 237, 262, 266, 283, 307, 319, 323, 328, 335, 342, 375, 502, 519, 544
parenthood, 341–343
parenting, 341, 342
part, 3, 4, 36, 43, 81, 85, 205–207, 242, 244, 264, 277, 397, 400, 436, 471, 509, 525
participant, 21, 210, 217–219, 283, 465, 530
participation, 175, 525, 550
partner, 4, 10, 29, 30, 43, 74–77, 86, 91, 94, 95, 97, 101, 127, 130, 131, 133, 151, 160, 171, 179, 180, 203, 205, 209, 214, 216, 217, 219, 236, 237, 242, 248, 249, 256, 263, 266, 267, 272, 276, 278, 283, 285, 319, 328, 330, 331, 333, 337, 340, 356, 373, 375, 376, 390, 391, 395, 399, 463, 525, 527, 539
party, 340
past, 47, 119, 130, 133, 180, 213, 218, 236, 239, 288, 294, 296, 301, 302, 314, 337, 371, 392, 441
patch, 154
path, 72, 229, 550
pathway, 234, 236, 243, 259, 438, 460, 520, 526
patience, 49, 75, 99, 107–109, 343
pause, 63, 74, 75, 80, 133, 216, 217, 219, 288, 375, 391
peer, 89, 310, 312, 313, 420–422, 509–511, 517
pelvis, 38
penetration, 9, 113, 248, 298, 333, 399
penis, 36, 105, 344
people, 10, 17, 333, 423, 540
perception, 5, 6, 17, 47, 48, 208, 333, 470, 474–476, 483, 497
performance, 236, 449
period, 6, 205
person, 62, 75, 98, 130, 207, 216, 233, 241, 248, 256, 314, 406, 413, 428, 472, 527, 540
perspective, 2, 5, 17, 44, 243, 250, 252, 268, 330, 377, 429, 449, 454, 469, 516, 540
phenomenon, 4, 299
philosophy, 254
photography, 449–451
physical, 2, 3, 5, 8, 13, 15–18, 20–24, 29, 40, 42–44, 46, 50, 52, 55, 57, 58, 62, 65, 68, 70, 73, 74, 78, 81–83, 86, 89–92, 94, 101, 104, 105, 109, 112, 117, 119, 132–134, 137, 138, 142, 144, 160, 163, 166, 167, 169, 172, 175, 180, 186, 188, 194, 197, 200, 203, 205, 208, 210–213, 215–218, 220, 221, 231, 233, 237, 238, 240, 242, 245, 247, 248, 250, 252, 254, 259, 265, 267, 273, 275, 278, 280, 290, 291, 294, 296–299, 305–308, 313, 314, 317, 327, 332, 336, 341–345, 348, 350,

359, 360, 367, 372, 373,
379, 381, 387, 388,
390–393, 397, 399, 400,
405, 425, 433, 437–439,
445, 447, 449, 456, 463,
470, 472, 473, 483–485,
492, 493, 497, 502, 516,
519, 520, 524, 539, 540,
545, 551
physicality, 16, 252, 295, 328, 352,
447, 539
physiology, 33, 35, 36, 38, 103, 530
picture, 333
place, 85, 219
plan, 197, 273, 283
planning, 83
platform, 430, 445, 456
play, 25, 26, 30, 38, 44, 85, 111, 112,
125, 135, 154, 160, 179,
187, 192, 194, 200–202,
206, 213, 215, 216, 219,
243, 247, 249, 257, 259,
261, 263, 269, 275, 277,
278, 280–283, 288, 299,
301, 310, 329–332, 340,
375, 380, 381, 387, 389,
390, 392–397, 399, 400,
425, 443, 447, 448, 451,
454, 471–474, 483, 486,
509, 517, 522, 529, 541,
551
playing, 28, 33, 85, 294, 314, 395
playlist, 91
pleasure, 3–5, 16, 17, 20, 26, 33, 36,
38, 41–47, 49, 57, 58, 61,
68, 70, 79, 92–95, 97, 99,
102, 104–106, 110, 112,
113, 119, 125, 127, 129,
134, 135, 147, 154,
206–208, 213, 215, 233,
242–245, 248, 249, 252,
286, 290, 291, 295, 299,
314, 322, 323, 327–329,
331, 333, 336, 342–345,
348, 359, 361, 365, 367,
368, 370–372, 380, 381,
387, 389, 392–394, 397,
399, 427, 436, 446,
449–451, 454, 464, 474,
489, 494, 500, 503, 506,
514, 515, 520, 521, 523,
527, 536, 539, 540, 544,
550, 551
plenty, 94
point, 105, 357
polyamory, 189, 338
polycule, 376
polyisoprene, 154
polyurethane, 154
pornography, 484–487
portrayal, 7, 17, 439, 447, 449, 450,
485
pose, 21, 514
position, 400
positioning, 17, 92, 94, 454
positivity, 48, 61, 131, 307, 310, 455,
521, 522, 539–541, 551
possessiveness, 374
post, 26, 194, 220, 265, 267, 273,
288, 315, 371, 418
postpartum, 343
potential, 2, 3, 5, 7, 17, 18, 24, 35,
37, 38, 44, 58, 66, 74, 78,
84, 91, 92, 103, 106, 107,
109, 119, 122, 125, 127,
129–131, 135, 137, 138,
142, 146, 153, 156, 160,
169, 171, 172, 175,

Index 577

178–180, 182, 186, 192, 194, 208–210, 221, 223, 237, 240, 249, 250, 252–254, 257, 259, 265, 273, 283, 284, 289–292, 294, 295, 297, 302, 305, 307, 308, 312, 314, 319, 328, 329, 337, 338, 340, 341, 352, 357, 370, 371, 381, 387, 391–393, 395, 401, 411, 418, 422, 433, 450, 464–466, 469–472, 477, 479, 483–485, 492, 494, 506, 513, 515, 517
power, 14, 15, 17, 29, 178–180, 192–194, 244, 248, 249, 260–266, 273, 275, 277–280, 284, 286–289, 295, 297, 306, 308, 329–332, 365, 379, 381, 388, 395, 397, 399, 419, 448, 449, 472, 474
powerlessness, 296, 298
practice, 1, 3–10, 13, 15, 17, 29, 30, 38, 59, 61, 64, 75, 80, 89, 92, 99, 101, 104, 107, 109, 114, 119, 122, 124, 131, 133, 137, 151, 161, 163, 177, 180, 186, 197, 223, 225, 231, 234, 250, 252, 254, 265, 266, 281, 287–290, 297–299, 305, 307–309, 313–315, 319, 321, 322, 328, 330, 332–334, 337, 340, 342, 345, 352, 370, 371, 373, 375, 381, 383, 390, 395, 397, 400, 405, 407, 412, 414, 420, 422, 425, 427, 430, 433, 436–438, 441, 443, 444, 446–448, 457, 460, 464, 474, 479, 480, 484, 485, 487, 494, 497, 500, 502, 503, 506, 511, 515, 517, 520–523, 525, 527, 539–541, 544, 546, 547, 550, 551
pre, 63, 131, 135, 136, 392
precaution, 81
prejudice, 353, 487–489
premise, 305
preparation, 8, 17, 23, 25, 26, 85, 86, 90, 122, 150, 153, 204, 210, 309, 314, 336, 337, 344
presence, 1, 250, 296, 315, 354, 465, 482, 524
present, 5, 18, 61, 64, 106, 190, 192, 201, 216, 217, 273, 277, 285, 290, 298, 337, 338, 371, 410, 425, 440, 448, 507, 538, 546
pressure, 13, 99–101, 103, 122, 125, 135, 331, 388, 510
prevent, 21, 84, 147, 154, 160, 166, 170, 174, 182, 319, 375, 391, 517
prevention, 119, 120, 129, 171
pride, 551
principle, 2, 73, 89, 94, 472, 544
priority, 155
privacy, 83, 467, 477, 479, 482
probability, 159
process, 34, 62, 83, 91, 92, 131, 133, 139, 140, 175, 176, 184, 186, 189, 191, 194, 197, 200, 212, 217, 218, 220, 223, 225, 227, 236, 241,

247–249, 252, 257, 259,
266, 272, 273, 287, 289,
294, 296–299, 302, 303,
305–309, 314, 315, 322,
332, 336, 386, 420, 430,
433, 443, 460, 464, 484,
508, 509, 511, 520, 522,
525, 527, 533, 539, 540,
545
processing, 297, 302, 304
procreation, 6
product, 384
production, 484
professional, 52, 54, 61, 86–89, 91,
133, 139–141, 214, 215,
217, 220, 221, 226–229,
455, 457, 495–497, 528
profit, 451, 454
progress, 525, 551
progression, 74, 137
prostate, 36, 105
protection, 160, 482, 483
provider, 135, 433, 435
psychoanalysis, 17
psychology, 290, 382, 441
public, 5, 200, 202, 467, 468,
474–476, 482
purpose, 267
pursuit, 487, 494
push, 139, 280, 471

quality, 84, 141, 344

range, 110, 117, 130, 139, 198, 208,
215, 218, 231, 245, 302,
305, 311, 335, 336, 395,
397, 428, 430, 458, 471,
495, 521, 536, 544
re, 133, 330

reach, 85
reaction, 130
read, 463
reader, 16
readiness, 23, 26, 281, 357
reading, 136, 288, 463
reality, 2, 29, 30, 137, 322, 448
realm, 13, 30, 61, 79, 86, 104, 107,
117, 159, 188, 192, 197,
200, 223, 233, 244, 262,
278, 308, 321, 323, 345,
365, 381, 389, 392, 451,
460, 469, 482, 519, 529,
533, 544, 546
reapplication, 154
reassurance, 131, 265, 288, 294, 332,
374, 406, 445
receiver, 13, 15, 92, 99, 102, 112,
379, 393
receiving, 95, 97, 151, 160, 283, 328,
333
recipient, 105
reciprocity, 10
reclaiming, 29, 289, 296, 297, 308,
309, 314, 353, 441, 492,
520, 540
reclamation, 30, 289, 291, 295, 298,
306, 351
recognition, 357, 429, 483
recovery, 224, 289, 305, 461, 496,
497, 506–509
rectum, 49, 105, 539
Reddit, 418, 462
reduction, 22, 118, 119, 136–138,
511–513
reflection, 64, 65, 203, 218, 278,
503–506, 516, 525, 526,
545, 550
regimen, 172, 174

region, 125
regression, 395
regulation, 226, 257
rejection, 136, 213, 237, 319
relation, 372
relationship, 2, 26, 29, 44, 48, 55, 73, 74, 89, 130, 183, 188, 189, 191, 197, 199, 206, 221, 223, 226, 237, 238, 240–242, 244, 248, 259, 280, 298, 306, 314, 317, 319, 334, 335, 337, 342, 343, 348, 353, 368, 375, 376, 419, 492, 500, 503, 504, 506, 509, 514–517, 527, 540
relaxation, 45, 51–55, 59, 81, 85, 89–91, 95, 131, 135, 136, 209, 216, 223, 226, 290, 306, 335, 336, 386
release, 2, 44, 244–247, 289–291, 299, 305–308, 314, 328, 393, 448, 493, 527, 540
reliability, 221
reliance, 443
relief, 290
reluctance, 324, 373, 419, 497
reminder, 353, 447
removal, 154
repertoire, 236, 310, 341, 400, 520, 521, 525, 527, 536–538, 551
repository, 443
representation, 15–18, 448–451, 485, 487
reprisal, 481
request, 331
research, 68–70, 432, 436, 441, 443, 446, 545

researcher, 73, 497
resentment, 249
resilience, 57, 89, 131, 141, 221–223, 254, 256, 257, 308, 342, 500, 502, 503
resistance, 17, 351
resolution, 199, 200, 302
resource, 229, 433, 447, 454, 460–464
respect, 17, 23, 28, 64, 72, 81, 86, 109, 115, 137, 144, 147, 175, 177, 183, 189, 191, 194, 197, 202, 203, 212, 217, 228, 239, 248, 262, 265, 266, 280, 294, 329, 332, 337, 350, 368, 373, 375, 381, 392, 394, 401–403, 439, 448, 479, 481, 521, 527, 530, 544, 552
response, 1, 2, 95, 132, 205, 208, 242
responsibility, 330, 471–473
responsiveness, 97
restraint, 399
restructuring, 511
result, 8, 122, 343, 443, 469, 525
reverence, 519
reversal, 179
review, 172
reward, 492
Richard Avedon, 451
richness, 236
right, 85, 86, 97, 112, 154, 226, 227, 509, 527, 551
rise, 4, 6, 406
risk, 22, 49, 57, 86, 95, 110, 117, 119, 121, 123, 126, 128, 133–137, 144, 148, 150, 152, 153, 156, 159, 160,

163, 170, 172, 174, 210, 374, 419, 450, 465, 471, 482
role, 16, 25, 26, 29–31, 33, 36, 38, 43, 52, 55, 62, 82, 92, 106, 125, 127, 135, 160, 166, 179, 187, 192, 206, 213, 226, 238, 243, 247, 270, 278, 285, 289, 297, 305, 310, 322, 331, 376, 386, 395, 399, 418, 443, 446, 448, 451, 453, 454, 461, 483, 486, 492, 494, 509, 522, 529, 530, 541, 546, 551
roleplay, 268–270, 397, 399
routine, 50, 55–58, 149, 159, 342
rule, 93

s, 4, 23, 30, 35, 44, 47, 58, 61, 62, 64, 85, 86, 101, 132, 135, 138, 142, 154, 172, 185, 186, 203, 206, 208, 210, 211, 217, 226, 234, 241, 242, 248, 266, 272, 287–289, 294, 296, 306, 309, 313, 330, 331, 352, 356, 367, 373, 375, 389, 390, 397, 408, 435, 437, 454, 455, 463, 482, 492, 498, 500, 506, 520, 525, 533, 539, 540
sacredness, 315
sadism, 387–389
sadness, 219, 290, 306
safe, 2, 3, 7, 8, 18, 23, 26, 28–30, 34, 35, 38, 61, 63, 64, 67, 68, 70, 73–75, 78–86, 89, 92, 94, 110, 112, 115, 117,

127, 130, 131, 133–137, 139, 141, 142, 144, 145, 147, 149, 150, 153, 154, 156, 157, 159, 166, 169, 177–180, 183, 185, 188, 192, 194, 195, 197, 200, 203–205, 207, 209–212, 215–218, 220, 221, 223, 226, 227, 232, 236, 237, 239, 247, 256, 259, 261, 262, 264–267, 270, 272, 277, 278, 280, 283, 285, 286, 288–290, 292, 294, 298, 299, 302, 306–308, 310, 311, 314, 315, 318, 319, 322–324, 327–329, 331, 332, 340, 342, 344, 352, 357, 367, 371–373, 375, 379, 381, 385, 390, 394, 395, 400, 403, 405, 406, 409, 412, 414, 418, 419, 422, 436, 438, 443, 448, 454, 456, 457, 466, 468, 471–474, 479, 483, 484, 510, 516, 520, 521, 524, 530, 539, 540, 546
safety, 3, 7, 8, 10, 15, 17, 21–24, 28, 31, 36, 38, 44, 52, 63, 68–70, 73, 74, 79, 80, 83, 89, 91, 92, 94, 97, 99, 106, 110–113, 117–119, 122, 125–127, 129, 131, 133, 134, 136–138, 147, 151, 154, 155, 159–161, 165, 166, 169, 172, 183, 197, 202, 205, 207, 208, 211, 213–215, 220, 221, 226, 240–242, 262, 265, 281, 283, 285, 287, 288, 294,

Index

296, 306–308, 313–315, 319, 322, 328, 333, 336–338, 344, 365, 367, 368, 371, 373–376, 380, 381, 384, 388, 389, 392, 394, 395, 397, 400, 403, 408, 414–416, 418–420, 422, 423, 425, 427, 431–433, 436, 437, 443, 445–447, 451, 454–456, 458, 461, 464, 468, 471, 473, 477, 482–484, 487, 502, 510, 517, 519, 521–523, 530, 544, 547, 550, 552
Sam, 340
Sarah, 259
satisfaction, 20, 55, 57, 73, 77, 106, 131, 186, 213, 275, 278, 345, 347, 348, 359, 397, 438, 500, 517, 524, 527, 536
Saudi Arabia, 468
scale, 206, 228
scan, 60
scanning, 216
scenario, 130, 171, 179, 185, 191, 197, 210, 217, 248, 256, 285, 294, 314, 331, 386
scene, 28, 79, 80, 131, 135, 136, 194, 197, 261, 265, 267, 270, 272, 273, 275, 283, 288, 392, 516
scrotum, 36
scrutiny, 465, 467
search, 227, 412, 427
section, 13, 15, 18, 21, 26, 33, 36, 41, 44, 47, 55, 58, 62, 65, 68, 70, 79, 81, 84, 86, 89, 92, 97, 99, 102, 105, 107, 110, 112, 119, 130, 139, 144, 147, 151, 153, 163, 166, 172, 175, 178, 180, 183, 186, 192, 197, 203, 205, 208, 218, 221, 226, 234, 237, 244, 247, 250, 252, 254, 257, 260, 262, 268, 275, 278, 281, 284, 286, 289, 292, 295, 297, 302, 305, 308, 310, 313, 323, 330, 334, 338, 341, 345, 365, 368, 370, 389, 392, 397, 400, 405, 408, 409, 412, 418, 420, 422, 425, 430, 433, 438, 441, 443, 446, 449, 460, 464, 466, 469, 472, 474, 479, 484, 487, 497, 500, 506, 509, 512, 514, 519, 523, 529, 533, 541, 544, 547, 550
secure, 21, 30, 70, 81, 84, 213, 216, 217, 259, 292, 340, 373, 502, 530
security, 226
self, 6, 17, 47–49, 57, 61, 65, 72, 131, 132, 141, 203, 205, 218, 221, 224, 225, 229, 234, 236, 247, 248, 252, 256, 289, 291, 295, 297, 299, 305, 308, 314, 319, 344, 345, 352, 353, 373, 400, 441, 448, 450, 451, 455, 477, 497, 502–506, 509, 514, 516, 517, 520, 521, 523–528, 531, 536, 539–541, 551, 552
sensation, 14, 41–44, 92, 95, 112, 125, 127, 135, 154, 160,

206, 210, 327–329, 360, 371, 372, 392, 539
sense, 2, 7, 13, 15, 30, 61, 70, 79, 91, 109, 130–132, 160, 161, 163, 172, 201, 220, 247, 248, 267, 285, 287, 289, 290, 295, 305, 307, 309, 313, 314, 337, 340, 344, 347, 350–352, 368, 375, 376, 388, 393, 395, 400, 412, 418, 420, 428, 431–433, 457, 517, 519, 520, 523–526, 530, 539, 540, 551, 552
sensitivity, 89, 119, 160, 228, 314, 344, 371, 448
sensory, 13, 111, 160, 242, 243, 252
series, 132, 444, 455
session, 94, 171, 185, 196, 209, 217–220, 224, 256, 294, 314, 315, 342
set, 28, 30, 58, 65, 67, 91, 180, 270, 306, 317
setting, 67, 73, 74, 81, 136, 169, 201, 283, 314, 322, 376
severity, 123
sex, 89, 154, 241, 308–310, 365–368, 444, 454–457
sexology, 382
sexuality, 4, 15–18, 24, 30, 131, 223, 234, 240–242, 248, 254, 268, 291, 295, 298, 308–310, 313–315, 319, 321, 323, 330, 332, 334, 345, 350, 351, 353, 368, 370, 376, 379, 414, 441, 443, 446–451, 457, 462, 468, 471, 476, 481, 487, 489, 498, 500, 509, 521, 524, 539, 543, 551
shame, 9–11, 47–49, 131, 136, 139, 216, 217, 226, 232, 239–242, 248, 256, 296, 308, 311, 322, 333, 335, 345, 352, 353, 366, 400, 419, 447, 451, 474, 487, 497–502, 520, 522, 524, 526, 527, 529, 531, 540, 551
shape, 4, 102, 104, 242, 243, 330, 539, 540
share, 15, 74, 256, 342, 376, 405, 409, 412, 418, 419, 423, 428, 429, 432, 445, 447, 454, 455, 457, 462, 477, 497, 510, 512, 520, 524, 525, 529–531, 545, 551
sharing, 72, 74, 75, 91, 259, 311, 313, 418–420, 422, 429, 430, 463, 523, 531
shift, 6, 289, 476, 486, 520, 522, 539, 540
shock, 448
shower, 91, 149
side, 85
Sigmund Freud, 387
sign, 219
signal, 3, 30, 208, 210, 216, 283, 328
significance, 26, 62, 107, 183, 225, 310, 352, 353, 396, 397, 432, 438, 446, 449, 461, 509, 529
silence, 333, 353
silicone, 84, 85, 112, 149, 154
site, 17, 330, 412, 445
situation, 171, 199
size, 95, 278, 539, 540
skill, 414, 521, 531

skin, 149, 151
slapping, 393
slickness, 84
soap, 149, 154
society, 4, 6, 7, 291, 295, 370, 379, 400, 479, 481, 497, 522, 527, 539, 541, 543, 552
sociology, 382, 441
solace, 15, 510
solidarity, 351, 481
song, 447
soreness, 332
source, 152, 302, 342, 371, 462, 494, 503, 506, 515, 523, 540, 551
space, 19, 62, 70, 81, 82, 85, 130, 133, 136, 139, 144, 147, 163, 166, 180, 220, 223, 227, 232, 290, 294, 306–308, 311, 314, 318, 324, 331, 344, 375, 389, 401, 403, 438, 456, 510, 524, 540
spanking, 392–394
specific, 10, 18, 57, 74, 75, 139, 154, 159, 167, 175, 200, 201, 205, 266, 269, 270, 290, 294, 356, 372, 395, 397, 425–427, 463, 467, 469, 544
spectacle, 16
spectrum, 243, 245, 290, 330, 376, 447, 457, 500, 519
spending, 516
sphincter, 1
spinal, 242
spirituality, 313
spot, 105
squeeze, 391

stability, 38
stage, 30, 58, 306, 497
standpoint, 242
start, 93, 112, 137
state, 206, 208, 213, 233, 290, 388
station, 146
status, 464, 465, 482
steel, 85
step, 58, 64, 65, 70, 72, 86, 89, 94, 117, 141, 147, 229, 264, 334, 403, 427, 433, 492, 496, 497, 500, 501, 509, 512, 515
sterilization, 156–159, 165
sterilizing, 157, 159
stigma, 7, 10, 17, 136, 213, 217, 227, 228, 232, 248, 256, 313, 318, 319, 332–335, 345, 352, 353, 362, 366, 378, 400, 409, 419, 420, 438, 443, 445, 448, 450, 451, 460, 465, 473–476, 479, 481, 483, 487, 498, 501, 519, 520, 522, 524, 529, 531, 541, 542, 546
stigmatization, 321, 451
stimulation, 4, 94, 104–106, 160, 372
stimulus, 205
stop, 63, 74, 94, 133, 138, 185, 210–212, 216, 261, 337, 375
storage, 158
story, 104, 242
storytelling, 457
strength, 58, 344, 523
strengthening, 51–55
stress, 346, 501
Stretch, 436

stretch, 1
stretching, 224, 328
structure, 38, 49, 371, 458
struggle, 217, 220, 331, 352, 419
study, 260
subject, 308, 448, 450, 457, 465
submission, 29, 259, 265, 267, 284, 285, 330, 331, 365, 379
submissive, 15, 179, 266, 267, 272, 285, 330, 400
substance, 512
suggestion, 159
suit, 91
sum, 525
summary, 7, 15, 35, 38, 81, 101, 119, 138, 191, 205, 262, 265, 291, 323, 348, 353, 370
supply, 84
support, 15, 26, 49, 57, 61, 70, 72, 89, 131, 133, 139, 141, 213, 215–217, 221, 226–229, 242, 257, 267, 273, 288, 294, 302, 306–308, 310–313, 350, 372, 375, 392, 403, 405, 406, 408, 409, 412, 419–422, 436, 454, 457, 460, 464, 465, 476, 479, 480, 482, 483, 486, 489, 492, 496, 497, 499, 500, 509–511, 513, 516, 517, 520, 523, 525, 530, 551
surface, 160, 273
surgery, 371
surrender, 17, 29, 314, 386
symbol, 438
system, 33, 36, 79, 213, 226, 492

taboo, 1, 2, 4, 6, 13, 15, 17, 18, 24, 29, 65, 138, 236, 248, 289, 295, 297, 308, 330, 333, 335, 351, 418, 438, 446, 447, 449, 450, 457, 465, 474, 497, 519, 527, 539, 546
Tantric, 254
tapestry, 29, 231, 332, 381, 389, 392, 397, 400, 455, 523
tapping, 391
Taylor, 339
tearing, 8, 84
technique, 2, 59, 60, 91, 101, 122, 135, 266, 287, 356, 360, 372, 454
technology, 510
temperature, 90
tension, 44, 51, 54, 60, 90, 91, 135, 224, 306, 365
term, 4, 63, 74, 79, 344, 368
Tessa Hughes-Freeland, 451
test, 154, 173
testament, 131
testing, 86, 172, 174
testosterone, 344
text, 436
texture, 160
the United States, 465
theme, 15
theory, 17, 26, 44, 178, 226, 278, 330, 373, 392, 447–449, 512
therapist, 52, 133, 217, 227, 228, 236, 241, 307, 309, 310, 516
therapy, 228, 306–311, 313, 455, 492, 509–511
thinking, 545
Thomas R., 437

Index 585

thought, 16, 540
threshold, 205
thrill, 15, 65, 388
thumb, 93
tightness, 135
time, 4, 18, 61, 63, 78, 83, 95, 112, 147, 171, 183, 189, 200, 208, 211, 225, 256, 259, 261, 289, 294, 335, 342, 375, 463, 469, 516, 525
tissue, 38, 122, 433
today, 454
tone, 53, 95
tool, 15, 60, 63, 79, 102, 133, 236, 259, 291, 295, 297, 305, 307, 308, 314, 328, 344, 352, 387, 412, 433, 513, 521, 523
topic, 1, 76, 339, 469
touch, 28, 305, 324, 395, 517
traffic, 79
training, 267, 425, 427
transfer, 164
transformation, 313
transgender, 370–373
transition, 94, 220
transmission, 159, 169, 299
transparency, 339
trauma, 29, 44, 61, 119, 122, 130, 132–135, 139, 180, 217, 218, 220, 221, 226, 236, 273, 289, 292–294, 296–299, 301, 305, 306, 308, 309, 314, 371, 392, 440, 461, 540
traumatization, 133
tray, 85
treatment, 129
trepidation, 180
triad, 375
trigger, 119, 130, 245, 306, 337, 374, 392
trust, 2, 4, 5, 14, 16, 17, 23, 24, 26–29, 48, 63, 64, 70, 76, 81, 84, 91, 101, 105, 107, 109, 112, 119, 130, 131, 133, 135, 137, 138, 142, 144, 160, 161, 163, 166, 169, 172, 175, 180, 183, 186, 188, 191, 194, 197, 199, 205, 206, 212, 213, 215, 217, 220–223, 226, 231, 234, 236–239, 241, 247, 249, 259, 262, 265–267, 278, 283, 285–289, 294–297, 299, 305, 310, 314, 322, 328–330, 332, 334, 335, 337, 343, 344, 348, 352, 356, 357, 367, 372, 374–376, 378, 379, 386, 388, 389, 392, 394, 395, 397, 400, 420, 433, 437, 439, 441, 446, 447, 511, 519, 521, 523–525, 527, 539, 547, 552
tube, 1
turmoil, 501
turning, 138
type, 154, 227, 317

UK, 467
umbrella, 368
understanding, 1, 4, 5, 7, 10, 14, 17, 18, 21, 26, 30, 31, 35, 38, 41, 43, 46, 48, 49, 58, 68, 70, 72, 74, 75, 81, 86, 92, 93, 101, 104, 107, 109,

119, 124, 131, 134, 136, 142, 154, 159, 161, 169, 172, 180, 186, 187, 189, 194, 200–203, 205, 208, 213, 215, 218, 221, 223, 231, 234, 241, 243, 244, 247, 257, 259, 265, 266, 270, 272, 278, 283, 284, 288, 291, 294, 297, 301, 305, 308, 310, 311, 322, 323, 329–332, 334, 338, 340, 341, 343, 345, 348, 352, 353, 356, 357, 368, 370, 372, 373, 378, 379, 381, 388, 389, 392, 394, 400, 405, 407, 408, 412, 414, 420, 422, 425, 427, 430, 431, 433, 441, 443, 445, 446, 448, 449, 451, 454, 457, 460, 462–465, 468, 473, 474, 476, 479, 483, 485, 487, 489, 492, 494, 500, 509, 514, 517, 519–523, 525, 535, 539, 541, 543, 546, 550, 552
up, 61, 89–92, 94, 95, 112, 115, 139, 154, 185, 209, 226, 324, 336, 386, 425, 447, 497
use, 63, 64, 74, 84–86, 110, 112, 133, 154, 156, 157, 159, 161, 170, 172, 185, 294, 328, 357, 374, 386, 391, 393, 395, 449, 450, 483
user, 418
uterus, 1, 49

vagina, 1, 3, 4, 97, 103, 203, 390, 393, 539
vaginoplasty, 371

vagus, 226
validation, 241, 517, 530, 551
validity, 522
value, 448
variety, 3, 8, 23, 90, 113, 127, 147, 226, 280, 332, 338, 368, 405, 416, 432, 433, 463
vehicle, 441
vera, 154
victimhood, 289
view, 11, 17, 330, 441, 522
viewpoint, 330
vigilance, 219
vinyl, 110
violation, 198, 199, 483
violence, 17, 132, 352
visibility, 2, 4, 17, 350, 425, 441, 448, 450, 451, 477, 479, 529
visual, 431, 448, 449, 462
voice, 325
volunteer, 419
vulnerability, 2, 16, 17, 24, 26, 28, 29, 48, 74, 109, 112, 130, 135, 136, 163, 180, 215, 217, 231, 232, 234, 236–239, 245, 247, 249, 254, 257, 259, 270, 290, 294, 295, 297, 310, 311, 314, 318, 324, 328, 330, 331, 336, 344, 348, 366–368, 372, 373, 375, 395, 399, 439, 449, 461, 497, 519, 523, 525, 527, 539, 541, 550
vulva, 105

wall, 105

Index 587

warm, 89–92, 94, 112, 209, 224, 324, 386
warming, 89, 91
warmth, 91
warning, 182, 208, 209
wash, 152
water, 91, 112, 154, 372
way, 10, 15, 78, 91, 104, 150, 153, 229, 234, 252, 254, 288, 294, 298, 319, 322, 323, 331, 332, 340, 343, 344, 370, 392, 395, 441, 449, 463, 464, 481, 494, 520, 552
weakness, 135
wealth, 405, 446, 454
web, 464
webinar, 419
weight, 331, 539
well, 23, 26, 40, 44, 49, 52, 55, 65, 107, 118, 124, 127, 137, 138, 142, 163, 169, 172, 174, 175, 180, 224, 242, 278, 288, 290, 294, 297, 305, 310, 337, 372, 397, 417, 433, 435, 436, 446, 471, 473, 479, 484, 495, 497, 500, 503, 514, 517, 520, 521, 531
wellbeing, 54, 55
wellness, 379
whole, 137, 188
will, 8, 13, 18, 20, 26, 36, 55, 58, 62, 70, 78, 81, 84, 89, 92, 97, 99, 105, 107, 139, 147, 151, 159, 163, 172, 175, 177, 183, 203, 205, 213, 228, 234, 237, 250, 252, 262–264, 275, 281, 286, 292, 295, 302, 313, 319, 323, 333, 334, 340, 373, 400, 409, 412, 418, 420, 425, 427, 433, 446, 451, 460, 463, 466, 472, 479, 497, 500, 506, 514, 522, 541, 547, 550
willingness, 30, 47, 101, 115, 237, 270, 337, 345, 348, 368, 419, 551
wish, 74, 191, 263, 335, 477, 484
withdrawal, 218
woman, 331
word, 3, 4, 28, 30, 63, 74, 79, 112, 133, 185, 216, 217, 256, 264, 283, 285, 288, 294, 340
work, 16, 48, 115, 180, 308, 354, 403, 436, 450, 451, 471, 476, 489, 522, 524
workshop, 210, 416, 419, 481, 530
world, 61, 70, 115, 144, 153, 351, 353, 408, 427, 464, 521, 523, 543
worth, 48, 132

zone, 298

www.ingramcontent.com/pod-product-compliance
Ingram Content Group UK Ltd.
Pitfield, Milton Keynes, MK11 3LW, UK
UKHW020733300125
454332UK00010B/400